CLAUDE TIHON, Ph.D.

BLEOMYCIN
CURRENT STATUS AND NEW DEVELOPMENTS

BLEOMYCIN

CURRENT STATUS AND NEW DEVELOPMENTS

Edited by

Stephen K. Carter
Northern California Cancer Program
Palo Alto, California

Stanford University Medical Center
Stanford, California

University of California
San Francisco, California

Stanley T. Crooke
Bristol Laboratories
Syracuse, New York

Baylor College of Medicine
Houston, Texas

Upstate Medical Center
Syracuse, New York

Hamao Umezawa
Institute of Microbial Chemistry
Tokyo, Japan

ACADEMIC PRESS   New York   San Francisco   London   1978
A Subsidiary of Harcourt Brace Jovanovich, Publishers

ACADEMIC PRESS, INC.
111 Fifth Avenue, New York, New York 10003

United Kingdom Edition published by
ACADEMIC PRESS, INC. (LONDON) LTD.
24/28 Oval Road, London NW1 7DX

Library of Congress Cataloging in Publication Data

Main entry under title:

Bleomycin, Current status and new developments.

"Papers . . . presented at a symposium held in Oakland,
California . . . jointly sponsored by the Northern Califor-
nia Cancer Program and Bristol Laboratories."
    1. Cancer—Chemotherapy—Congresses. 2. Bleomycin—
Congresses. I. Carter, Stephen K. II. Crooke, Stanley
T. III. Umezawa, Hamao, Date IV. Northern
California Cancer Program. V. Bristol-Myers Company.
Bristol Laboratories. [DNLM: 1. Bleomycin—Congresses.
2. Neoplasms—Drug therapy—Congresses. QV269 B647 1977]
RC271.B57B58   616.9′94′061   8-21561
ISBN 0-12-161550-2

CONTENTS

CONTRIBUTORS

Numbers in parentheses indicate the pages on which authors' contributions begin.

FUMINORI ABE (311), *Research Laboratory, Pharmaceutical Division, Nippon Kayaku Company Ltd., 3–31, Shimo, Kita-ku, Tokyo, Japan*

DAVID S. ALBERTS (131), *Section of Hematology–Oncology, Department of Internal Medicine, University of Arizona Health Sciences Center, Tucson, Arizona 85724*

NORIKO AMANO (35), *Research Laboratory, Pharmaceutical Division, Nippon Kayaku Company Ltd., 3–31, Shimo, Kita-ku, Tokyo, Japan*

LAURENCE H. BAKER (173), *Department of Oncology, Wayne State University School of Medicine, Detroit, Michigan 48201*

S. C. BARRANCO (81), *Division of Cell Biology, Department of Human Biological Chemistry and Genetics, University of Texas Medical Branch, Galveston, Texas 77550*

WILLIAM T. BRADNER (333), *Antitumor Biology, Bristol Laboratories, Thompson Road, Syracuse, New York 13201*

ALAN BROUGHTON (107, 131), *Department of Pathology and Laboratory Medicine, University of Texas Health Science Center, Houston, Texas 77025*

STEPHEN K. CARTER (9), *Northern California Cancer Program, 1801 Page Mill Road, Palo Alto, California 94304; Department of Medicine, Stanford University, Stanford, California; Department of Medicine, University of California, San Francisco, California*

HSIAO-SHENG CHEN (131), *Section of Hematology–Oncology, Department of Internal Medicine, University of Arizona, Tucson, Arizona 85724*

JOSEPH CHEN (131), *Section of Hematology–Oncology, Department of Internal Medicine, University of Arizona Health Sciences Center, Tucson, Arizona 85724*

CHARLES A. COLTMAN, JR. (227), *Department of Medicine, University of Texas Health Science Center at San Antonio, San Antonio, Texas 78284*

ROBERT L. COMIS (279), *Hematology–Oncology Section, State University of New York, Upstate Medical Center, Syracuse, New York 13210*

STANLEY T. CROOKE (1, 117, 343, 357), *Bristol Laboratories, P.O. Box 657, Syracuse, New York 13201; Department of Pharmacology, Baylor College of Medicine, Houston, Texas 77025; Department of Pharmacology, Upstate Medical Center, Syracuse, New York 13210*

YERACH DASKAL (57), *Department of Pharmacology, Electron Microscopy Unit, Baylor College of Medicine, Houston, Texas 77030*

EDWARD DePERSIO (227), *Oklahoma Medical Research Foundation, 825 Northeast 13th, Oklahoma City, Oklahoma 73104*

KAZUO EBIHARA (299, 311), *Research Laboratory, Nippon Kayaku Company Ltd., 3–31, Shimo, Kita-ku, Tokyo, Japan*

LAWRENCE H. EINHORN (201), *Department of Medicine, Indiana University School of Medicine, Indianapolis, Indiana 46202*

HISAO EKIMOTO (299, 311), *Research Laboratory, Nippon Kayaku Company Ltd., 3–31, Shimo, Kita-ku, Tokyo, Japan*

MICHAEL A. FRIEDMAN (191), *Cancer Research Institute, University of California School of Medicine, San Francisco, California 94143*

ABRAHAM GOLDIN (91), *International Treatment Research, Division of Cancer Treatment, National Cancer Institute, National Institutes of Health, Bethesda, Maryland 20014*

THEODORE E. GRAM (293), *Laboratory of Toxicology, National Cancer Institute, Bethesda, Maryland 20014*

JOSEPH GROSS (131), *Section of Hematology–Oncology, Department of Internal Medicine, University of Arizona Health Sciences Center, Tucson, Arizona 85724*

PETRE N. GROZEA (227), *Oklahoma Medical Research Foundation, 825 Northeast 13th, Oklahoma City, Oklahoma 73104*

FERENC GYORKEY (57), *Department of Laboratory Service, Veterans Administration Hospital, Houston, Texas 77030*

CHARLES W. HAIDLE (21), *University of Texas System Cancer Center, M. D. Anderson Hospital and Tumor Institute, Houston, Texas 77030*

YOSHIMASA HASHIMOTO (311), *Research Laboratory, Pharmaceutical Division, Nippon Kayaku Company Ltd., 3–31, Shimo, Kita-ku, Tokyo, Japan*

KLAUS HÖFFKEN (215), *Innere Universitätsklinik und Poliklinik (Tumorforschung), West German Tumor Center, Essen, Federal Republic of Germany*

DANIEL HOTH (243), *Division of Medical Oncology, Vincent T. Lombardi Cancer Research Center, Georgetown University School of Medicine, Washington, D.C. 20007*

YUKIO INUYAMA (267), *Department of Otorhinolaryngology, School of Medicine, Keio University, 35 Shinano machi, Shinyu-ku-ku, Tokyo, Japan*

STEPHEN E. JONES (227), *Department of Internal Medicine, University of Arizona Health Sciences Center, Tucson, Arizona 85724*

IRA KLINE (91), *International Treatment Research, Division of Cancer Treatment, National Cancer Institute, National Institutes of Health, Bethesda, Maryland 20014*

MONTAGUE LANE (143), *Department of Pharmacology, Clinical Cancer Research, Baylor College of Medicine, Houston, Texas 77030*

DANIEL E. LEHANE (143), *Department of Pharmacology, Clinical Cancer Research, Baylor College of Medicine, Houston, Texas 77030*

ROSA LIU (131), *Section of Hematology–Oncology, Department of Internal Medicine, University of Arizona Health Sciences Center, Tucson, Arizona 85724*

ROBERT B. LIVINGSTON (165), *Department of Medicine, University of Texas Health Science Center, Audie Murphy Memorial Veterans Administration Hospital, San Antonio, Texas 78284*

R. STEPHEN LLOYD (21), *University of Texas Health Science Center, Graduate School of Biomedical Sciences, Houston, Texas 77030; University of Texas System Cancer Center, M.D. Anderson Hospital and Tumor Institute, Houston, Texas 77030*

AKIRA MATSUDA (35, 299, 311), *Research Laboratory, Pharmaceutical Division, Nippon Kayaku Company Ltd., 3–31, Shima, Kita-ku, Tokyo, Japan*

MICHAEL MAYERSOHN (131), *Section of Hematology–Oncology, Department of Internal Medicine University of Arizona Health Sciences Center, Tucson, Arizona 85724*

EDWARD G. MIMNAUGH (293), *Laboratory of Toxicology, National Cancer Institute, Bethesda, Maryland 20014*

TADAAKI MIYAMOTO (185), *Division of Hospitals, National Institute of Radiological Sciences 4-9-1, Anagawa, Chiba City, Japan*

THOMAS E. MOON* (131, 227), *Department of Biomathematics, The University of Texas System Cancer Center, M.D. Anderson Hospital and Tumor Institute, Houston, Texas 77025*

FRANCO M. MUGGIA (151), *Cancer Therapy Evaluation Program, Division of Cancer Treatment, National Cancer Institute, National Institutes of Health, Bethesda, Maryland 20014*

RAINHARDT OSIEKA (215), *Innere Universitätsklinik und Poliklinik (Tumorforschung), West German Tumor Center, Essen, Federal Republic of Germany*

DONALD PERRIER (131), *Section of Hematology–Oncology, Department of Internal Medicine, University of Arizona Health Sceinces Center, Tucson, Arizona 85724*

ARCHIE W. PRESTAYKO (117), *Bristol Laboratories, P.O. Box 657, Syracuse, New York 13201; Department of Pharmacology, Baylor College of Medicine, Houston, Texas 77025*

MARCEL ROZENCWEIG (151), *Cancer Therapy Evaluation Program, Division of Cancer Treatment, National Cancer Institute, National Institutes of Health, Bethesda, Maryland 20014*

SYDNEY SALMON (131), *Section of Hematology–Oncology, Department of Internal Medicine, University of Arizona Health Sciences Center, Tucson, Arizona 85724*

PHILIP SCHEIN (243), *Division of Medical Oncology, Vincent T. Lombardi Cancer Research Center, Georgetown University School of Medicine, Washington, D.C. 20007*

MAX E. SCHEULEN (215), *Innere Universitätsklinik und Poliklinik (Tumorforschung), West German Tumor Center, Essen, Federal Republic of Germany*

---

*Currently at Cancer Center Division, College of Medicine, University of Arizona Health Sciences Center, Tucson, Arizona 85724

CARL G. SCHMIDT (215), *Innere Universitätsklinik und Poliklinik (Tumorforschung)*, *West German Tumor Center, Essen, Federal Republic of Germany*
SIEGFRIED SEEBER (215), *Innere Universitätsklinik und Poliklinik (Tumorforschung)*, *West German Tumor Center, Essen, Federal Republic of Germany*
BRANIMIR IVAN SIKIC (293), *Laboratory of Toxicology, National Cancer Institute, Bethesda, Maryland 20014*
FREDERICK P. SMITH (243), *Division of Medical Oncology, Vincent T. Lombardi Cancer Research Center, Georgetown University School of Medicine, Washington, D.C. 20007*
JAMES E. STRONG (343), *Department of Pharmacology, Baylor College of Medicine, Houston, Texas 77025*
KATSUTOSHI TAKAHASHI (35, 311), *Research Laboratory, Pharmaceutical Division, Nippon Kayaku Company Ltd., 3–31, Shimo, Kita-ku, Tokyo, Japan*
ANDREW T. TURRISI III (151), *Cancer Therapy Evaluation Program, Division of Cancer Treatment, National Cancer Institute, National Institutes of Health, Building 37, Room 6E12, Bethesda, Maryland 20014*
HAMAO UMEZAWA (15, 35, 299, 311), *Institute of Microbial Chemistry 4–23, Kamiosaki 3-Chome, Shinagawa-ku, Tokyo, Japan*
DANIEL D. VON HOFF (151), *Cancer Therapy Evaluation Program, Division of Cancer Treatment, National Cancer Institute, National Institutes of Health, Bethesda, Maryland 20014*
TODD H. WASSERMAN (253), *Department of Radiation Oncology, University of California Medical Center, San Francisco, California 94143*
TAKUMI YAMASHITA (299, 311), *Research Laboratory, Nippon Kayaku Company Ltd., 3–31, Shimo, Kita-ku, Tokyo, Japan*
OSAMU YOSHIOKA (35, 299, 311), *Research Laboratory, Pharmaceutical Division, Nippon Kayaku Company Ltd., 3–31, Shimo, Kita-ku, Tokyo, Japan*

PREFACE

Bleomycin is a drug with unique pharmacologic characteristics that plays an important role in the therapy of a wide range of human malignancies. This book reviews both the preclinical studies and the clinical role of this important compound and also gives data on analogs under development. The papers in this book were all presented at a symposium held in Oakland, California and jointly sponsored by the Northern California Cancer Program and Bristol Laboratories.

It is hoped that this book will be of interest to all scientists involved in both the preclinical and clinical aspects of drug development since the papers on bleomycin also explore the critical broad flow of steps that any drug must pass through in its evaluation. This volume will look at chemistry, mechanism of action, bioassay pharmacology, toxicology, pathology, and clinical evaluation in relation to the bleomycins.

Chapter 1

BLEOMYCIN: A BRIEF REVIEW

Stanley T. Crooke

Bleomycin will be discussed in detail in subsequent papers. Thus, the purpose of this paper is to provide a brief overview of bleomycin and analogs, and to introduce the papers that will follow.

I. CHEMISTRY

The bleomycins are a group of complex glycopeptides extracted from a strain of *Streptomyces verticillus*. Figure 1 shows the general structure of the bleomycins, and the terminal amines of several of the analogs, which may be purified by ion-exchange chromatography. Most of the bleomycin species are soluble in water and methanol, and insoluble in other organic solvents (Umezawa *et al.*, 1966). A closely related group of compounds, the phleomycins, also has antitumor activity (Bradner and Pindell, 1971).

Bleomycin analogs can be divided into three groups. First generation analogs include the 13 analogs comprising the clinically employed bleomycin, Blenoxane . Second generation bleomycin analogs are those prepared since the original 13 were

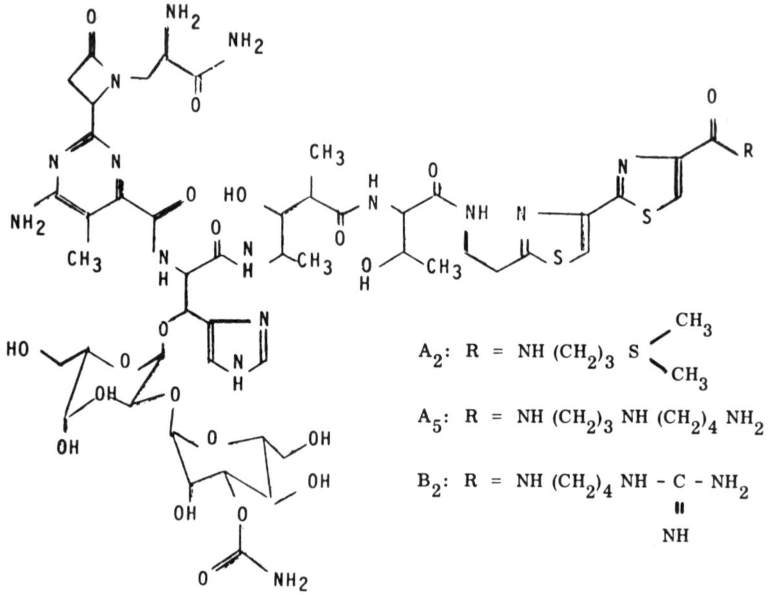

Fig. 1. The structure of bleomycin.

isolated, which differ from others only by differences in the terminal amine. Third generation analogs are those which differ from other analogs in the bleomycinic acid nucleus.

II. MECHANISM OF ACTION

That bleomycin binds to DNA has been demonstrated by studies with tritiated bleomycin (Umezawa, 1974) and by studies on circular dichroism. The circular dichroism studies suggested that bleomycin binds to DNA without causing extensive changes in secondary structure (Krueger *et al.*, 1973). Binding of bleomycin is thought to be a partial intercalation in the major groove, and the inhibiting effect of copper ions is suggested to be due to an alteration in the secondary structure of bleomycin such that binding to DNA is not efficient (Murokami *et al.*, 1973).

After binding, bleomycin excises free bases, resulting in single-strand breaks (Haidle *et al.*, 1972; Koyama *et al.*, 1968; Muller *et al.*, 1972; Saunders *et al.*, 1975; Suzuki *et al.*, 1969). Double-stranded scission occurs at higher concentrations of bleomycin, and is thought to occur when a number of single-strand breaks occur proximally enough to result in double-strand breaks (Saunders *et al.*, 1975). An active center, similar to esterase active centers, in which the threonine hydroxyl and the histidine imidazole groups participate in the reaction with DNA has been proposed. The pH optima suggest that the α-amino group of the β-amino-alanine moiety of bleomycin is involved in the reaction, and studies on enzymatically inactivated bleomycin have suggested that the carboxyamide portion of the β-aminoalanine moiety is also involved (Umezawa, 1974).

Bleomycin has been observed to inhibit the replication of viruses, bacteria, and mammalian cells, and a broad range of tumor cells (Crooke and Bradner, 1977).

Bleomycin treatment of sensitive cells *in vitro* has resulted in degradation of preformed DNA (Cox *et al.*, 1974; Miyaki *et al.*, 1975), and inhibition of DNA synthesis (Suzuki *et al.*, 1968; Muller *et al.*, 1975). Inhibition of RNA and protein synthesis have been reported to be somewhat less sensitive to bleomycin than DNA synthesis (Crooke *et al.*, 1975; Watanabe *et al.*, 1973).

Eukaryotic cells are reported to be most sensitive to bleomycin during the G_2 and M in phases of the cell cycle (Barranco and Humphrey, 1971; Terasima and Umezawa, 1970). Whether cycling or noncycling cells are more sensitive to bleomycin is unclear, but most studies suggest that noncycling cells are more sensitive (Twentyman and Bleehen, 1973; Terasima *et al.*, 1972).

III. CLINICAL PHARMACOLOGY

Bleomycin is absorbed rapidly after intramuscular administration, resulting in peak plasma concentrations approximately one-third to one-half of those obtained after rapid intravenous administration (Fujita, 1971). Bleomycin is also absorbed following subcutaneous administration, but the extent of absorption is imprecisely defined. Only minute quantities of bleomycin are absorbed after intravesical administration of as much as 120 u (Johnson *et al.*, 1976).

Plasma clearance of bleomycin following rapid intravenous administration is rapid. The $t_{1/2} \beta$ in patients with normal renal function is approximately 115 min. In patients with creatinine clearances less than 25-35 ml/min the $t_{1/2}\beta$ of bleomycin increases exponentially as the creatinine clearance decreases (Crooke *et al.*, 1977b; Crooke *et al.*, 1977a).

Although the principal mechanism of detoxification of bleomycin is renal excretion, a bleomycin inactivating enzyme has been described (Umezawa *et al.*, 1972). It is possible that this enzyme accounts for intracellular inactivation and perhaps a portion of the total detoxification in patients with compromised renal function.

IV. CLINICAL TOXICOLOGY

A. Pulmonary

The usual dose-limiting toxicity of bleomycin is pulmonary fibrosis. Although the reported incidence of pulmonary toxicities has varied from 0-40% with 0-6% toxicity-related deaths, the incidence of clinically significant pulmonary toxicities is approximately 10%. The incidence and severity of pulmonary toxicities are related to age and total dose. Patients > 70 years old, or those receiving > 400 u are clearly at greater risk than younger patients treated with lower doses (Blum *et al.*, 1973). Radiotherapy to the thorax probably increases the incidence of bleomycin pulmonary toxicities.

The development of pulmonary toxicities is ususally delayed, typically occurring between 4 and 10 weeks after initiation of therapy. Physical findings, rales and rhonchi and occasionally pleural friction rubs, usually precede radiographic changes, and may progress to signs and symptoms of respiratory failure. The radiographic presentation is typical of interstitial pneumonitis which may progress to pulmonary fibrosis (Agre, 1974; Blum *et al.*, 1975; Blum *et al.*, 1973; E.O.R.T.C., 1970; Yagoda *et al.*, 1972). It has been suggested that patients with bleomycin pulmonary toxicity may present in one of two ways: a minimal form with exertional dyspnea, minimal radiographic changes, and a normal resting arterial partial pressure of oxygen; and a severe form with prominent roentgenographic findings and hypoxemia at rest (Samuels *et al.*, 1976).

The histopathologic manifestations of bleomycin lung toxicity in humans are comparable to those noted in animals, and do not differ significantly from interstitial pneumonitis and fibrosis associated with many other lung toxins. The lesions are found more frequently in the lower lobes and subpleural areas and consist of a fibrinous exudate, atypical proliferation of alveolar cells, hyaline membranes, interstitial and intraalveolar fibrosis and squamous metaplasia of the distal air spaces (Blum, 1974; Daskal *et al.*, 1976; Livingston *et al.*, 1973). Electron microscopic studies suggest Type I alveolar cell destruction followed by Type II cellular proliferation (Bedrossian, 1974). In addition, nucleolar fibrillar centers and granular nuclear bodies have been shown in Type I and Type II alveolar epithelial cells and fibroblasts (Daskal *et al.*, 1976).

It is clear that bleomycin pulmonary toxicity is associated with changes in pulmonary function tests. It has not been established, however, that pulmonary functions tests are predictive, i.e., that by performing serial pulmonary function tests on a patient it is possible to detect early bleomycin toxicity, and discontinue the drug in time to avoid progressive pulmonary involvement.

In a study of 150 patients vital capacity was noted to be decreased in patients with bleomycin lung toxicity, but it was felt that clinical parameters provided a better index of toxicity than pulmonary function tests in many patients (Blum *et al.*, 1973). A decrease in total lung capacity and vital capacity was noted in approximately 20, and a decrease in diffusion capacity was found in 7 of 40 patients in another study. However, no correlation between changes in pulmonary functions and advent of pulmonary toxicity or dose of bleomycin could be ascertained (Yagoda *et al.*, 1972).

A statistically significant decrease in forced vital capacity was found in five of six patients treated with bleomycin who had abnormal chest x rays at the initiation of the study, but the change in forced vital capacity noted in eight patients with normal chest x rays was not statistically significant, and no correlation between the total dose of bleomycin and pulmonary function tests could be determined (Pasqual *et al.*, 1973). Similarly, a decrease in total lung capacity was found in a series of 26 patients, but the nature and extent of the changes seemed to correlate best with the type of tumor rather than the developments of toxicity (Rudders, 1973).

Recently, it has been suggested by two groups that serial determinations of carbon monoxide diffusion capacity may allow earlier detection of pulmonary toxicities than other methods (Baker, personal communication; Comis *et al.*, 1978).

B.   Other Toxicities

Bleomycin induces a febrile response in 20-50% of patients treated. Hyperpyrexia is more common in patients with lymphomas (Agre, 1974). Moreover, in approximately 6% of these patients acute fulminant reactions (hypotensive response) are reported in association with hyperpyrexia (Agre, 1974).

Mucocutaneous toxicities are common in patients treated with bleomycin. These toxicities include alopecia, hyperpigmentation of skin, erythema, hyperkeratosis, and muscositis, and are total-dose related. The incidence and severity of mucositis are increased when bleomycin is employed in combination with radiotherapy to the head and neck (Crooke and Bradner, 1977).

Neither clinically significant myelosuppression nor immunosuppression has been reported to be associated with bleomycin. However, subclinical myelosuppression induced by bleomycin may contribute to the myelosupression in markedly marrow-toxic regimens (Baker *et al.*, 1975).

V.   CLINICAL ACTIVITY

As a single agent bleomycin has demonstrated activity against the tumors indicated in Table I. Response rates $\geqslant 15\%$ in 40 or more patients have been reported for these tumors.

TABLE I.   Tumors Responsive to Bleomycin As a Single Agent

Squamous cell carcinoma
Head and neck
Larynx
Cervix
Vulvo-vaginal
Skin
Penis
Lymphomas
Mycoses fungoides
Testicular carcinomas

In general, combinations in which bleomycin is employed are active against a spectrum of tumors similar to those sensitive to bleomycin as a single agent. In squamous cell carcinoma of the head and neck bleomycin-containing combinations are definitely active, and most active regimens employ both bleomycin and methotrexate (Crooke and Bradner, 1977). In squamous cell carcinoma of the cervix, mitomycin C, vincristine, and bleomycin is one of the more active regimens (Baker *et al.*, 1975).

Bleomycin has been employed in two types of regimens in Hodgkins disease. It has been combined with MOPP at a dose of 2 or 10 u/m^2 iv on days 1 and 8 of each course. Data from a randomized comparative trial suggest that low-dose bleomycin is as good as high-dose bleomycin, and that the response rates obtained are improved by the addition of bleomycin (Carter and Blum, 1976). Additionally, bleomycin has been employed in various combinations thought to be non-cross-resistant to MOPP, such as ABVD, and these combinations have been shown to be active (Bonadonna et al., 1975).

In the treatment of testicular carcinomas bleomycin clearly is part of first-line therapy. The combinations employing bleomycin generally include vinblastine, and may include actinomycin D or cis-platinum, and result in a high response rate (Crooke and Bradner, 1977).

VI. BLEOMYCIN AND RADIOTHERAPY

Although bleomycin has been administered in combination with radiotherapy in animal systems and in patients, the proper dose, the proper schedule relative to radiotherapy, and a precise definition of the risk-to-benefit ratio remain poorly defined. Studies to be discussed during this symposium may better answer some of these questions.

VII. OTHER ACTIVITIES

Bleomycin has been employed in several ways which will not be discussed during this symposium. Since it chelates a variety of potentially radioactive metals, and is reported to localize in certain tumors, bleomycin has been studied as a tumor-scanning agent. Of the metal chelates prepared, ^{111}In and ^{57}Co-bleomycin have been studied most thoroughly. Although both have been reported to be superior to other scanning compounds in various studies, many of the studies have not been reproduced, and the role of bleomycin as a tumor-scanning agent remains poorly defined (Silberstein et al., 1976; Crooke and Bradner, 1977).

Bleomycin has been employed topically for the treatment of a variety of dermatologic diseases. Injected intradermally, it has demonstrated activity against several types of verrucae (Crooke, unpublished data, 1977). It has also been employed in the local treatment of various skin cancers and in psoriasis (Ihedd et al., 1976). In none of these diseases has the role of bleomycin been established.

Bleomycin has also been administered intravesically for the treatment of recurrent superficial bladder tumors. The response rate was approximately equal to the response rate induced by thiotepa, but only minimal absorption occurred, and no systemic toxicities were observed (Johnson et al., 1976)

VIII. CONCLUSIONS

In conclusion, then, bleomycin is an antibiotic with a unique structure, mechanism of action, and toxicologic profile. It has clinical activity against several tumors, and, in addition, it has potential utility when administered topically, and as a tumor-scanning agent. Moreover, an extensive analog development program has resulted in a number of analogs which may extend the utility of the bleomycins.

REFERENCES

Agre, K. A. (1974). In *Proceedings of the New Drug Seminar on Bleomycin*, Soper, W. T., and Gott, A. B. (Eds.), pp. 66–81. Automation Industries, Inc., Vitro Laboratories Div., Silver Spring, MD.

Baker, L. H., Opipari, M., and Izbicki, R. (1975). *Proc. Am. Assoc. Cancer Res. 16*, No. 138.

Barranco, S. C., and Humphrey, R. M. (1971). *Cancer Res. 31*, 1218–1223.

Bedrossian, C. W. M. (1974). In *Proceedings of the New Drug Seminar on Bleomycin*, Soper, W. T., and Gott, A. B. (Eds.), pp. 169–186. Automation Industries, Inc., Vitro Laboratories Div., Silver Spring, MD.

Blum, J., and Brodovsky, H. S. (1975). *Proc. Am. Assoc. Cancer Res. 16*, No. 1107.

Blum, R. H. (1974). In *New Drug Seminar on Bleomycin*, Soper, W. T., and Gott, A. B. (Eds.), pp. 151–162. Automation Industries, Inc., Vitro Laboratories Div., Silver Spring, MD.

Blum, R. H., Carter, S. K., and Agre, K. A. (1973). *Cancer 31*, 903–904.

Bonadonna, G., Zucali, R., Monfardini, S., DeLena, M., and Uslenghi, C. (1975). *Cancer 36*, 252–259.

Bradner, W. T., and Pindell, M. H. (1971). *Nature 196*, 682–684.

Carter, S. K., and Blum, R. H. (1976). *Prog. Biochem. Pharmacol. 11*, 158–171.

Comis, R. L., Ginsberg, S., Prestayko, A. W., Auchinclaus, J. H., and Crooke S. T. (1978). In *Current Chemotherapy: Proceedings of the 10th International Congress of Chemotherapy Vol. II*, Siegenthaler, W., and Luthy, R. (Eds.), pp. 1135–1137.

Cox, R., Daoud, A. H., and Irving, C. C. (1974). *Biochem. Pharmacol. 23*, 3147–3151.

Crooke, S. T., and Bradner, W. T. (1977). *J. Med. 7*, 333–428.

Crooke, S. T., Stiz, T. O., Bannon, M., and Busch, H. (1975). *Physiol. Chem. Phys. 7*, 177–190.

Crooke, S. T., Comis, R. L., Einhorn, L. H., Strong, J. E., Broughton, A., and Prestayko, A. W. (1977a). *Cancer Treatment Rep. 61*, 1631–1636.

Crooke, S. T., Luft, F. T., Broughton, A. W., Strong, J. L., Casson, K., and Einhorn, L. (1977b). *Cancer 39*, 1430–1434.

Daskal, Y., Gyorkey, F., Gyorkey, P., and Busch, H. (1976). *Cancer Res. 36*, 1267–1272.

E.O.R.T.C. (1970). *Br. Med. J. 2* 643–645.

Fujita, H. (1971). *Jpn. J. Clin. Oncol. 12*, 151–162.

Haidle, C. W., Weiss, K. K., and Kuo. M. T. (1972). *Mol. Pharmacol. 8*, 531–537.

Ihedd, S., Kawamaru, T., Hammamatsu, T., Nakayama, H., Ishihara, K., and Sato, A. (1976). (Unpublished data).

Johnson, D. E., Bracken, R. B., Prestayko, A. W., Brown, T. E., and Crooke, S. T. (1976). *J. Am. Med. Assoc. 236*, 1353–1354.

Koyama, G., Nakamura, H., Muraoka, Y., Takita, T., Maeda, K., Umezawa, H., and Iitaka, Y. (1968). *Tetrahedon Lett. 44*, 4635–4638.

Krueger, W. C., Pschigoda, L. M., and Reusser, F. (1973). *J. Antibiot. 26*, 424–428.

Livingston, R. B., Bodey, G. P., Gottlieb, J. A., and Frei, E. (1973). *Cancer Chemother. Rep. 57*, 219–224.

Miyaki, M., Ono, T., Hori, S., and Umezawa, H. (1975). *Cancer Res. 35*, 2015–2019.

Muller, W. E. G., Yamazaki, Z., Breter, H., and Zahn, R. K. (1972). *Eur. J. Biochem. 31,* 518–525.

Muller, W. E. G., Totsuka, A., Nusser, I., Zahn, R. K., and Umezawa, H. (1975). *Biochem. Pharmacol. 24,* 911–915.

Murokami, H., Mori, H., and Taira, S. (1973). *J. Theor. Biol. 42,* 443–460.

Pasqual, R. S., Mosher, M. B., Sikand, R. S., DeConti, R. C., and Bou Huys, A. (1973). *Ann. Rev. Resp. Dis. 108,* 211–217.

Rudders, R. A. (1973). *Ann. Intern. Med. 78,* 618–620.

Samuels, M. L., Johnson, D. E., Holoye, P. Y., and Lanzotti, V. J. (1976). *J. Am. Med. Assoc. 235,* 1117–1120.

Saunders, G. F., Haidle, C. W., Saunders, P. P., and Kuo, M. T. (1975). In *Pharmacological Basis of Cancer Chemotherapy.* Williams & Wilkins, Baltimore, pp. 507–529.

Silberstein, E. B. (1976). *Am. J. Med. 60,* 226–237.

Suzuki, H., Nagai, K., Yamaki, H., Tanaka, N., and Umezawa, H. (1968). *J. Antibiot. 21,* 379–386.

Suzuki, H., Nagai, K., Yamaki, H., Tanaka, N., and Umezawa, H. (1969). *J. Antibiot. 22,* 446–449.

Terasima, T., and Umezawa, H. (1970). *J. Antibiot. 23,* 300–304.

Terasima, T., Takabe, Y., Katsumata, T., Watanabe, M., and Umezawa, H. (1972). *J. Natl. Cancer Inst. 49,* 1093–1100.

Tobey, R. A. (1972). *J. Cell. Physiol. 79,* 259–266.

Twentyman, P. R., and Bleehen, N. M. (1973). *Br. J. Cancer 28,* 500–507.

Umezawa, H. (1973). *Biomedicine 18,* 459–475.

Umezawa, H. (1974). *Fed. Proc., Fed. Am. Soc. Exp. Biol., 33,* 2296–2301.

Umezawa, H., Surhara, Y., Takita, T., and Maeda, K. (1966). *J. Antibiot., Ser. A. 19,* 210–219.

Umezawa, H., Takeuchi, T., Hori, S., Sawa, T., Ishizuka, M., Ichikawa, T., and Komai, T. (1972). *J. Antibiot. 25,* 409–420.

Watanabe, M., Takabe, Y., and Katsumata, T. (1973). *J. Antibiot. 26,* 417–423.

Yagoda, A., Mukherji, B., Young, C., Etchubana, E., LaMonte, C., Smith, J. R., Tan, C. T., and Krakoff, I. H. (1972). *Ann. Intern. Med. 77,* 861–870.

Chapter 2

THE CURRENT ROLE OF
BLEOMYCIN IN CANCER THERAPY

Stephen K. Carter

I. INTRODUCTION

Bleomycin was a drug eagerly awaited by investigators in the United States. The early clinical reports by Ichikawa (1970) indicated that this antitumor antibiotic, which had been discovered by Umezawa, was active against a range of solid tumors as well as lymphomas. To Ichikawa belongs the credit of first discovering that bleomycin appeared to have specific effects against squamous cell tumors, and he reported activity against squamous cell tumors of the head and neck, cervix, lung, esophagus, and penis (Ichikawa, 1970; Ichikawa et al., 1970). Kimura et al. (1972) were the first to describe activity against the entire range of malignant lymphomas. From the first reports out of Japan two crucial aspects of the toxicity of this drug were obvious. One was a positive factor and the other was a negative factor. The positive aspect was the fact that bleomycin did not have significant myelosuppressive effects. This opened up many prospects for combination approaches which still dominate the clinical trials with this agent to date. The second aspect of the toxicity was pulmonary side effects which began as a pneumonitis and progressed to pulmonary fibrosis which could be fatal. Many studies since then have attempted to predict the toxicity or ameliorate it while vigorous analog development has been pursued with the aim of finding a compound which would not have this toxicity.

II.   STUDIES IN THE UNITED STATES

Studies in the United States confirmed most of the original Japanese findings (Blum et al., 1973; Carter, 1976; Carter and Blum, 1976). The overall similarity of results is just one example of how the two countries have more similarities than differences within the framework of their major commitments to new anticancer drug development. These similarities form the basis of the U.S.–Japan agreement on cancer research which has cancer chemotherapy as one of its major programs.

The phase I studies in the United States elucidated a toxicity pattern identical to that reported by the Japanese. Skin toxicity was often dose-limiting while bone marrow toxicity was rarely severe if it occurred at all. The pulmonary toxicity was also rapidly recognized as the factor which would limit chronic usage of the drug and which would also make high doses not clinically cost-effective.

The phase II studies in the United States confirmed the previously reported activity in squamous head and neck tumors, squamous lesions of the cervix, and in the lymphomas. The single-agent activity was characterized by remissions that were mostly partial in character and which were of short duration. While these remissions were not of dramatic clinical benefit they did indicate the potential value for combination studies. Activity in lung cancer and esophageal cancer was minimal in the U.S. studies and as a single agent this drug has to be deemed inactive within the clinical setting in which it was evaluated. Activity in testicular cancer was found to be an additional indication for bleomycin and combination studies with vinblastine have proven to be one of the most significant effects found with the compound.

When any new drug is found to be active against a given tumor type in phase II studies the phase III strategy can move in a variety of ways. These can include comparative trials with other active drugs, combination studies with other active drugs, combination with other therapeutic modalities, or attempts at schedule, dose level, and route manipulations. All of these have been attempted with bleomycin for some tumor types but combination chemotherapy attempts would have to rank as the most prominent.

III.   TESTICULAR CANCER

Testicular cancer would have to rank as perhaps the tumor in which the greatest triumph with bleomycin in combination has occurred. Samuels (1975; Samuels et al., 1973) was the first to combine bleomycin with vinblastine and he observed a significant increase in response rate. This increase in response rate included complete remissions, some of which gave disease-free durations of such length that the achievement of cure became a reasonable assumption. This was followed by the studies of Golbey (Silvay *et al.*, 1973) and Cvitkovic *et al.* (1974), which first added actinomycin D to velban and bleomycin (VAB I), then platinum to the three (VAB II), and then adriamycin and cytoxan to the four (VAB III). The VAB III (Cvitkovic *et al.*, 1975) regimen also was shown to be highly effective, with nearly everyone treated responding to some degree and with a high percentage of complete responding. Both Samuels and Golbey found that giving bleomycin by continuous infusion in this setting appeared to enhance its effectiveness. Einhorn *et al.* (1976) were able to demonstrate dramatic effects with just velban, bleomycin, and platinum, and others have studied additional approaches. Several papers in this symposium will detail the exciting data that have been generated in this area. What is clear is that advanced testicular cancer is now a potentially curable lesion with highly aggressive combination chemotherapy. These regimens need to be administered by experienced oncologists within a therapeutic framework of adequate supportive care. If utilized by inexperienced clinicians there is the dual risk of either excessive drug-related mortality and/or loss of a potential cure possibility.

IV.   MALIGNANT LYMPHOMAS

The malignant lymphomas represent another group of malignancies for which bleomycin has been incorporated into many combinations. In Hodgkin's disease bleomycin has been integrated into primary therapy in two major ways. One approach has been to add bleomycin to the MOPP combination. This has been studied by the Southwest Oncology Group (SWOG) under the study chairmanship of Coltman (personal communication). Published reports have indicated a higher complete response rate with low dose bleomycin plus MOPP as compared to a concomitant control of MOPP alone. A third arm of high-dose bleomycin plus MOPP was dropped for excessive toxicity. Since this large group study has three different maintenance arms there are nine different induction–maintenance possibilities which will have to be analyzed for remission duration, survival, and chronic toxicity, which are the ultimate end points for analysis of such studies. Currently the SWOG is studying two regimens of MOPP plus low-dose bleomycin plus adriamycin, compared to MOPP and low-dose bleomycin alone.

A second thrust in Hodgkin's disease has been to utilize bleomycin in combinations that would be non-cross-resistant with MOPP. Bonadonna *et al.* (1975) devised a four-drug regimen called ABVD which utilized adriamycin, bleomycin, vinblastine, and dacarbazine (DTIC). They have shown ABVD to be equivalent to MOPP for induction and non-cross-resistant. Current studies involve fixed sequences of MOPP and ABVD. The cancer and leukemia group B (CALGB) has a combination under study in which streptozotocin is substituted for dacarbazine in the ABVD combination.

In the non-Hodgkin's lymphomas the same two trends can be observed. Bleomycin has been added to the three-drug regimen of cyclophosphomide, vincristine, and prednisone which is called either CVP or COP depending upon how the alkylating agent is given. Several groups have added adriamycin as a fifth drug and high complete response rates are reported in diffuse histiocytic lymphomas and others with poor risk histologies (Schein *et al.*, 1975). It appears that these more aggressive five-drug regimens can give a higher percentage of long-term complete responses, which can be considered cures, than was observed with COP or CVP. Non-bleomycin-containing regimens such as CHOP and non-bleomycin- and adriamycin-containing combinations such as C-MOPP also give excellent results and so a range of highly active combinations exists. Bonadonna and Manfardini (1974) have reported on an ABV combination which can be seen as interacting with CVP in a similar manner to ABVD and MOPP. ABV is ABVD without the dacarbazine.

V.   HEAD AND NECK CANCER

In head and neck cancer, combinations have not been so extensively evaluated (Goldsmith and Carter, 1975). Only a few series of aggressive combinations with bleomycin have been reported and none of them has been established as clearly superior to methotrexate alone, which has to be considered as the standard for this disease. The combination of bleomycin with radiation for these tumors has been evaluated in many countries. This has an experimental as well as a clinical rationale and both experimental and clinical studies will be reported in this symposium.

VI.   UTERINE CERVIX TUMORS

Uterine cervix has been a tumor in which chemotherapy has been relatively neglected until recently (Wasserman and Carter, 1977). Bleomycin has been placed into a three-drug combination including mitomycin C and vincristine. Studies in the United States by Baker and in Japan by Miyamoto indicate that this regimen is significantly more active in terms of regression than single-agent therapy.

VII.   BRONCHOGENIC CARCINOMA

Despite the fact that single-agent activity in bronchogenic carcinoma was disappointing, many combinations have been attempted because of the marrow-sparing properties of bleomycin. Highly aggressive regimens such as COMB (Livingston *et al.*, 1975) and BACON (Livingston *et al.*, 1974) in squamous lesions gave a higher response rate than single-agent therapy but without any survival gain, so that these regimens cannot be recommended.

VIII.   DOSE LEVEL, ROUTE, AND SCHEDULE

Studies with bleomycin that have looked at dose level, route, and schedule have given some indications but nothing that can be considered definitive. Bleomycin does not appear to have a steep dose-response curve as is commonly found with myelosuppressive drugs. In the malignant lymphoma there appears to be no dose-response effect as low doses do just as well as high doses with lessened toxicity. The validity of this statement in solid tumors is less clearly demonstrated. Livingston *et al.* report on three dose levels of bleomycin in his COMB regimen (1975). At 30 mg/m^2 the highest response rate was observed but toxicity was prohibitive. As the dose was lowered to 15 and 7.5 mg/m^2 the toxicity became tolerable but the response rate dropped. Baker has modified the bleomycin level in the MOB regimen for uterine cervix with equivocal results.

When route is scrutinized the IM appears to be equally effective when compared to the IV but this is not clearly established within any individual tumor type. Studies in Japan have indicated that bleomycin in oil given IM mimics continuous IV infusion and may be more effective. Studies in testicular carcinoma in the United States appear to favor continuous infusions of bleomycin but this has not been definitively established by controlled comparison and has not been extensively evaluated in other tumor types.

IX. SUMMARY

Bleomycin is clearly established as an active drug with an interesting and important spectrum of activity. In testicular cancer and the lymphomas it is an integral part of combinations which have curative potential. In head and neck cancer its combination with radiation offers the potential of increased local control and ultimate survival enhancement. In cervical cancer combinations are generating exciting preliminary data. The drug is part of a wide range of investigative protocols. It has proven to be an important weapon to be added to the arsenal of the clinical oncologist.

REFERENCES

Blum, R. H., Carter, S. K., and Agre, K. (1973). *Cancer 31,* 903–914.

Bonadonna, G., and Manfardini, S. (1974). *Cancer Treatment Rev. 1,* 167–181.

Bonadonna, G., Zucali, R., Manfardini, S., *et al.* (1975). *Cancer 36,* 252–259.

Carter, S. K. (1976). *Gann Monogr. Cancer Res. 19,* 285–299.

Carter, S. K., and Blum, R. H. (1976). *Prog. Biochem. Pharmacol. 11,* 158–171.

Cvitkovic, E., Currie, V., Ochoa, M., Pride, G., and Krakoff, I.H. (1974). *Proc. Am. Assoc. Cancer Res. 15,* 179.

Cvitkovic, E., Currie, V., Krakoff, I. H., and Golbey, R. (1975). *Proc. Am. Assoc. Cancer Res. 16,* 273.

Einhorn, L. H., Furnas, B. E., and Powell, N. (1976). *Proc. Am. Soc. Clin. Oncol.-AACR 17,* 240.

Goldsmith, M. A., and Carter, S. K. (1975). *Cancer Treatment Rev. 2,* 137–158.

Ichikawa, T. (1970). *Progress in Antimicrobial and Anticancer Chemotherapy (Proc. 6th Int. Congr. Chemother.), Vol. II.* University of Tokyo Press, Tokyo, pp. 228–290.

Ichikawa, T., Nakano, I., and Krokawa, I. (1970). *Progress in Antimicrobial and Anticancer Chemotherapy (Proc. 6th Int. Congr. Chemother.), Vol. II.* University of Tokyo Press, Tokyo, pp. 304–308.

Kimura, K., Sakai, Y., Konda, C., *et al*. (1972). *Proc. 7th Int. Congr. Chemother., 1972.* Prague 2, 667–668.

Livingston, R. B., Einhorn, L. H., Bodey, G. P., Burgess, M. A., Freireich, E. J., and Gottlieb, J. A. (1975). *Cancer 36*, 327–332.

Livingston, R. B., Burgess, M. A., Gottlieb, J. A., Bodey, G. P., and Rodriguez, V. (1974). *Proc. Am. Assoc. Cancer Res. 15*, 173.

Samuels, M. L. (1975). *Proc. Am. Assoc. Cancer Res. 16*, 112.

Samuels, M. L., Johnson, D. E., and Holoye, P. Y. (1973). *Proc. Am. Assoc. Cancer Res. 14*, 23.

Schein, P. S., Chabner, B. A., Cannellos, G. P., *et al*. (1975). *Br. J. Cancer 31* (Suppl. II), 465–473.

Silvay, O., Yagoda, A., Wittes, R., Whitmore, W., and Golbey, R. (1973). *Proc. Am. Assoc. Cancer Res. 14*, 68.

Wasserman, T. A., and Carter, S. K. (1977). *Cancer Treatment Rev. 4*, 25–46.

Chapter 3

RECENT STUDIES ON BIOCHEMISTRY
AND ACTION OF BLEOMYCIN

Hamao Umezawa

I. INTRODUCTION

The author discovered bleomycin in 1966 in his study of phleomycin-type anti-biotics (Umezawa, 1976) and Ichikawa (1976) noted its therapeutic effect on squamous cell carcinoma. The clinical study was thus extended and this antibiotic was found to exhibit strong therapeutic action against the malignant lymphomas. It was also recently found that this antibiotic, used in combination with a vinca alka-loid or a platinum compound, can exhibit therapeutic action against testis tumors. On the other hand, the chemistry and biochemistry of the antibiotic have been studied in relation to its mechanism of cytotoxic and therapeutic actions and this has contributed to development of more effective derivatives or analogs. In this paper the author reports his recent studies on chemistry and biochemistry of mech-anisms of actions of bleomycin, its structure–activity relationships, and its action in combination with a microbial product enhancing immune responses.

II. STUDIES

As first found by the author and his collaborators (Umezawa, 1976), bleomycin binds with DNA, and the chemical reaction between bleomycin and DNA results in single-strand scission. Recently, Asakura *et al.* (in press) have proven that double-stranded structures of DNA were the requirement for the binding with bleomycin. ^{3}H-SV40 DNA sediments with 53 S in alkaline sucrose density gradient centrifugation, and the product, after the reaction with bleomycin, sediments with 16 S and 18 S, to produce a combined single peak. We studied the inhibition of this bleomycin action by oligodeoxynucleotides in the reaction condition where about 60% of SV40 superhelical DNA was converted by bleomycin to the nicked open circular form. Single-stranded octadeoxynucleotides such as d(pTpG)$_4$ or d(pCpA)$_4$ (d means deoxy, p means phosphate, and T, G, C, and A mean thymidine, deoxyguanosine, deoxycytosine, and deoxyadenosine, respectively) alone did not inhibit the bleomycin action. The bleomycin action was also not inhibited by addition of d(pTpG)$_{6-9}$ or d(pCpA)$_{6-9}$ alone. However, the addition of the mixtures d(pTpG)$_4$ and d(pCpA)$_4$ or d(pTpG)$_{6-9}$ and d(pCpA)$_{6-9}$, which could form double strands, inhibited the bleomycin action against SV40 DNA. The mixture of hexadeoxynucleotides such as d(pTpG)$_3$ and d(pCpA)$_3$, which seemed to form double strands over four base pairs also easily inhibited the bleomycin action, although the mixture of such tetranucleotides [the mixture of d(pTpG)$_2$ and d(pCpA)$_2$] did not inhibit the bleomycin action. These tetradeoxynucleotides are thought to be able to make double strands over four complete base pairs if the partner deoxynucleotides are large enough. In fact, the mixtures of d(pTpG)$_2$ and d(pCpA)$_{6-9}$ or d(pTpG)$_{6-9}$ and d(pCpA)$_2$ inhibited the bleomycin action. These results indicate that the double-stranded structures of DNA are the requirement for the binding with bleomycin and the region of DNA in binding with a bleomycin molecule is extended over four base pairs along a DNA double strand. Single-stranded DNA such as heat- or alkaline-denatured DNAs has been known to be susceptible to the action of bleomycin. These DNAs also inhibited the bleomycin action against SV40 DNA. There is no doubt that double-stranded structures can be formed in some regions of macromolecular DNA and these parts can bind with bleomycin. The chemistry of the binding will be elucidated by physicochemical study of the binding of bleomycin with double-stranded oligodeoxynucleotides.

The structure of bleomycin proposed by Umezawa in 1972 has been revised in 1978 (Fig. 1). Various bleomycins produced by fermentation consist of the same disaccharide moiety and the complicated peptide parts which are different from one another in their terminal amine moiety. The terminal amine moiety is not essential for the action to cause DNA strand scission, because bleomycin B1, which contains ammonia as the terminal amine, causes single-strand scission of DNA. (Umezawa, 1976).

The amino group of the d-carboxamide moiety and the adjacent secondary amino group in the first amino acid residue of the pyrimide chromophore of the first amino acid residue, N^4 of the imidazole group, the d-amino group of the β-hydroxyhistidine moiety, and the carbamoyl group in the sugar moiety have been shown recently to be copper ligands of the bleomycin molecule. The first amino acid residue consisting of a side chain and the 4-amino-6-carboxy-5-methylpyrimidine moiety may be tentatively called blactaminopyramidine acid. Recently, Takita *et al.*, at the Institute of Microbial Chemistry isolated (demethylblaminopyrimidyl) histidine from

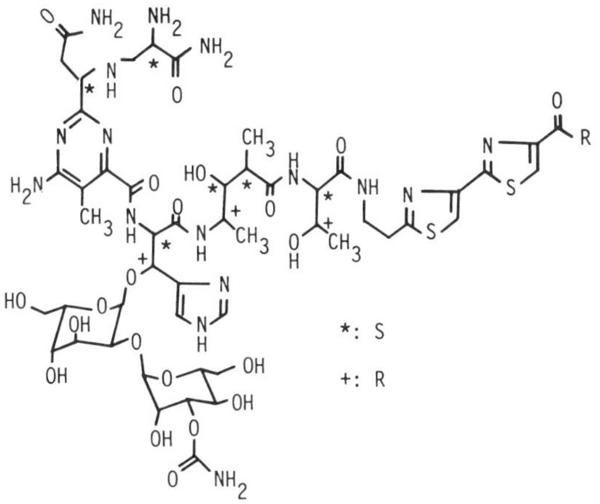

Bleomycins:

A1: R = NH-$(CH_2)_3$-SO-CH_3;   Demethyl-A2: R = NH-$(CH_2)_3$-S-CH_3;

A2: R = NH-$(CH_2)_3$-S$\overset{CH_3}{\underset{+}{\overset{}{\diagdown}}}CH_3$;   A2'-a: R = NH-$(CH_2)_4$-$NH_2$;

A2'-b: R = NH-$(CH_2)_3$-NH_2;   A2'-c: R = NH-$(CH_2)_2$$\begin{array}{c}\diagup N\\ \diagdown N\diagup\\ H\end{array}$

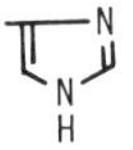

, A5: R = NH-$(CH_2)_3$-NH-$(CH_2)_4$-NH_2;   A6: R = NH-$(CH_2)_3$-NH-$(CH_2)_4$-NH-$(CH_2)_3$-NH_2;

B1': R = NH_2;   B2: R = NH-$(CH_2)_4$-NH-$\overset{\overset{\displaystyle NH}{\|}}{C}$-$NH_2$;

B4: R = NH-$(CH_2)_4$-NH-$\overset{\overset{\displaystyle NH}{\|}}{C}$-NH-$(CH_2)_4$-NH-$\overset{\overset{\displaystyle NH}{\|}}{C}$-$NH_2$;   Bleomycinic acid: R = OH

Fig. 1. Structures of bleomycins.

culture filtrates of the bleomycin-producing strain. This peptide forms a copper complex. This supports the idea that the main copper ligands of the bleomycin molecule must be located in the blactaminopyrimidyl-β-hydroxyhistidyl moiety of the bleomycin molecule. Bleomycin copper complex does not cause strand scission of DNA, although there are observations which show the binding of the bleomycin copper complex with DNA. As reported by Yoshioka and Umezawa *et al.* (this volume), in animal cells the cupric ion of the bleomycin copper complex is reduced to the cuprous ion and the cuprous ion is transferred to a cellular protein which has the ability to bind with cuprous ion. This type of cellular protein was first found by the study of bleomycin behavior *in vivo*.

As found by the author (1976), bleomycin hydrolase, which hydrolyzes the carboxamide group in the blactaminopyrimidyl moiety of the bleomycin molecule, is widely distributed in animal tissues. Copper-free bleomycin is susceptible to this enzyme reaction but the bleomycin copper complex is resistant. The volume of experimental data indicating that the therapeutic action of bleomycin against squamous cell carcinoma is due to a low content of this enzyme in this type of tumors is increasing. Moreover, bleomycin is distributed at a high concentration in this type of tumor.

In order to develop more effective bleomycins or more effective antibiotics of a similar type it may be necessary to study the mode of the biosynthesis of bleomycin in detail. Recently, Fujii *et al.* at the Nippon Kayaku Co. succeeded in isolating peptides which could be thought to be the biosynthesis intermediates. From culture filtrates, (demethylblactaminopyrimidyl) histidine, (demethylblactamino-pyrimidyl) histidylalanine, (demethylblactaminopyrimidyl) histidyl-4-amino-3-hydroxy-2-methyl)]pentanoic acid, and (demethylblactaminopyrimidyl) histidyl-(4-amino-3-hydroxy-2-methyl)pentanoylthreonine were isolated. The methylation product of the last one, that is, blactaminopyrimidylhistidyl-(4-amino-3-hydroxy-2-methyl)pentanoylthreonine, was also isolated from culture filtrates. This indicates that the biosynthesis of the bleomycin peptide was started from the synthesis of (demethylblactaminopyrimidyl) histidine on a multienzyme and the demethylblact-aminopyrimidyl moiety is methylated when the methylation point is separated from the multienzyme by a great enough distance. The hydroxylation of the histidyl part to produce the β-hydroxyhistidine moiety occurs in a later step, because blactaminopyrimidylhistidyl-(4-amino-3-hydroxy-2-methyl)pentanoylthreonyl-2',2-aminoethyl-2',4'-bithiazole acid was obtained.

As found by Hori *et al.* at the Institute of Microbial Chemistry, leupeptin acid (acetyl-L-Leu-L-Leu-L-L-Arg) is biosynthesized from acetate, leucine, arginine, and ATP on a multienzyme, and, as found by Umezawa *et al.* (1978), the biosynthesis of this multienzyme is controlled by a plasmid which can be transferred from a leu-peptin-producing methionine-requiring mutant to a leupeptin-nonproducing and arginine-requiring mutant. It is possible that a plasmid is involved in the biosynthesis of the multienzyme for the synthesis of bleomycin peptides. In order to find more effective, bleomycin–phleomycin-type antibiotics the biosynthesis may be worth studying in detail.

Various bleomycins which have unique terminal amine moieties can be prepared by fermentation or by derivation of bleomycinic acid, which can be obtained by enzymic hydrolysis of bleomycin B2 or chemically from bleomycin demethyl-A2. As reported by Matsuda *et al.* (this volume), various bleomycins are different in their degree of renal and pulmonary toxicities and the one named pepbleomycin has been selected as the one most deserving clinical study. It is also possible to develop derivatives in which the amino group of the α-aminocarboxyamide part of the blactaminopyrimidyl moiety may yield antibiotics that show different antitumor spectrum from the present bleomycin. This study is being done in collaboration with Dr. Tanaka and others in the Nippon Kayaku Co. Research Institute.

Bleomycin is one of the antitumor chemotherapeutic agents which can cure some types of human tumors. Studies of its derivatives or analogs may yield ones that will increase the rate of cure. On the other hand, combination with an agent

which can reestablish the depressed immune response in cancer patients may increase the rate of cure by bleomycin. The author is now conducting studies of this possibility.

It might be thought that compounds which bind to the surface of cells involved in immunity may enhance or decrease immune responses. Such compounds can be found by searching for those which inhibit the enzymes on the cellular surface. The method has been established by the author. Aoyagi *et al.* (1976) found that intact animals cells including macrophages and lymphocytes hydrolyze the N-terminal peptide bond of peptides, and the enzymes involved in this hydrolysis, that is, aminopeptidases, are not released extracellularly. We found bestatin [(3S, 4S)-3-amino-4-phenylbutanoyl-L-leucine] in culture filtrates of streptomyces (Umezawa *et al.*, 1976a). Bestatin inhibits aminopeptidase B and leucine aminopeptidase. This microbial product enhanced delayed-type hypersensitivity in a wide range of its doses (0.1-100 μg/mouse) (Umezawa *et al.*, 1976b). Bestatin suppressed the growth of experimental animal tumors in which the growth could be tested for 30 or more than 30 days. By enhancing delayed-type hypersensitivity, bestatin in the dose increased the effect of bleomycin on Ehrlich carcinoma (Umezawa, 1977). Bestatin has extremely low toxicity. The preliminary study by Ichikawa and Fukushima indicated that bestatin increased T-cell population in the depressed patients and the preliminary clinical study by Ichikawa and Hirokawa indicated that bestatin was worth the clinical study in treatment of cancer in detail.

III.   CONCLUSION

Chemical and biochemical studies of bleomycin are interesting in the field of chemistry of natural products. But the studies in relation to the cancer treatment are far more important. Bleomycin is one of the antitumor agents that can cure some type of human tumors. Further detailed study on mechanisms of actions and on development of more effective analogs or derivatives will contribute to the approach to the goal of successful cancer therapy.

REFERENCES

Aoyagi, T., Suda, H., Nagai, M., Ogawa, K., Suzuki, J., Takeuchi, T., and Umezawa, H. (1976). *Biochim. Biophys. Acta 452,* 131-143.

Asakura, H., Umezawa, H., and Hori, M. (in press). *J. Antibiot.*

Ichikawa, T. (1976). *Gann Monogr. Cancer Res. 19,* 99-116.

Kunishima, M., Fujii, T., Nakayama, Y., Takita, T., and Umezawa, H. (1976). *J. Antibiot. 29,* 853-856.

Umezawa, H. (1976). *Gann Monogr. Cancer Res. 19,* 3-36.

Umezawa, H. (1977). *Biomedicine 26,* 236-249.

Umezawa, H., Aoyagi, T., Suda, H., Hamada, M., and Takeuchi, T. (1976a). *J. Antibiot. 29,* 97-99.

Umezawa, H., Ishizuka, M., Aoyagi, T., and Takeuchi, T. (1976b). *J. Antibiot. 29,* 857-859.

Umezawa, H., Okami, Y., and Hotta, K. (1978). *J. antibiot. 31,* 95-98.

Chapter 4

ACTION OF BLEOMYCIN ON DNA[1]

Charles W. Haidle
R. Stephen Lloyd

I. INTRODUCTION

During the past 10 years there has been a great deal of research on the action of bleomycin on isolated, purified DNA including bacterial DNAs, DNAs from both bacterial and mammalian viruses, mammalian DNAs, and synthetic deoxypoly-nucleotides (Umezawa *et al.*, 1966; Haidle, 1971; Haidle *et al.*, 1972a,b; Haidle and Bearden, 1975; Umezawa, 1975, 1976; Miyaki and Ono, 1976; Müller *et al.*, 1976; Müller and Zahn, 1976, 1977; Bearden *et al.*, 1977; Kuo *et al.*, 1977). In all cases the drug causes extensive damage to the DNAs including the release of free bases. Thymine appears to be preferentially released at low drug concentrations (Müller *et al.*, 1972); however, at high drug concentrations the release of all bases can be detected (Haidle *et al.*, 1972b). Also the phosphodiester backbone is broken predominantly on the $3'$-side of the deoxyribose (Kuo and Haidle, 1973). Another possible consequence of the drug action is a breakage of the deoxyribose itself. In addition the drug causes a decrease in the melting temperature of the DNA (Nagai *et al.*, 1969a).

[1] This research was supported in part by grant No. CA 13246 awarded by the National Cancer Institute, DHEW, and grant No. G-441 awarded by the Robert A. Welch Foundation.

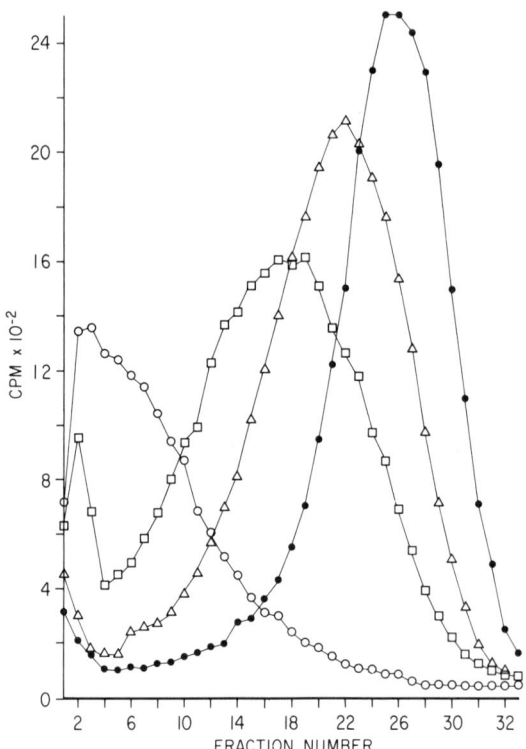

Fig. 1.   Fragmentation of bacterial DNA as a function of increasing bleomycin concentration. Alkaline sucrose gradients; sedimentation was to the left. The reaction mixtures contained 25 mM 2-mercaptoethanol, 15 μg/ml of ^{3}H-thymidine-labeled DNA, and bleomycin as follows: ○, control (no bleomycin); □, 10 μg/ml; △, 40 μg/ml; ●, 60 μg/ml. The reaction mixtures were incubated for 1 hr at 37°. Redrawn from Haidle, 1971.

This DNA breakage reaction proceeds very slowly in the presence of the drug alone, but is greatly stimulated by the presence of thiol compounds such as 2-mercaptoethanol or dithiothreitol (Haidle, 1971; Nagai *et al.*, 1969b); oxidizing agents such as hydrogen peroxide also stimulate the reaction (Onishi *et al.*, 1975).

The main purpose of studying this extracellular reaction is to attempt to correlate it with the intracellular effects leading to cell death. Of course, from the biochemist's point of view, this extracellular reaction is of great interest in itself.

Most of the work on this reaction has employed alkaline sucrose gradients to assay the decrease in the molecular weight of the DNA in the presence of the drug. Figure 1 shows such an alkaline gradient in the presence of increasing drug concentrations using *Bacillus subtilis* DNA in the presence of 25 mM 2-mercaptoethanol. Using high drug concentrations (5-10 mg/ml) one can achieve about 80% solubilization of the DNA.

Bleomycin is a potent inhibitor of most bacterial and mammalian cell cultures

(Crooke and Bradner, 1976). It is also very effective in the induction of bacterio-phage from the lysogenic strain of *E. coli* (λ) and also of certain phages from *B. subtilis* (Haidle *et al.*, 1972c).

Bleomycin, with a molecular weight of only 1500, displays a high degree of sub-strate specificity. There is no action on RNA, as demonstrated by the inability of the drug to cause any decrease of the molecular weight of RNA (Haidle *et al.*, 1972a). In addition, if one prepares an RNA/DNA hybrid using reverse transcrip-tase, the drug degrades the DNA strand while leaving the RNA strand intact (Haidle and Bearden, 1975). Also, if one pretreats globin mRNA with high concentrations of bleomycin, followed by the removal of the drug by extensive dialysis, the mRNA is

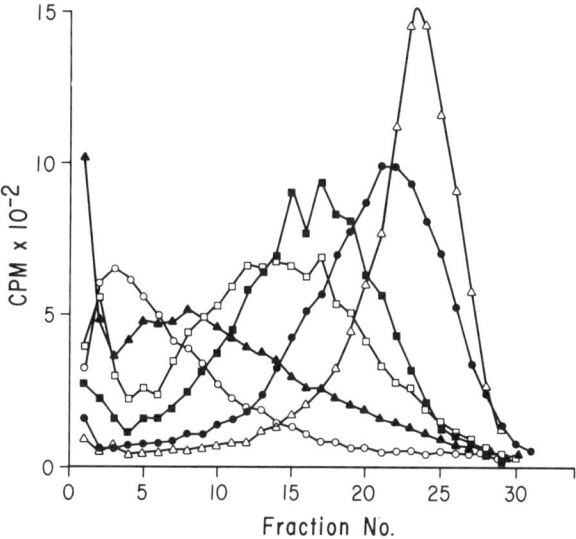

Fig. 2. Inactivation of the bleomycin-induced DNA fragmentation by EDTA, CDTA, and EGTA in the presence of 2-mercaptoethanol. Alkaline sucrose gradients; sedimentation was to the left. The standard reaction mixtures contained: 50 g/ml (0.0333 mM, assuming a molecu-lar weight of 1500) of bleomycin; 25 mM 2-mercaptoethanol, 50 μg/ml (0.1501 mM) of *B. subtilis* DNA in a total volume of 0.4 ml of 12.5 mM Tris-Cl pH 8.0. The mixtures were incu-bated for 1 hr at 21° ; 0.1 ml of 1.5 N NaOH, 3.5 N NaCl was added to stop the reaction prior to layering on alkaline sucrose gradients. The bleomycin was mixed with the chelating agent to be tested (dissolved in 0.05 M Tris-Cl, pH 8.0) and preincubated under the indicated conditions prior to addition to the standard reaction mixture. Preincubation reactions performed at 80° were allowed to cool for 10 min prior to use in the reaction mixtures. After the incubations described, the reaction mixtures were layered onto 4.5 ml 5–20% (w/v) sucrose gradients con-taining 0.3 N NaOH and 0.7 N NaCl (7). The gradients were centrifuged in the Beckman SW 50.1 rotor (Beckman Instruments, Palo Alto. Calif.) at 40,000 rpm (149,000 g) for 4 hr at 5°. The gradients were collected, samples treated with trichloroacetic acid, and radioactivity deter-mined. The bleomycin was preincubated at the indicated temperatures and times with 0.25 mM of the indicated chelating agents or 0.05 M Tris-Cl, pH 8.0 prior to addition to the standard reaction mixtures. All concentrations were those of the final reaction mixtures. ○ , DNA con-trol, no bleomycin, no chelator; △, bleomycin control, no chelator □ , preincubated with EDTA for 10 min at 80°; ●, preincubated with EGTA for 10 min at 80°; ▲, preincubated with DCTA for 10 min at 80° ; ■ , preincubated with CDTA for 20 min at 21°.

γ

fully functional in synthesizing globin using a wheat-germ embryo translation system (Kuo *et al.*, 1977). Since bleomycin can degrade DNA derived from the bacteriophage PBS1, which contains deoxyuridine in place of thymidine, it would appear that the specificity for DNA atack lies in the presence of deoxyribose in DNA since the base composition of RNA versus DNA or the secondary structure does not seem to confer the specificity (Haidle *et al.*, 1972a).

II.   EFFECT OF CHELATING AGENTS

More recently we have been examining the effect of EDTA on the extracellular reaction. Conflicting reports have appeared in the literature concerning the effect of EDTA. There have been claims for both an inhibitory effect and a noninhibitory effect. Since there is a possibility for the involvement of metal ions in the bleomycin–DNA reaction, we thought it important to examine the effect of various chelating agents on the reaction.

As illustrated in Fig. 2, bleomycin was inactivated by the chelating agents 1,2-diaminocyclohexane-N, N'tetraacetic acid (CDTA), ethylenediamine tetraacetic acid (EDTA), and [ethyleneglycol-bis] (p-aminoethylether)-N,N' tetraacetic acid (EGTA). The inactivation reaction was dependent upon both the concentration of the chelating agents and the time and temperature of the incubation of the chelating agents with bleomycin. CDTA was the most effective in the inactivation reaction,

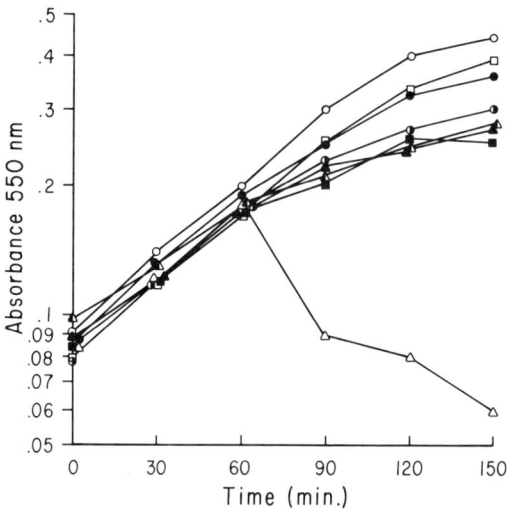

Fig. 3.   Loss of growth inhibition of *B. subtilis* after reaction of bleomycin with chelating agents. The bleomycin (20 μg/ml, 0.0133 m*M*) was preincubated with the indicated chelators (0.1 m*M*) or 0.05 *M* Tris-Cl, pH 8.0 for 10 min at 80° prior to addition to the cell culture. All concentrations were those of the final cell cultures. ○, control, no bleomycin, no chelating agent; △, bleomycin only; □, EGTA only; ●, CDTA only; ▲, EDTA only; ■, EGTA preincubated with bleomycin; ◑, CDTA preincubated with bleomycin; ▲, EDTA preincubated with bleomycin.

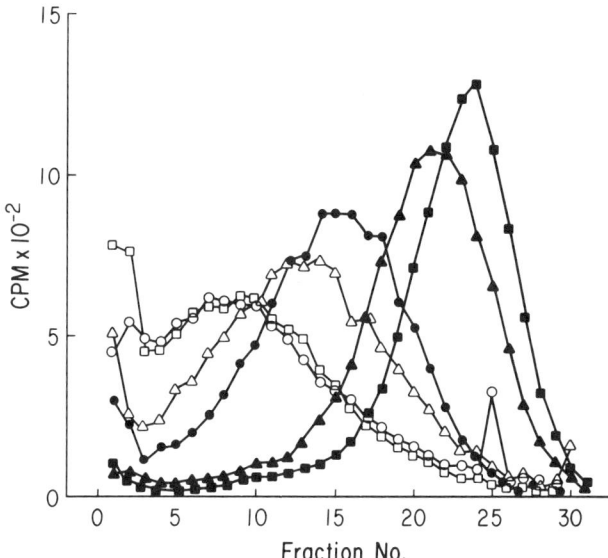

Fig. 4. Stimulatory effect of Mg^{2+} on the bleomycin-induced fragmentation of DNA. Alkaline sucrose gradients; sedimentation was to the left. The bleomyicn (1.0 μg/ml, 0.666 μM) was preincubated with the indicated concentrations of Mg^{2+} for 20 min at 21° prior to addition to the final reaction mixtures. All concentrations were those of the final reaction mixtures. ○, DNA control, no bleomycin, no Mg^{2+}; △, bleomycin control, no Mg^{2+}; □, 2.5 mM Mg^{2+} no bleomycin; ●, 0.25 mM Mg^{2+}, 1 μg/ml of bleomycin; ▲, 1.25 mM Mg^{2+}, 1 μg/ml of bleomycin; ■, 2.5 mM Mg^{2+}, 1 μg/ml of bleomycin.

and EGTA was the least effective. Although the experiment represented by Fig. 2 was performed in the presence of 2-mercaptoethanol, very similar profiles were obtained in the absence of the reducing agent using a long incubation period (16–17 hr). After reaction with the chelators the bleomycin was inactive in both the extracellular DNA fragmentation reaction (Fig. 2) and the inhibition of the growth of a *Bacillus subtilis* system. This loss of the ability to inhibit the bacterial growth is shown in Fig. 3. Lysis of the bacterial population was observed in the absence of any chelating agent (open triangles). In all of the other curves, representing samples containing chelating agents, there was only a slight inhibition of bacterial growth. When purified DNA was preincubated with EDTA followed by the addition of bleomycin, little inhibition of the fragmentation of the DNA was observed. Thus the chelating agents are assumed to be reacting with the active site(s) on the bleomycin molecule. Since Mg^{2+} and Ca^{2+} stimulated the extracellular DNA fragmentation reaction and since the chelators used have a high affinity for these ions, the possibility exists that metal ions are required for bleomycin activity. Figure 4 shows the stimulatory effect of Mg^{2+} on the extracellular reaction.

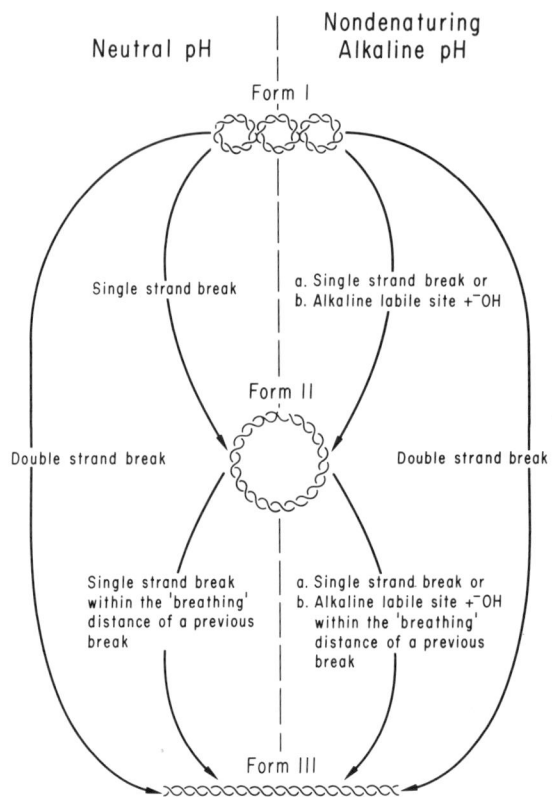

Fig. 5.   A schematic representation showing the effects of damage to the PM2 DNA molecule when assayed under either neutral or nondenaturing alkaline conditions.

III.   ALKALINE LABILE DAMAGE USING PM2 DNA AS THE SUBSTRATE

All of the experiments described in the previous section have been based on the changes in sedimentation velocity using sucrose gradients of fragmented linear DNA after reaction with bleomycin. In order to increase the sensitivity of the detection of breakage of isolated DNA, the experimental design for the remainder of this research was based on the use of the superhelical covalently closed-circular DNA isolated from the bacteriophage PM2 (Espejo and Canelo, 1968) (Fig. 5). This method is based on the differences in electrophoretic mobilities of the three topological forms of PM2 DNA: form I a native superhelical molecule; form II, a nicked relaxed circular molecule; and form III, a double-standed linear molecule. In order to test for alkaline labile sites which could be introduced by the action of the drug, bleomycin-treated DNA samples were assayed either under neutral conditions or nondenaturing alkaline conditions; the nondenaturing alkaline assay effectively hydrolyzes alkaline labile sites (e.g., sites at which bases have been removed) but does not denature the DNA. Using this method, the neutral assay only measures direct single- and double-strand breaks. The amount of DNA in each band was determined by ethidium bromide intercalation in double-stranded DNA and fluorescence scanning as previously described (Bearden *et al.*, 1977).

In order effectively to analyze alkaline labile damage in the PM2 DNA, it was necessary to determine the conditions at which known alkaline labile sites could be hydrolyzed without irreversibly denaturing the DNA. A method utilizing acid–heat-treatment of the DNA to selectively remove purines was used to generate an alkaline labile DNA population (Lindahl and Nyberg, 1972). When analysis for strand breakage was performed at neutral pH, the percentage of surviving form I DNA with increasing time of acid incubation at 60°C showed a very slow rate for the

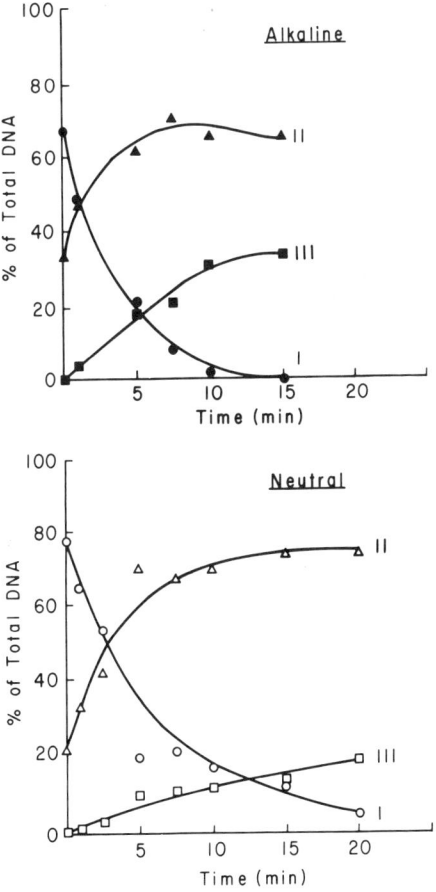

Fig. 6. Effect of bleomycin on PM2 DNA with increasing reaction time. The bottom panel shows the percentage of DNA in each form as a function of reaction time analyzed at neutral pH: ○, form I; △, form II; □ , form III, The top panel shows the same reaction analyzed at pH 11.7: ●, form I; ▲, form II; ■, form III.

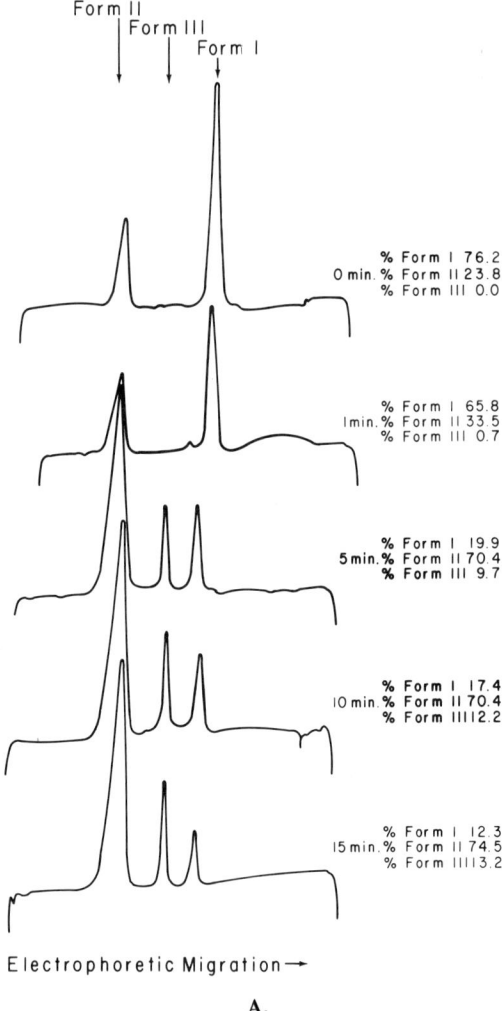

Form II
Form III
Form I

% Form I 76.2
0 min. % Form II 23.8
% Form III 0.0

% Form I 65.8
1 min. % Form II 33.5
% Form III 0.7

% Form I 19.9
5 min. % Form II 70.4
% Form III 9.7

% Form I 17.4
10 min. % Form II 70.4
% Form III 12.2

% Form I 12.3
15 min. % Form II 74.5
% Form III 13.2

Electrophoretic Migration →

A.

Fig. 7. Tracings of fluorescent gel scans. These scans show the changes in the areas under the DNA peaks after increasing bleomycin–DNA reaction time. Electrophoresis was from left to right with form I migrating the fastest, followed by form III and then form II. Panels A and B show analyses under the neutral and alkaline conditions, respectively.

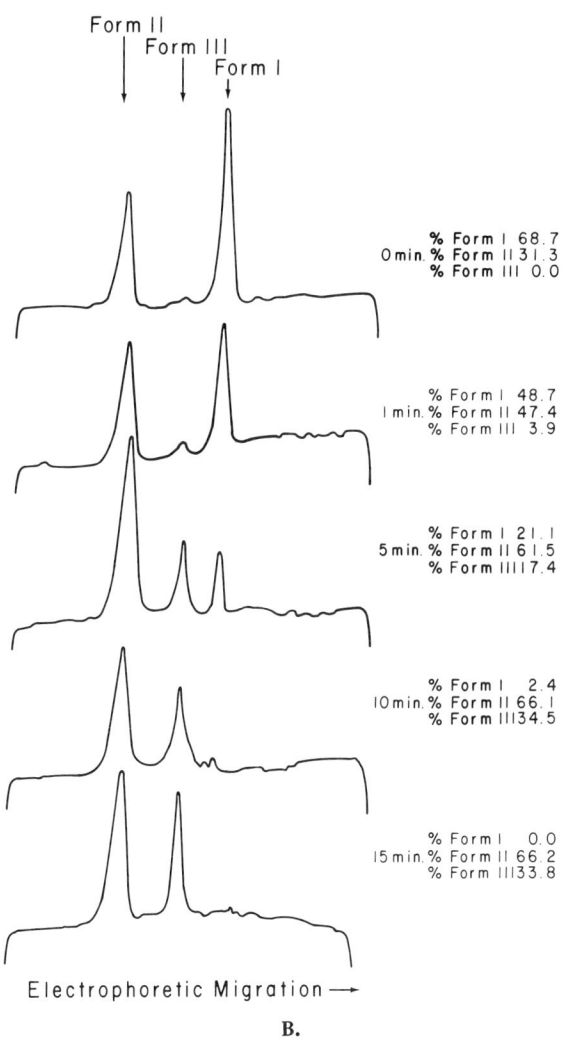

Fig. 7. continued.

introduction of single-strand breaks. However, when the pH from aliquots of the same population of acid–heat-treated DNA was raised to 11.7 for 2.5 hr, neutralized and analyzed on the agarose gels, an exponential loss of form I DNA with a corresponding increase in form II DNA was detected. This demonstrates that the alkaline labile damage in the form of purine base removal can be effectively assayed using PM2 DNA at pH 11.7 without irreversibly denaturing the DNA. Alkaline treatment beyond 2.5 hr showed no further alkaline hydrolysis, indicating complete hydrolysis of alkaline labile sties.

Figure 6 shows a composite of a time course reaction using 0.5 μg/ml of bleomycin, 2-mercaptoethanol, and PM2 DNA analyzed under both neutral and nondenaturing alkaline conditions. It is evident that low doses of bleomycin (0.5 μg/ml) caused extensive damage to the DNA in a short time. The percentage of form I DNA at the zero time point (before bleomycin was added) was 76.2 in the neutral analysis and 68.7 after alkali treatment. This indicates that approximately 7.5% of the starting DNA population contained sites which were hydrolyzable under the nondenaturing alkaline conditions. At the start of the experiments, there was 23.8 and 31.3% of form II DNA in the neutral and alkaline analyses, respectively; form III DNA was present at time zero in amounts not detectable by fluorescence scanning. Under neutral conditions, form I DNA (open circles) decreased to less than 5% after 20 min of reaction with bleomycin. In contrast, in analyses by nondenaturing alkaline conditions in which both breaks and hydrolyzed alkaline labile sites contribute to the loss of form I DNA (closed circles), less than 5% of superhelical DNA remained after only 10 min of incubation. Form II DNA (open triangles) increased rapidly to approximately 70% after 10 min of reaction and remained fairly constant throughout the remainder of the neutral pH experiment. However, form II DNA, when analyzed with nondenaturing alkali (closed triangles), reached a fairly constant precentage after 5 min of reaction but began to diminish gradually toward the end of the experiment. Form III DNA analyzed under neutral conditions was observed immediately after the start of the reaction and steadily increased with increasing time of fragmentation to approximately 15% at 20 min. Analyses using the nondenaturing alkaline assay showed an increase in form III DNA to nearly 35% after 15 min of reaction. Figure 7 illustrates tracings of gel scans for both neutral (Panel A) and nondenaturing alkaline (Panel B) analyses and the calculated planimetered areas of the peaks. These results show that: (a) form I DNA is lost with bleomycin treatment; (b) bleomycin is inducing direct single-strand breaks and also causing double-strand breaks; (c) the rate at which form I DNA is lost is greater when analyzed under nondenaturing alkaline pH, thus indicating hydrolysis of alkaline labile sites which were induced by bleomycin treatment. In this experiment the rate of loss of form I DNA proceeded approximately twice as fast when analyzed under nondenaturing alkaline conditions, or approximately one detectable hydrolyzable site introduced for every direct single-strand break. Over a wide range of bleomycin concentrations and temperatures the average rate at which damage was introduced into isolated DNA in the form of single-strand breaks and alkaline labile sites shows that the reaction proceeds 1.9 times faster when analyzed under alkaline conditions compared with neutral conditions. Therefore in the bleomycin–DNA fragmentation reaction for every single-strand break directly introduced by the drug, a second alkaline labile site is also formed.

The rate of appearance of form III DNA molecules was also studied under the neutral and nondenaturing alkaline conditions. Over a wide range of bleomycin concentrations and reaction temperatures approximately two linear DNA molecules were produced when analyzed under alkaline conditions for each linear molecule produced under neutral conditions.

IV.   ACCUMULATION OF DOUBLE-STRAND BREAKS IN FORM I PM2 DNA

As demonstrated in the previous section, the action of bleomycin on isolated DNA results in the formation of alkaline labile sites, single-strand breaks, and double-strand breaks. Since we wished to determine if the appearance of linear form III DNA molecules was the result of a random accumulation of single-strand breaks or was the result of direct double-strand cleavage, an experiment was run in which 0.5 μg/ml of bleomycin was incubated for varying times with PM2 DNA in the presence of 2-mercaptoethanol. Approximately 93% of the total DNA population at time zero consisted of form I DNA, but this value decreased rapidly to approximately 20% after 25 min of incubation with bleomycin. The orginal DNA preparation (at time zero) also contained approximately 7% of form II DNA; form III was present at the start of the experiment in amounts not detectable by fluorescence scanning. Form II DNA increased rapidly to about 70% after 25 min of reaction and remained fairly constant throughout the remainder of the experiment. Form III DNA increased with increasing time of exposure to bleomycin from less than 1% at time zero to nearly 13% after 45 min. The increase in the amount of both the form II DNA and the form III DNA was derived from the conversion of the original form I DNA. Even though the original DNA population was not pure superhelical form I DNA, the appearance of form III DNA could not have arisen exclusively from even a very highly damaged form II DNA population in the original DNA preparation. This was evident because after 25 min there was 10.6% linear DNA (form III), while the starting amount of nicked open circles was only 6.9%. Since more form III DNA was observed after 25 min of incubation than form II DNA present at the start of the experiment, some of the form III DNA must have been derived from the form I DNA present at time zero. The average number of breaks per molecule was calculated for the 25 min time point to be 1.05, where the average number of breaks per molecule is equal to the mass fraction of form I DNA at any time point divided by twice the mass fraction of form III at that time (D. L. Robberson, personal communication). Thus, it can be seen that the form III DNA could not have arisen as the result of the accumulation of *random* single-strand breaks. For purposes of discussion a double-strand break is defined as a single-strand break in one strand close enough to a second break in the opposite strand to result in the formation of a double-strand break. Since the calculated average number of breaks per molecule is approximately one after 25 min of reaction, it is not possible to account for the large number of linear molecules present by a mechanism involving the accumulation of *random* single-strand breaks.

The specificity of bleomycin to induce double-strand breaks on altered PM2 DNA substrates was tested. Purines were selectively removed by acid–heat-treatment as previously described. Standard bleomycin–DNA reaction mixtures were performed as previously described. The loss of form I DNA from which purines were removed and the subsequent increase of forms II and III directly paralleled the reaction with PM2 which had not been partially depurinated. This result illustrates that bleomycin will not preferentially bind and cause a break at those sites on the DNA where bases have been removed and that the accumulation of double-strand breaks is not enhanced by an alkaline labile substrate.

The effect of the superhelical structure on the introduction of direct double-strand breaks by bleomycin was tested. The form I° DNA is a relaxed covalently closed circle; the number of superhelical turns in the molecule is a normal distribution around zero at the same temperature and salt concentration in which the DNA was relaxed. The results of a $37°C$ incubation in the presence of 0.5 μg/ml of bleomycin using a form I DNA population and a form I° DNA population showed that the decrease in the percentage of form I was somewhat faster in the initial part of the experiment but that after 30 min of reaction the percentages of form I and form I° DNA were essentially the same. Even though the loss of form I versus form I° was not identical, the production and increase in form III was identical for the two substrates. This shows conclusively that bleomycin does not require major helical distortions in the form of superhelical turns to induce double-strand breaks.

ACKNOWLEDGMENTS

We gratefully acknowledge the gift of PM2 DNA and use of laboratory equipment from Dr. Roger R. Hewitt, and the helpful discussions with Dr. Donald L. Robberson.

REFERENCES

Bearden, J. C., Jr., Lloyd, R. S., and Haidle, C. W. (1977). *Biochem. Biophys. Res. Commun. 75*, 442.
Crooke, S. T., and Bradner, W. T. (1976). *J. Med. 7*, 333.
Espejo, R. T., and Canelo, E. S. (1968). *Virology 34*, 738.
Haidle, C. W. (1971). *Mol. Pharmacol. 7*, 645.
Haidle, C. W., and Bearden, J., Jr., (1975). *Biochem. Biophys. Res. Commun. 65*, 815.
Haidle, C. W., Kuo, M. T., and Weiss, K. K. (1972a). *Biochem. Pharmacol. 21*, 3308.
Haidle, C. W., Weiss, K. K., and Kuo, M. T. (1972b). *Mol. Pharmacol. 8*, 531.
Haidle, C. W., Weiss, K. K., and Mace, M. L., Jr. (1972c). *Biochem. Biophys. Res. Commun. 48*, 1179.
Kuo, M. T., and Haidle, C. W. (1973). *Biochem. Biophys. Acta 385*, 109.
Kuo, M. T., Auger, L. T., Saunders, G. F., and Haidle, C. W. (1977). *Cancer Res. 37*, 1345.
Lindahl, T., and Nyberg, B. (1972). *Biochem. 11*, 3610.
Miyaki, M., and Ono, T. (1976). *Gann Monogr. Cancer Res. 19*, 37-50.

Müller, W. E. G., and Zahn, R. K. (1976). *Gann Monogr. Cancer Res. 19,* 51-62.

Müller, W. E. G., and Zahn, R. K. (1977). *Prog. Nucl. Acid Res. Mol. Biol. 40,* 21.

Müller, W. E. G., Yamazaki, Z., Breter, H. J., and Zahn, R. K. (1972). *Eur. J. Biochem. 31,* 518.

Müller, W. E. G., Rohde, H. J., and Zahn, R. K. (1976). *J. Mol. Med. 1,* 173.

Nagai, K., Suzuki, H., Tanaka, N., and Umezawa, H. (1969a *J. Antibiot. (Tokyo) 22,* 569.

Nagai, K., Yamaki, H., Suzuki, H., Tanaka, N., and Umezawa, H. (1969b). *Biochim. Biophys. Acta 179,* 165.

Onishi, T., Iwata, H., and Takagi, Y. (1975). *J. Biochem. 77,* 745.

Umezawa, H. (1975). In *Antibiotics. Mechanism of Action of Antimicrobial and Antitumor Agents,* Vol. III, Corcoran, J. W., and Hahn, F. E. (Eds.). Springer, New York, pp. 21-33.

Umezawa, H. (1976). *Gann Monogr. Cancer Res. 19,* 3-36.

Umezawa, H., Maeda, K., Takeuchi, T., and Oakami, Y. (1966). *J. Antibiot. (Tokyo), Ser. A 19,* 200.

Chapter 5

INTRACELLULAR FATE AND
ACTIVITY OF BLEOMYCIN

Osamu Yoshioka
Noriko Amano
Katsutoshi Takahashi
Akira Matsuda
Hamao Umezawa

I.   INTRODUCTION

Professor Umezawa has proposed the following principle concerning the selective effect of bleomycins (BLM): that BLM is distributed in tumors in a higher concentration than in normal tissues, and that BLM is not inactivated in those tumors, or that it is activated in those tumors.

In this paper we will report about the inactivation of BLM which is one factor of the above-mentioned principle.

There are two types of inactivation activities of BLM, in the case of various tissues of the rat and the transplantable tumor cells in animals. One of the inactivating activities is due to the inactivating enzyme called BLM-hydrolase, and the other is due to low molecular components in the normal tissues or tumor cells.

II. INACTIVATION OF BLM BY BLM-HYDROLASE

A. Methods for Determining BLM-Hydrolase Activities

BLM-hydrolase has already been reported to be a new member of the amino-peptidase B group. This enzyme has been found to hydrolyze the amide group of the β-aminoalanine amide moiety in the BLM molecule (Umezawa *et al*, 1974). Hereafter, this hydrolyzed BLM will be described as deamide-BLM.

Two methods have already been established for the determination of BLM inactivating activities. Although studies on the selective effect of BLM have been made using these two methods, it is as yet impossible to measure specifically enough the BLM-hydrolase activity (Müller *et al*., 1975; Umezawa *et al*., 1972).

For determining this BLM-hydrolase activity we have developed a high-pressure liquid chromatographical method (which we shall call the HPLC method).

The preparation procedures of the dialyzed crude enzyme of rat liver (called enzyme-D) used for basic studies and its reaction conditions are shown in Table I.

TABLE I. Determination of BLM-Hydrolase Activity in the Cytosol of Rat Liver

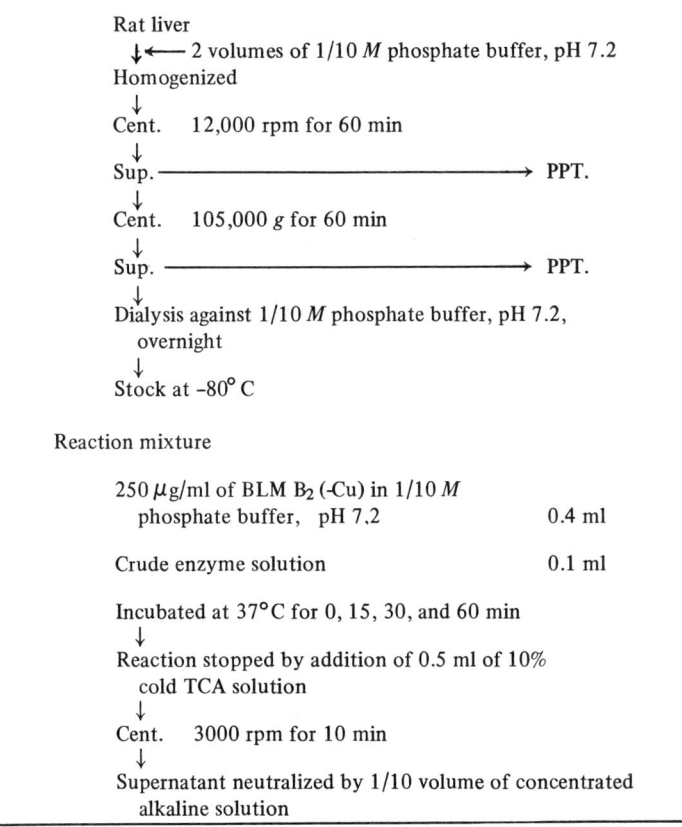

Preparation of crude enzyme from rat liver

Rat liver
$\downarrow$$\longleftarrow$ 2 volumes of 1/10 M phosphate buffer, pH 7.2
Homogenized
$\downarrow$
Cent.   12,000 rpm for 60 min
$\downarrow$
Sup. $\longrightarrow$ PPT.
$\downarrow$
Cent.   105,000 g for 60 min
$\downarrow$
Sup. $\longrightarrow$ PPT.
$\downarrow$
Dialysis against 1/10 M phosphate buffer, pH 7.2,
   overnight
$\downarrow$
Stock at $-80°$ C

Reaction mixture

250 μg/ml of BLM B_2 (-Cu) in 1/10 M
   phosphate buffer, pH 7.2   0.4 ml

Crude enzyme solution   0.1 ml

Incubated at 37°C for 0, 15, 30, and 60 min
$\downarrow$
Reaction stopped by addition of 0.5 ml of 10%
   cold TCA solution
$\downarrow$
Cent.   3000 rpm for 10 min
$\downarrow$
Supernatant neutralized by 1/10 volume of concentrated
   alkaline solution

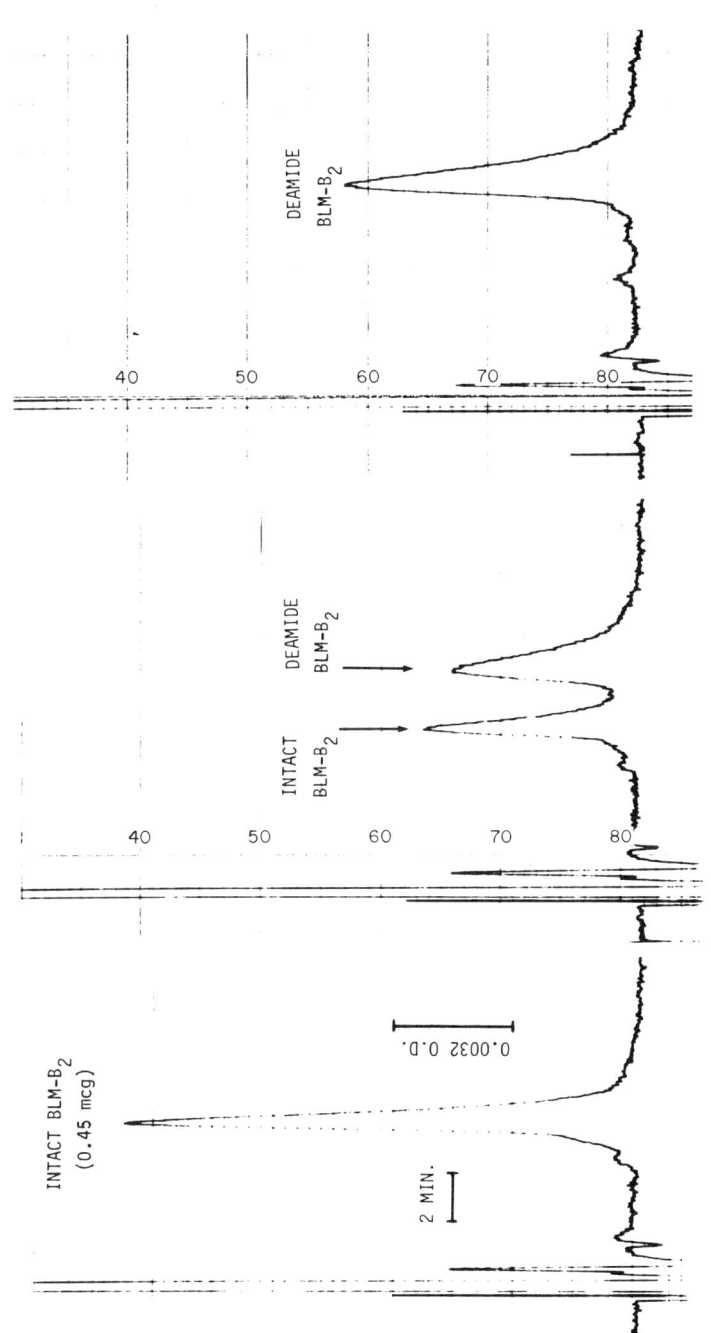

Fig. 1. Separation of intact and deamide BLM-B$_2$ by HPLC method.

BLM B_2 (-Cu) was used as the substrate for determining BLM-hydrolase in all experiments. The intact BLM and the deamide BLM in the reaction mixture were both measured by the methods shown in Table II (bioassay and HPLC methods).

TABLE II.   Assay of BLM in Reaction Mixture

Bioassay
> A neutralized sample was diluted to the concentration of 10 μg/ml by 1/10 M phosphate buffer, pH 7.2, and remaining potency was determined by bioassay.

High-pressure liquid chromatographical analysis
> Intact and deamide-BLM in the neutralized solution were changed to the copper chelated form by the addition of 2–3 mg of cupric carbonate (basic) and then 5 μl of each sample was injected to HPLC column to measure each peak area.

Condition of HPLC analysis
> Column: 2.1 ϕ x 330 mm
> Lichrosorb SI 60, particle size = 5 μm (Merck)

> Mobile phase: methanol:acetonitrile:20% ammonium acetate Aq. sol.:acetic acid
> for BLM B_2: 525:475:50:0.5
> BLM A_2: 700:300:50:0.5

The deamide BLM B_2 that is formed from the BLM-hydrolase and the intact BLM B_2 were both separated satisfactorily using the HPLC method as shown in Fig. 1. This HPLC method can be used in analyzing the various BLMs that differ from the BLM B_2 in their terminal amine moiety by adjusting the ratio of methanol and acetonitrile in their mobile phase.

In order to ascertain whether this HPLC method coincides with the conventional bioassay method, the aforementioned enzyme-D of rat liver was used for determining inactivation. As shown in Fig. 2, the decrease of biopotency correlated well with the decrease of intact BLM B_2. Furthermore, the rate of formation of deamide BLM B_2 fits exactly with the above two rates of decrease.

It was also ascertained that BLM B_2 (-Cu) was inactivated only by BLM-hydrolase in the dialyzed crude enzyme (enzyme-D) of rat liver.

B.   Comparison of BLM-Hydrolase Activities in Various Tissues

Female Donryu strain rats, 9 weeks old, were used for experiments. The tissues were excised from the rats after they were sacrificed by decapitation, and were chilled on ice. These chilled tissues were homogenized with 1/10 M phosphate buffer (pH 7.2) twice their weight in an Ultra-Turrax homogenizer.

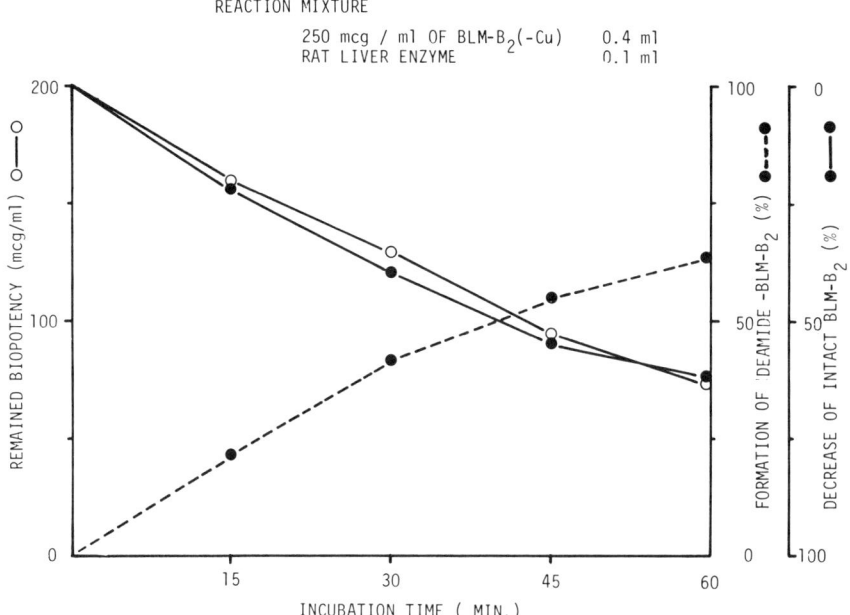

Fig. 2.   Inactivation of BLM B$_2$ (-Cu) by rat liver 105,000 g supernatant (Dialyzed).

The supernatants of 105,000g centrifugation for 60 min were collected and 2 ml of these supernatants were further centrifuged with Centriflo, CF-25 (Amicon) at 1000g for 30 min. This ultrafiltration was used in place of dialysis because of the instability of BLM-hydrolase. The ultrafiltrates thus obtained were frozen at -80°C for further experiments.

The high molecular fractions remaining in the Centriflo cones were washed again twice by centrifugation, each time with 2 ml of the same buffer solution, and finally resolved in the same buffer solution to 2 ml. These high molecular fractions were used a enzyme solutions. For the reaction mixture, 0.2 ml of BLM B$_2$ (-Cu) (2000 μg/ml) solution was added to 0.2 ml of the enzyme solution. These were then incubated for 0, 15, 30, and 60 min, respectively, at 37°C, and then 0.4 ml of 10% TCA was added at each respective time to terminate the reaction. The results are shown in Fig. 3.

Great differences of BLM-hydrolase activity were observed among the tissues. Tissues that showed higher BLM-hydrolase activity were the lymph node, bone marrow, and kidney. Medium activities were shown in the liver, fore-stomach, lung, esophagus, brain, spleen, and pancreas, whereas lower activities were shown in the large intestine, muscle, caecum, skin, small intestine, and glandular stomach.

The high activity in the lymph node and the bone marrow is interesting. Bleomycin is well known as an anticancer drug with no bone-marrow toxicity and immunosuppressive action.

The main reason these tissues did not receive any damage from BLM is probably the inactivation of BLM due to their high enzymatic activity.

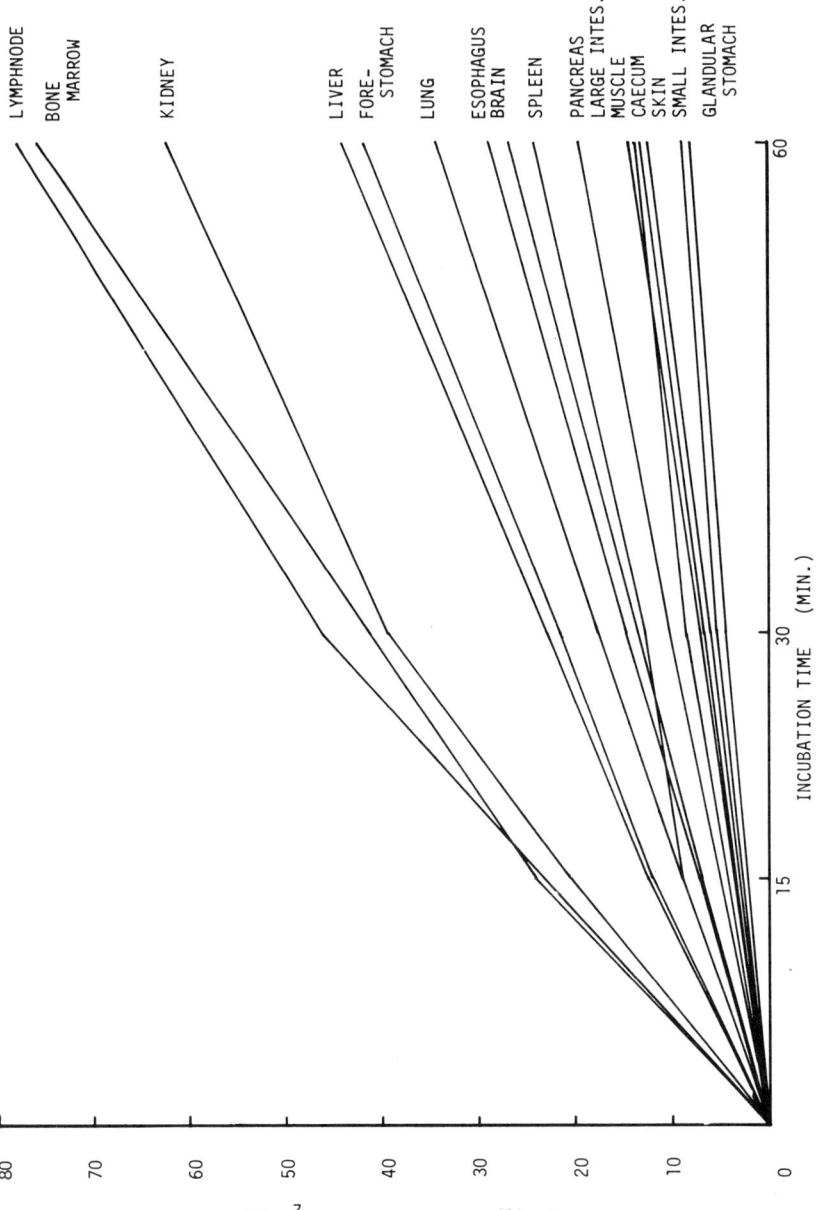

Fig. 3. BLM-hydrolase activity in high molecular fractions of various tissues of rat.

C. Studies on the Inhibitor of BLM-Hydrolase

The study of the inhibitor of BLM-hydrolase was undertaken in the hope that it may be a useful way for proving the resistance mechanism in the tissues and cells thought to have acquired BLM resistance for the aforementioned reasons.

As reported by Umezawa (1976), partially purified BLM-hydrolase of mouse and rat liver was competitively inhibited by L-lysyl-β-naphthylamide, L-arginyl-β-naphthylamide and bestatin.

Compounds as shown in Table III were used to study the inhibitory activity. Here the inhibition rate is shown in 60 min incubation at 37°C, after 0.1 ml of inhibitor solution and then 0.2 ml BLM solution (2000 μg/ml) were further added to 0.1 ml of enzyme solution.

In the aforementioned L-arginyl-β-napthylamide and bestatin, even in the high concentration of 10 mM, inhibitions were recognized only to the degree of 62.6% and 6.4% respectively. Among compounds examined it was found that leupeptin had the strongest inhibition activity.

Leupeptin, acetyl-L-leucyl-L-leucyl-DL-argininal, discovered by Aoyagi *et al.* (1969), is a specific inhibitor of plasmin, trypsin, and papain.

TABLE III. Effect of Various Compounds on the BLM-Hydrolase of Rat Liver

Compounds	Concentration	% of inhibition
L-arginyl-β-NA	10 mM	62.6
L-DAPA-OMe	50	42.6
	10	21.2
L-Lysyl-NH$_2$	10	45.9
L-DAPA-NH$_2$	10	21.6
BLM A$_2$(-Cu)	1 mg/ml	21.6
epi-B$_4$ (-Cu)	1	21.0
BLM A$_2$ (+Cu)	1	17.5
Phenylalanyl-NH$_2$	10 mM	17.0
L-Alanyl-β-NA	10	15.8
L-DAPA	10	12.8
epi-A$_2$ (-Cu)	1 mg/ml	13.3
Hydroxy-bestatin	10 mM	10.6
Bestatin	10	6.4
L-Lysine	10	4.7
L-Arginine	10	3.9
AHPA-arginine	10	12.6
Leupeptin	10	97.4
	6.42	97.1
	2.14	93.1
	0.71	87.9
	0.24	73.1
	0.05	20.1

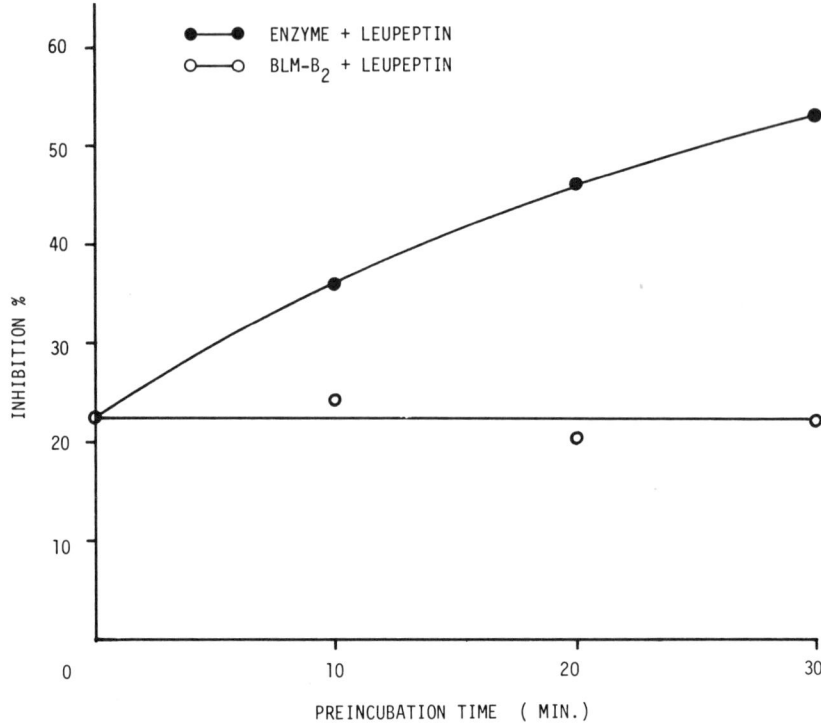

Fig. 4. Effect of preincubation on the inhibition of BLM-hydrolase by leupeptin.

The inhibition percentage on BLM-hydrolase, as shown in Fig. 4, was increased when enzyme-D was preincubated with leupeptin. There was, however, no change when BLM was preincubated with leupeptin. This result differs from the case of the competitive inhibition of leupeptin for trypsin. The mode of inhibition of leupeptin for BLM-hydrolase is now under investigation.

The dose-inhibition relationship for leupeptin is shown in Fig. 5. In this case 0.1 ml of leupeptin solution was added to 0.1 ml of enzyme-D solution and preincubated at 37°C for 30 min, after which 0.2 ml of BLM B_2 (-Cu) (2000 $\mu g/ml$) solution was added and then incubated for 60 min. Under this condition the ID_{50} of leupeptin was 35 μM.

D.   Sensitivity of Bone-Marrow Cells to BLM and the
Effect of Leupeptin on BLM Sensitivity *in Vitro*

As described above, the bone marrow of rats had high BLM-hydrolase activity and also proved resistant to BLM. Studies were therefore made concerning the inhibition of DNA synthesis induced by BLM A_2(-Cu) in primary cultured bone-marrow cells, along with studies on the effect of leupeptin on that inhibition.

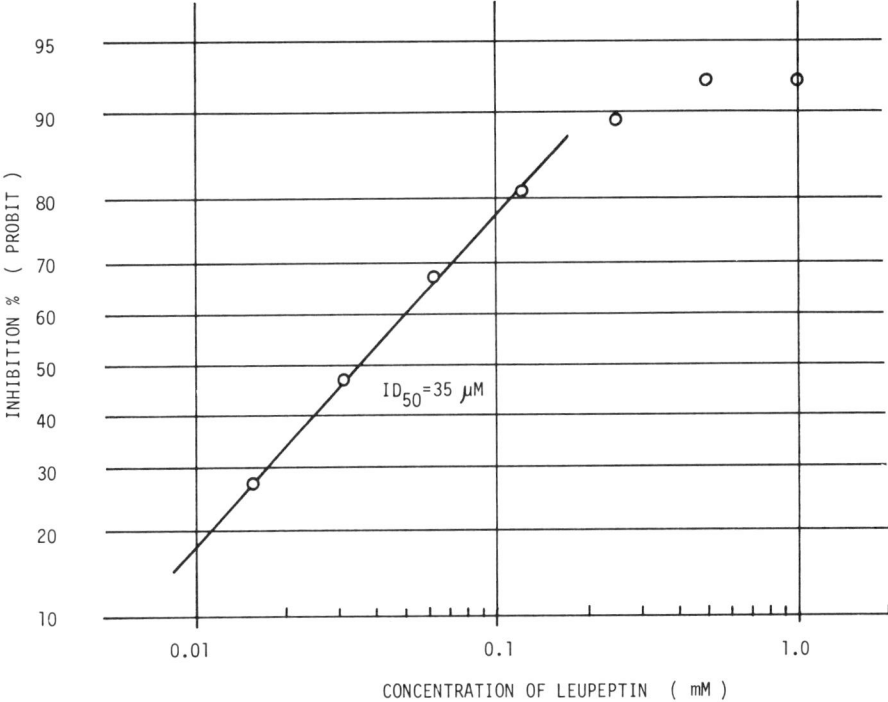

Fig. 5. Inhibition of BLM-hydrolase by leupeptin.

Bone-marrow cells were harvested from rat femur and suspended in the MEM containing 10% calf serum.

A volume of 0.5 ml of leupeptin solution was added to 2 ml of cell suspension (1.3 x 10^6 cells/ml) and incubated at 37°C for 2 hr. Then 0.1 ml of BLM A_2(-Cu) solutions were added to the incubation mixture and incubated for 3 hr.

To this incubation mixture [^{3}H]-thymidine (2 μCi/0.05 ml) solution was added and incubated for an additional 1 hr, after which the radioactivity of the acid-insoluble fraction was counted. As shown in Fig. 6, the DNA synthesis was not inhibited (1.6%) by BLM A_2(-Cu) at the highest concentration of 100 μg/ml. Under the same conditions, however, inhibition of DNA synthesis up to 60 to 70% was regularly obtained in AH 66 cells which are sensitive to BLM.

But in the presence of leupeptin DNA synthesis is clearly inhibited, and the dose-response relationship was observed for each BLM A_2(-Cu) concentration. This result suggested that the cause of resistance to BLM in bone-marrow cells may be mainly the higher activity of BLM-hydrolase in these cells than in other tissues.

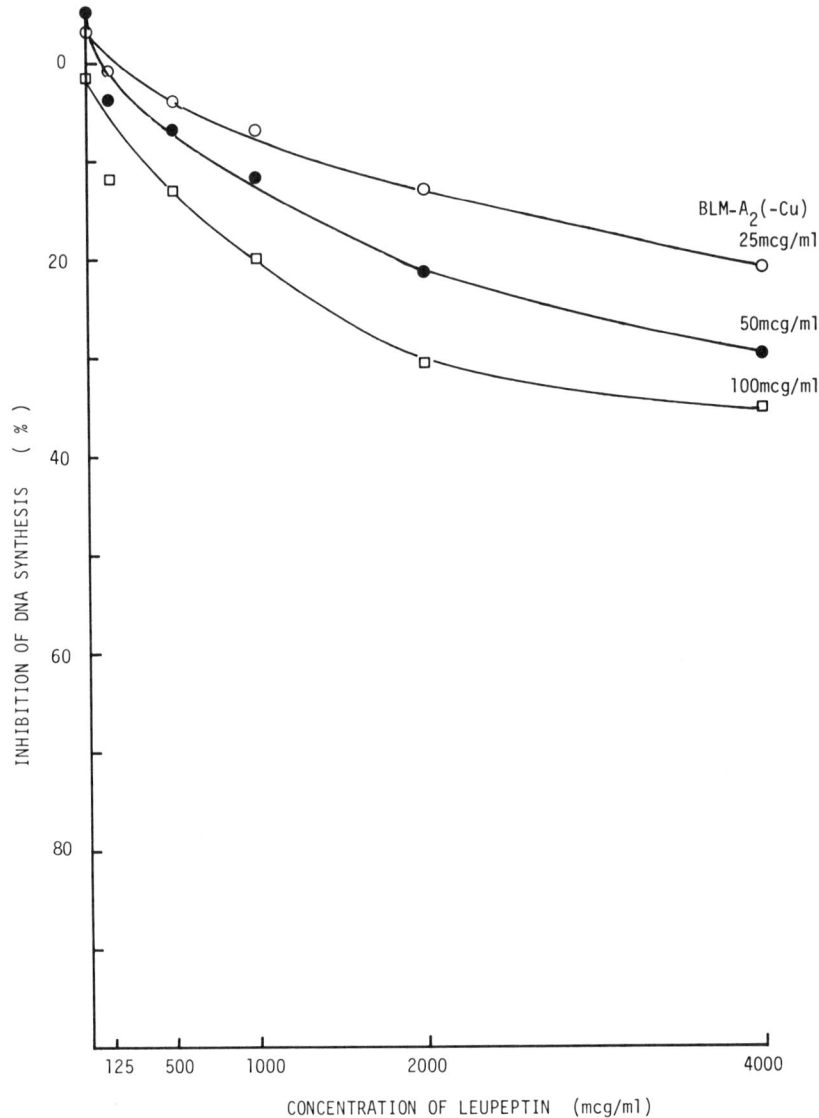

Fig. 6. Effect of leupeptin on the inhibition of DNA synthesis by BLM A₂ (-Cu) in rat bone-marrow cells *in vitro*.

E.   BLM-Hydrolase Activity in Transplantable Tumor Cells in Animals

Although it has already been pointed out that BLM-hydrolase dictates the sensitivity difference between squamous cell carcinoma and sarcoma, further studies to compare three transplantable tumor cells have been made in order to see if this can be proved generally in other transplantable tumor cells.

TABLE IV.   BLM-Hydrolase Activity of Transplantable Tumor Cells and Rat Liver

Cells	Enzyme activity (μg/mg protein/min)	Relative ratio
AH 66	0.189	1.00
AH 66F	0.557	2.95
L1210	1.398	7.39
Rat liver	1.113	5.89

As shown in Table IV, the activity was the lowest in BLM-sensitive AH 66 and higher in AH 66F and L1210 which were resistant. It has been suggested that the sensitivity difference in these three tumors is also due to BLM-hydrolase.

III.   INACTIVATION OF BLM BY LOWER COMPONENTS OF TISSUES AND TUMOR CELLS

A.   Detection of Inactivation of BLM by Low Molecular Fraction in AH 66 F Cells

When nondialyzed 105,000g supernatant of AH 66 and AH 66F cells (2×10^8 cells/ml) were used as enzyme solutions to measure the BLM-hydrolase activity by the HPLC method, the following phenomena were observed.

As shown in Fig. 7, in AH 66 cells the decrease of intact BLM B_2 and the formation of deamide BLM B_2 were well correlated and the sum of these components was kept at approximately 100%.

In contrast to this, in AH 66F cells there was a discrepancy between the two components with the formation of deamide BLM B_2 showing a lower rate than the decrease rate of intact BLM B_2. Moreover the sum of these two components decreased with the lapse of time. These results suggested the presence of another degradation process of BLM B_2 (-Cu) in the supernatants of AH 66F cells, and also pointed to the fact that degradation products that could not be detected by the HPLC were present. Accordingly, the low molecular components of the supernatant of AH 66F cells were removed by ultrafiltration with Centriflo.

When the high molecular fraction was analyzed by the HPLC method under the same conditions, there was no decrease in the sum of the two components (intact and deamide) as shown in Fig. 8, and rates of degradation and formation were well correlated.

These results suggest that the BLM degradation activities other than the BLM-hydrolase activity occurred in the low-molecular-weight fraction of AH 66F cells. Degradation activity did not occur with copper-chelated BLM B_2 in this low-molecular-weight fraction.

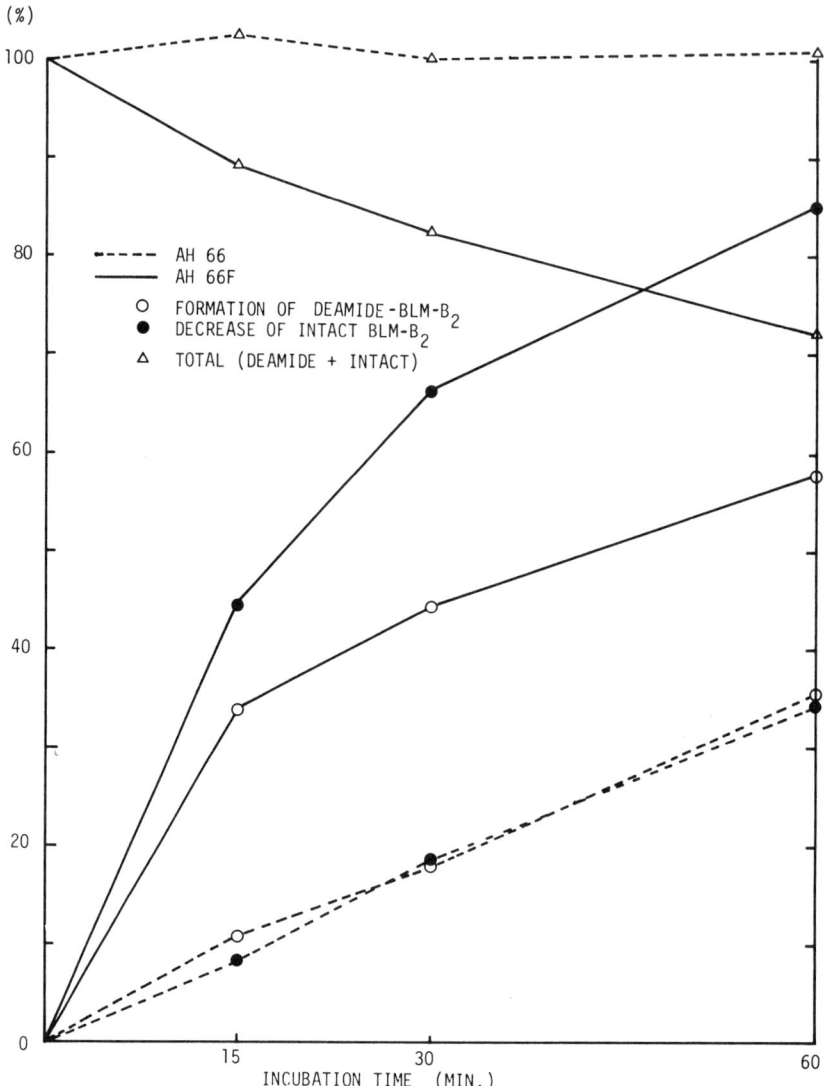

Fig. 7.   Degradation of BLM B$_2$ by Cytosol of AH 66 and AH 66F Cells.

B.   Correlation between the BLM-Inactivating Activities and the Ascorbic Acid Concentration in Low Molecular Fraction in Various Rat Tissues and Tumor Cells

Onishi *et al.* (1975) have reported that the inactivating activities of various rat tissues were proportioned to their concentrations of ascorbic acid. We therefore studied the correlation between the inactivating activities and the ascorbic acid concentration in the low molecular fraction in various rat tissues and tumor cells.

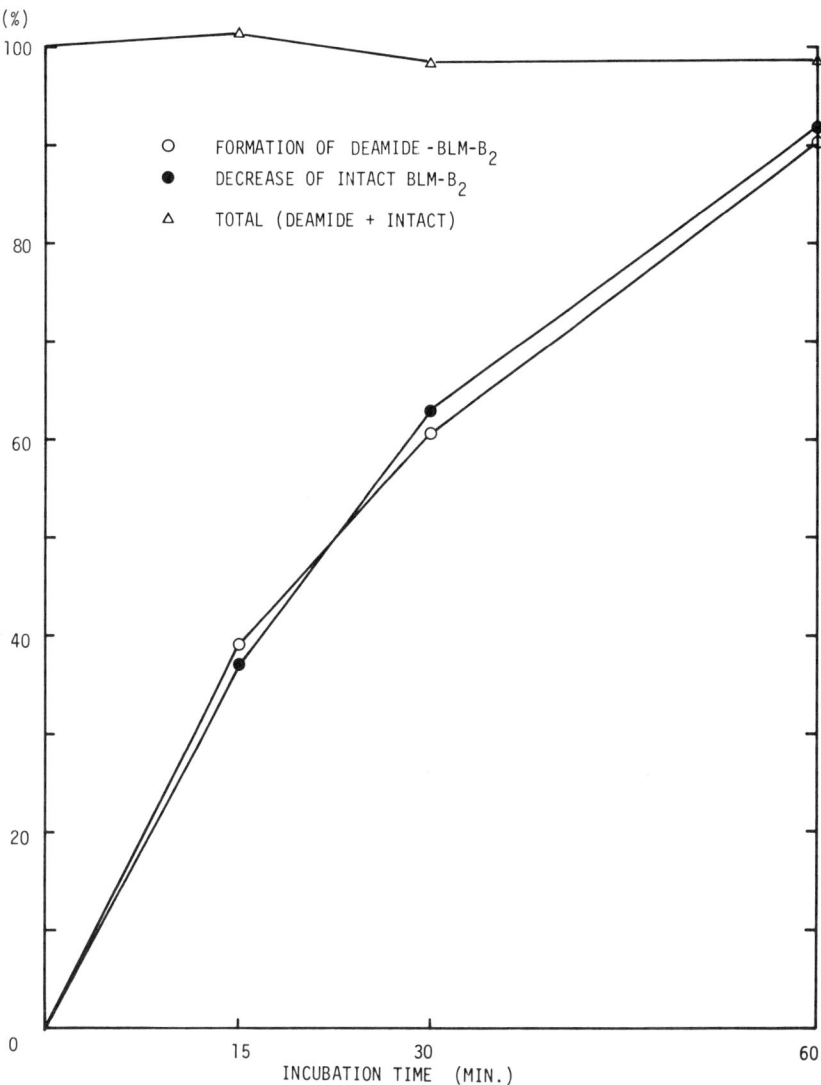

Fig. 8. Degradation of BLM B_2 by high molecular fraction of cytosol of AH 66F cells.

The frozen ultrafiltrates that had been preserved were used. 0.1 ml of BLM B_2 (-Cu) (100 μg/ml) solutions were added to 0.1 ml of ultrafiltrates and incubated at 37°C. After 0 and 30 min the reaction was stopped by the addition of 0.05 ml of 200 mM CuSO$_4$ solution. The remaining biopotency was determined by bioassay.

As shown in Fig. 9, it was observed that BLM was inactivated by the low molecular fraction in rat tissues and tumor cells. A correlation was also observed between the rate of this inactivation and the concentration of ascorbic acid in almost all

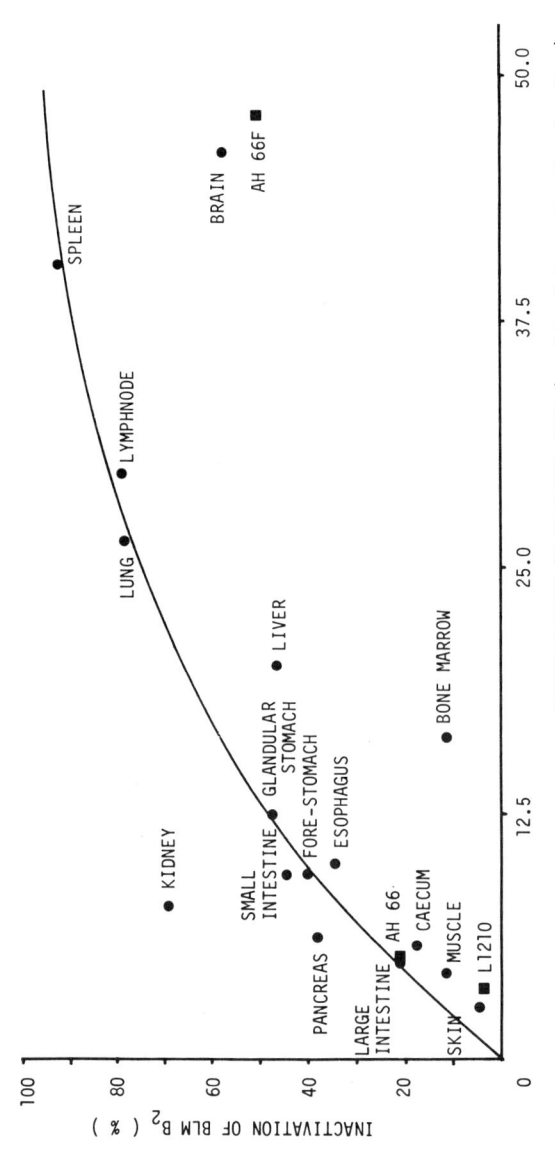

Fig. 9. Correlation between BLM inactivation activity and ascorbic acid concentration in low molecular fraction of various rat tissues and tumor cells.

tissues and tumor cells. In kidney, bone marrow, liver, brain, and AH 66F cells, however, this correlation does not seem to exist.

The tissues showing higher BLM inactivating activities due to low molecular fractions were the spleen, lymph node, lung, and kidney. The tissues showing lower inactivation were skin, L1210, muscle, bone marrow, AH 66, and large intestine.

When the results for bone marrow and lymph node are compared it has been suggested in the case of bone marrow that low molecular inactivation was small and that the BLM resistance was due to BLM-hydrolase, whereas in the case of lymph node both low molecular inactivation and high molecular inactivation were observed.

C.   Inactivation of BLM by Ascorbic Acid and Inhibition of Its Inactivation by EDTA

Further studies were made on this inactivation which was thought to be caused by ascorbic acid. As shown in Table V, BLM B_2(-Cu) was inactivated when $1/15\,M$ phosphate buffer was used as vehicle, but was not inactivated when distilled water was used as a vehicle even though it contained ascorbic acid. Inactivation also did not occur in $1/15\,M$ phosphate buffer containing 1mM EDTA.

TABLE V.   Inactivation of BLM B_2 (-Cu) by Ascorbic Acid and Effect of EDTA[a]

Conc. of ascorbic	% of inactivation		
Acid (mM)	A	B	C
2.0	0	39.7	0
1.0	7.4	39.9	4.6
0.5	1.2	25.8	0
0.25	0	21.1	4.8

Sources of	% of inactivation	
ultrafiltrate	-EDTA	+1 mM EDTA
AH 66F cells	31.9	2.4
Lymph node	63.5	0

[a] Reaction mixture:
    Ascorbic acid sol. or ultrafiltrate   0.1 ml
    BLM B_2 (-Cu) 100 μg/ml   0.1 ml
Vehicle:
    A. Distilled water
    B. $1/15\,M$ phosphate buffer, pH 7.2
    C. $1/15\,M$ phosphate buffer, pH 7.2 with 1 mM EDTA

Incubated for 30 min at $37°$ C, reaction stopped by addition of
50 μl of 0.2 M CuSO$_4$

Furthermore, in the case of ultrafiltrates prepared from lymph node and AH 66F cells, the inactivation of BLM B_2(-Cu) was completely inhibited by the presence of 1mM EDTA. From these results it can be deduced that certain metals are essential for low molecular inactivation and that ascorbic acid seems to stimulate this reaction. The reason for the low inactivation in brain, AH 66F, liver, and bone marrow tissues in relation to the amount of ascorbic acid seems to be the small amount of these metals present. In the case of kidney, on the other hand, the rate of inactivation seems to be high because of the presence of a large amount of these metals. According to our preliminary results, one of these metals seems to be Fe^{2+}, but further details of this reaction are now under investigation.

IV. THE ROLE OF HIGH AND LOW MOLECULAR FRACTIONS ON INACTIVATION OF BLM

A. In 105,000G Supernatant of Rat Liver

So far, observations have been made about the high molecular and low molecular inactivation activities. But in order to verify the rates at which these two contribute to inactivation in 105,000g supernatant, the following experiments have been done.

105,000g supernatant of rat liver was separated in high and low molecular fractions with Centriflo, CF-25. The inactivation activities of each fraction and the whole 105,000g supernatant were determined against various concentrations of BLM B_2 (-Cu), using the bioassay method for measurement. As shown in Fig. 10, the ratio of inactivation by high molecular fractions decreased as the concentration of BLM became lower. In contrast, the ratio by low molecular fractions increased. At 30 μg/ml the ratio of inactivation by both fractions became equal. The sum of

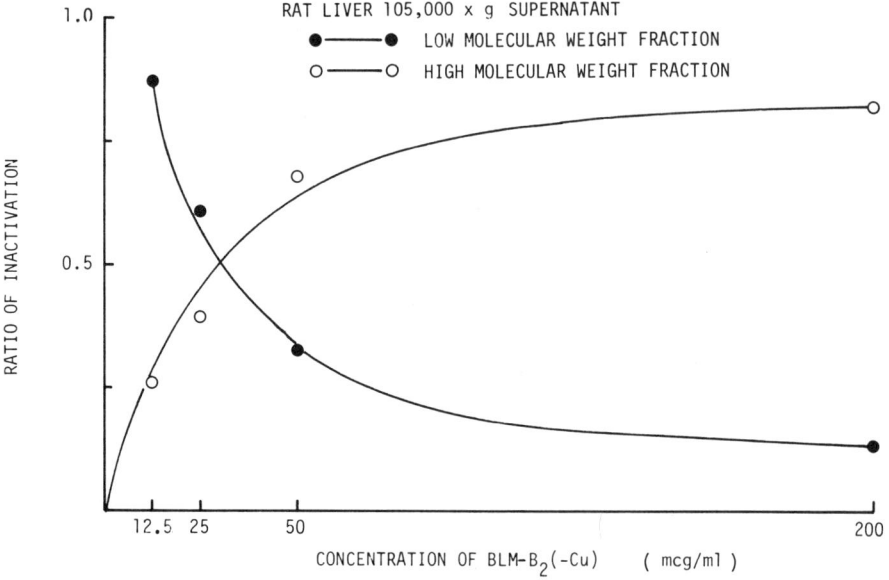

Fig. 10.   The role of high and low molecular weight fractions on the inactivation of BLM B_2 (-Cu).

the amount of inactivation by each fraction was well correlated with the amount of inactivation observed in whole 105,000g supernatant.

These results suggest that each inactivation proceeds independently, and also that the contribution of inactivation by low molecular fraction increases in the range of low BLM concentration.

The same results were obtained in the case of AH 66F cells.

B. The Role of High or Low Molecular Fractions on BLM Sensitivity at the Cell Level

Studies were next made on each inactivating activity at the cell level. As described above, in AH 66F cells both the BLM-hydrolase activity and the low molecular inactivation activity were high, and they were resistant to BLM. It is important in order to clarify their role at the cell level to know whether or not one or both inactivating activities at cell level is the real cause for resistance to BLM.

It was found that when AH 66F cells were cultured in MEM containing 10% calf serum, the intracellular ascorbic acid and the inactivating activities due to low molecular fraction were minimized within 24 hr without changing the cellular growth rate. This process is shown in Fig. 11. The BLM-hydrolase activity was, however, kept at more than 80% of the original cells. These states could be maintained even in long-term cultivations.

Comparative studies were, therefore, made of the BLM sensitivity between primary (day 0) and cultured (day 11) cells. The study was carried out under the same condition as when bone marrow cells were studied by inhibition of DNA synthesis. As shown in Fig. 12, in cultured cells deficient in low molecular inactivating activities the increase of inhibition of DNA synthesis in BLM A_2(-Cu) was small.

However, with HR-BLM(-Cu), which is one of the BLM-hydrolase-resistant BLMs, the inhibition of DNA synthesis at 100 μg/ml increased about 3.4 times in primary culture cells and about 2 times in cultured cells.

As shown in Fig. 13, the same results obtained in survival on BLM-treated primary and 13th-day cultures of AH 66F cells. These results suggest that BLM resistance in AH 66F cells were due mainly to BLM-hydrolase and not to low molecular inactivating activity.

C. The Role of High and Low Molecular Components in Rat Tissues and Tumor Cells upon BLM Sensitivity

All the results discussed in this paper are shown in Fig. 14. The chart indicates each inactivating activity in ratio to 1.0 activity for the liver.

1. The tissues showing high activity for BLM-hydrolase alone are bone marrow and skin. The bone marrow clearly shows resistance due to BLM-hydrolase. In the skin, although BLM-hydrolase activity is low, when BLM B_2 (-Cu) and bestatin are applied together in a mouse the skin concentration rises about 3 to 10 times, and therefore it is suggested that BLM-hydrolase is effective mainly in the skin.

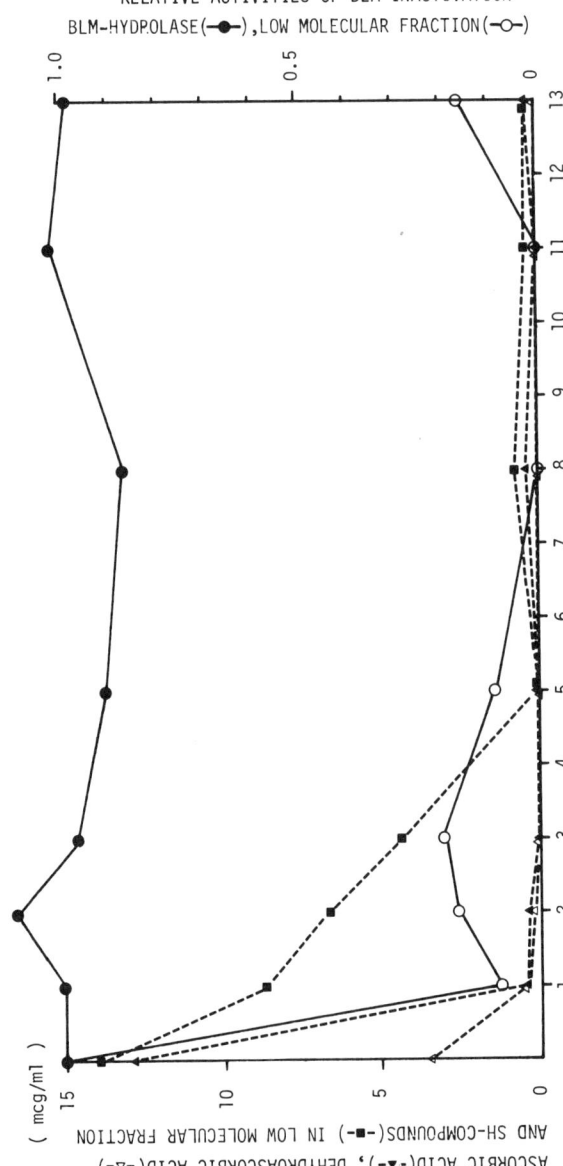

RELATIVE ACTIVITIES OF BLM-INACTIVATION
BLM-HYDROLASE(—●—),LOW MOLECULAR FRACTION(—○—)

DAYS OF CULTIVATION

(mcg/ml)

AND SH-COMPOUNDS(—■—) IN LOW MOLECULAR FRACTION
ASCORBIC ACID(—▲—), DEHYDROASCORBIC ACID(—△—)

Fig. 11. Fluctuation of quantities of intracellular reducing agents and activities of BLM inactivation in cultured AH 66F cells.

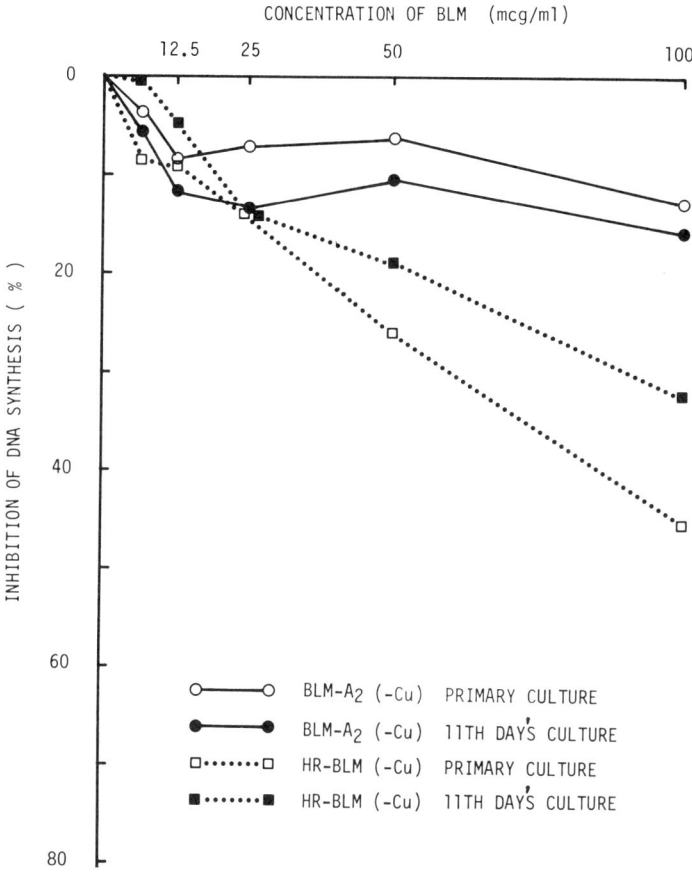

Fig. 12. Comparison of primary and 11-day culture of AH 66F cells on BLM-induced inhibition of DNA synthesis.

2. The tissues in which hydrolase activities and low molecular inactivation activities are approximately the same are lymph node, kidney, liver, and fore-stomach. In these tissues both activities are thought to contribute to the BLM inactivation. This problem in connection with the lymph node still needs to be investigated.

3. The tissues in which inactivation is due mainly to low molecular fraction are spleen, lung, esophagus, brain, small intestine, and glandular stomach.

In general, a high concentration of BLM is distributed in the lung, but low molecular inactivating activity is high and the hydrolase activity is also relatively high. One reason for this seems to be that young rats (9 weeks old) were used. In the lung it is thought that hydrolase contributes mainly to the inactivation. This is deduced from the fact that the rise in distribution in the lung occurred with the parallel use of bestatin. Inactivating activity in the lung needs also to be investigated in the future.

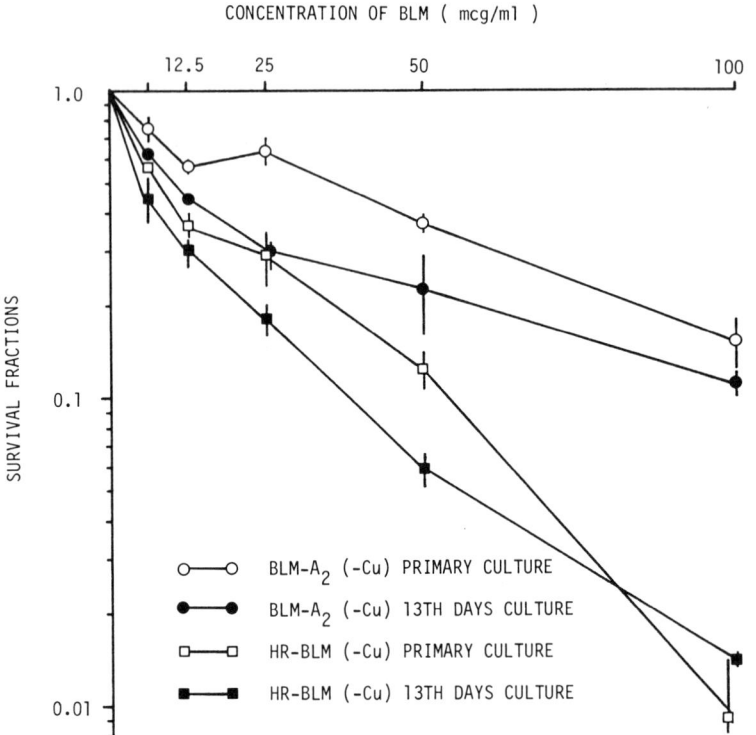

Fig. 13. The effect of BLMs on survival of primary and 13-day cultures of AH 66F cells.

V. CONCLUSION

The following results have been obtained from the studies of inactivating activities of BLM B_2(-Cu), which dictates the selective effects of BLM in the various tissues of rat and tumor cells.

1.   The HPLC method for determining the BLM-hydrolase activities was developed and the activities of various tissues and tumor cells were studied. Higher activities were observed in the lymph node and bone marrow, which are insensitive to BLM.

2.   It was observed that leupeptin was a strong inhibitor of BLM-hydrolase. It was also shown that the resistance to BLM in bone-marrow cells was due mainly to BLM-hydrolase activity from the increase of sensitivity by the parallel application of leupeptin and BLM.

3.   The presence of metals is essential in the inactivation reaction of BLM by low molecular components and ascorbic acid stimulates this reaction. The tissues in which these inactivating activities were higher were the spleen, lymph node and lung, whereas in the bone marrow this activity was lower.

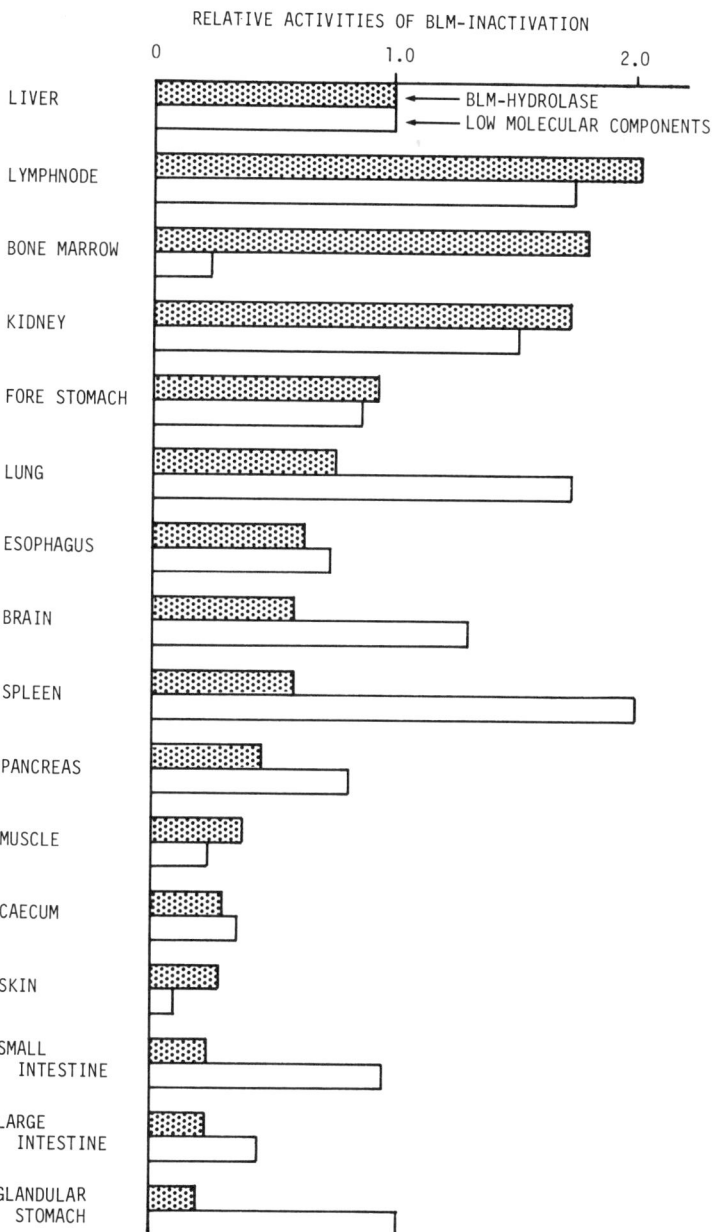

Fig. 14. Effective role of high and low molecular components on inactivation of BLM in various organs.

4.   The effect of BLM-hydrolase and low molecular components on BLM inactivation was studied. It was observed that, in 105,000g supernatant of rat liver the inactivation occurred mainly in low concentration of BLM by low molecular components and in high concentration of BLM by BLM-hydrolase.

Comparative studies of the roles played in BLM sensitivity at the cell level were made: Observations were made on cultured AH 66F cells which had deficient inactivating activity of low molecular fraction and primary cultured cells. It was shown that in the AH 66F cells the BLM-hydrolase activity was the main cause for resistance to BLM, rather than the intracellular low molecular inactivating activity.

The possible role of each inactivating activity in various tissues was also discussed.

REFERENCES

Aoyagi, T., Miyata, S., Nanbo, M., Kojima, F., Ishizuka, M., Takeuchi, T., and Umezawa, H. J. (1969). *J. Antibiot. 22,* 558–568.

Müller, W. E. G., Totsuka, A., Zahn, R. K., and Umezawa, H. (1975). *Z. Krebsforsch. 83,* 151–162.

Onishi, T., Iwata, H., and Takagi, Y. (1975). *Biochem. Biophys. Acta 378,* 439–449.

Umezawa, H. (1976). *Gann Monogr. Cancer Res. 19.*

Umezawa, H., Takeuchi, T., Hori, S., Sawa, T., Ishizuka, M., Ichikawa, T., and Komai, T. (1972). *J. Antibiot. 25,* 409–420.

Umezawa, H., Hori, S., Sawa, T., Yoshioka, T., and Takeuchi, T. (1974). *J. Antibiot. 27,* 419–424.

Chapter 6

MORPHOLOGICAL MANIFESTATIONS
OF BLEOMYCIN TOXICITY[1]

Yerach Daskal
Ferenc Gyorkey

I. INTRODUCTION

A wide variety of studies have been reported on the effects of bleomycin on cell growth *in vitro* as well as on cellular ultrastructure. Clinically, bleomycin has been used in the treatment of a variety of tumors, particularly squamous cell carcinomas and lymphomas. However, as will be shown in greater detail later, pulmonary toxicity is apparently the major fatal complication of bleomycin therapy. As early as 1971, Rilke and Pilotti, as well as Simosato *et al.* (1971) reported on histological aberrations in the distribution of Type II pneumocytes concomitant to the onset of pulmonary fibrosis in patients with malignant tumors treated with bleomycin. Electron-microscopic studies on lung biopsies obtained from cancer patients treated with bleomycin were reported by Bedrossian *et al.* (1973) and essentially confirmed the earlier observations. It was concluded that bleomycin induces a pulmonary lesion with a potential target in the Type I alveolar epithelial cells. It was postulated (Bedrossian *et al.*, 1973) that bleomycin may impair surfactant production by the Type II cells, thus leading to alveolar collapse and ultimately resulting in diffuse fibrosis. It is important, however, to determine unequivocally that the reported

[1]These studies were supported in part by Cancer Center Research Grant CA 10893, P5, from the National Cancer Institute, a grant from the Wolf Memorial Foundation, and a generous gift from Mrs. Jack Hutchins.

reduction in the number of the Type I cells is indeed a manifestation of bleomycin treatments rather than a general phenomenon related to pulmonary fibrosis of random etiology.

II. STUDIES

In a recent follow-up study of experimentally induced pulmonary toxicity with bleomycin in pheasants, Bedrossian et al. (1977) have confimed their earlier studies and have suggested that the primary targets of the drug are the epithelial rather than the alveolar endothelial cells, as suggested by Simosato et al. (1971).

Figure 1 is a scanning electron micrograph of an untreated human lung. The presence of Kuhn's pores in the background facilitates specimen orientation, whereby the alveolar septum can be identified. Several alveolar sacs may be seen in this field and a characteristic terminal bronchiole opening into an alveolar sac can be easily identified (Fig. 1b).

This particular alveolar septum shows a minimal amount of associated connective tissue that is considered as a normal component of the untreated lung (Fig. 2).

Examination of similar biopsies from patients who have been treated with various doses of bleomycin ranging from 360 to 400 mg total dose revealed significant deviation from the normal pattern observed above. A direct comparison of a treated alveolar septum (Fig. 3) to a similar region of an untreated one (Figs. 1 and 2) shows the greatly increased thickness of the septal wall, the presence of large amounts of connective tissue, a significant decrease in the luminal spaces, and cellular hyperplasia (Fig. 3 pointers). Despite these striking effects observed after bleomycin treatments, these morphological manifestations as observed with scanning electron microscopy (SEM) were not different from biopsy specimens of patients diagnosed with pulmonary fibrosis of etiologies other than bleomycin. Therefore, it was concluded that at the cellular level there were no distinct morphological markers unique to bleomycin toxicity. Thus attempts must be made to detect and define characteristic subcellular lesions that are uniquely associated with bleomycin toxicity.

Figure 4 is a transmission electron micrograph of the specimen observed earlier with scanning electron microscopy (Fig. 3). In addition to the Type II cell hyperplasia characteristic of diffuse interstitial fibrosis (DIF), changes were observed in the nucleoplasm and nucleoli of these cells. Similar changes were also noted in Type I cells that were also greatly reduced in number as well as in interstitial fibroblasts. At low magnifications (Fig. 4) it was quite difficult to resolve those morphological aberrations. With respect to the nucleoli, these contained well defined fibrillar centers. Although these fibrillar centers were surrounded by nucleolar fibrillar components as in Type I cells (Fig. 5b), they were of greater electron density and further separated from the main nucleolar body. The nucleoplasm of Type II cells contained a larger number of nuclear bodies (Bouteiile et al., 1974; Buttner and Horstmann, 1967) than Type I cells (Table I). These bodies were of the BNB, MNB,

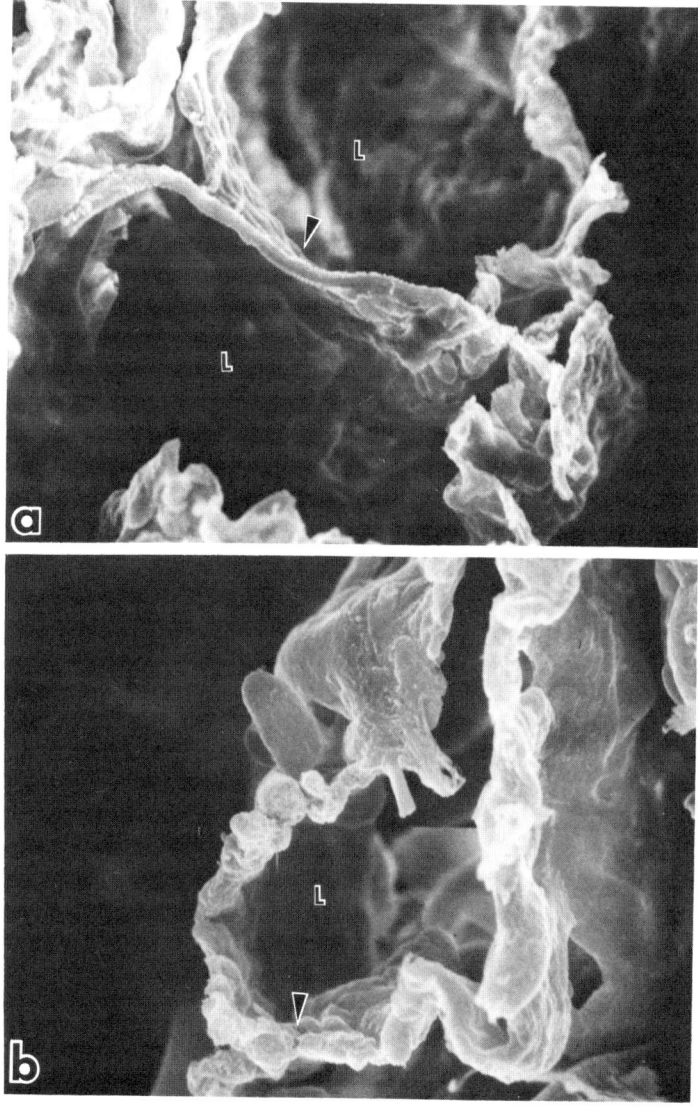

Fig. 1. Scanning electron micrographs of normal human lung. (a) Kuhn's pores in the background facilitate orientation. Alveolar cells form a cobblestone-like pattern. (b) A different view of a terminal bronchiole opening into an alveolar sac. Alveolar lining with epithelial cells (pointers). L–luminal space. (a) x357 (b) x442.

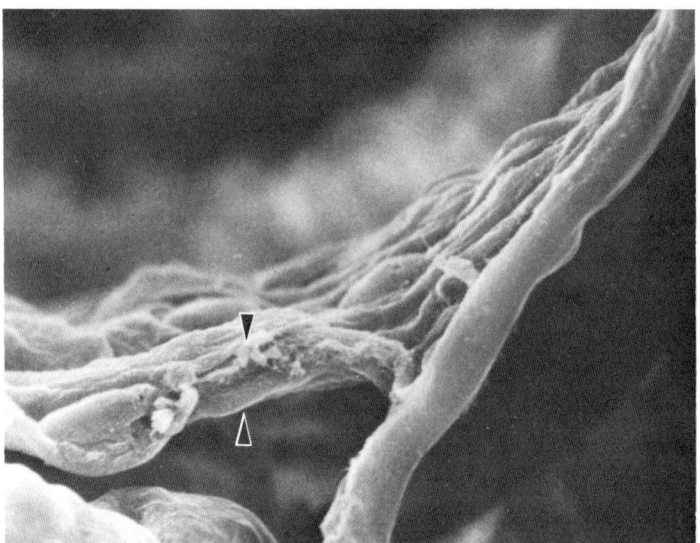

Fig. 2. Electron micrograph of normal human lung alveolar septum, observed in Fig. 1a with cobblestone arrangement of the epithelial cells lining the alveolus. Note the overall thickness of the septal wall (demarcated by pointers) that contains also some connective tissue components. x14,450.

and GNB[2] varieties (Figs. 4 and 6). Their sizes ranged from 0.3 to 0.7 μm. The core of the GNB contained granules similar in size and morphology to nucleolar granular components, but of higher electron density. All three varieties could be found within a single nucleus (Fig. 6). Nuclei containing as many as nine nuclear bodies were observed. Frequently, only those nuclear sections containing nucleoli also contained nuclear bodies. GNBs were commonly enclosed by a capsule of low electron density. Morphologically, this capsule was similar to components of the BNBs or MNBs. Frequently, the BNBs contained a highly granular core and a lamellated capsule or cortex (Fig. 6).

TABLE I. Distribution of Nuclear Bodies in Human Alveolar Cell Nuclei after Bleomycin Treatments.

	Type I cells, $n^a = 24$	Type II cells, $n = 52$	Septal fibroblasts, $n = 27$
Bleomycin	2.3 ± 1.2^b	4.8 ± 0.8^b	2.8 ± 1.1^b
Control	< 1	< 1	< 1

[a] n, number of nuclei examined.
[b] Mean ± S.D.

[2] The abbreviations used are: BNB, beaded nuclear body; MNB, membranous nuclear body; GNB, granular nuclear body.

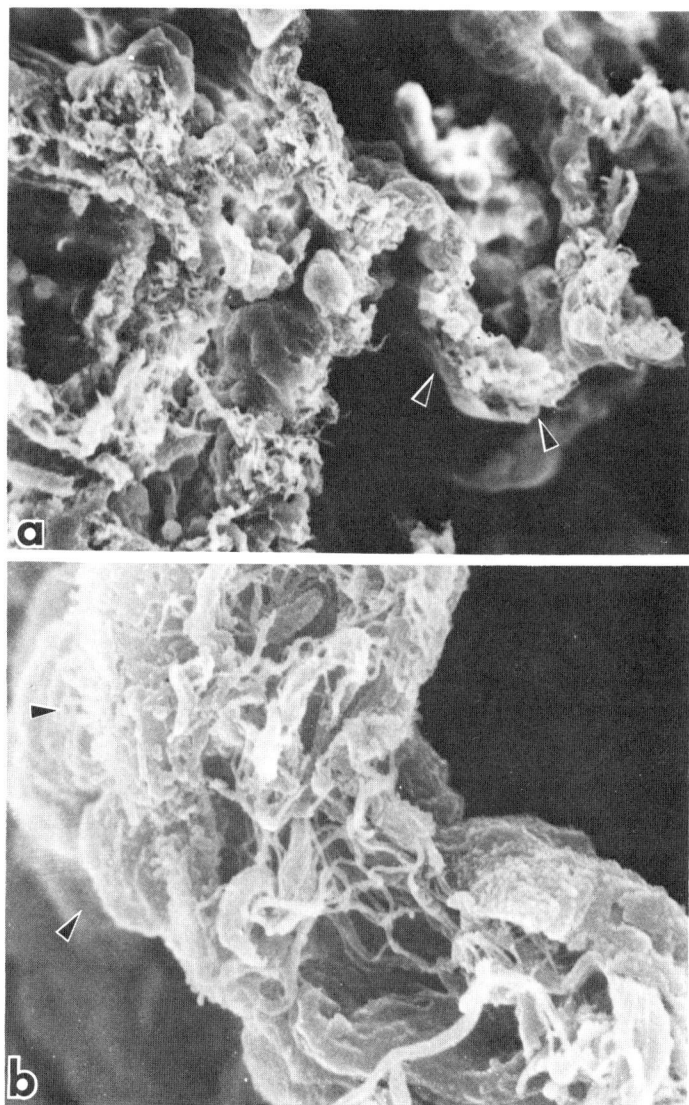

Fig. 3. Micrographs of bleomycin-treated human lung (390 mg total dose). (a) Significant increase in the connective tissue components resulting in an overall increase in the thickness of the alveolar septum (pointers). At higher magnifications (b), alveolar cell hyperplasia is evident (pointers) as well as the interstitial fibrous components within the septum. (a) x433.5. (b) x14.450.

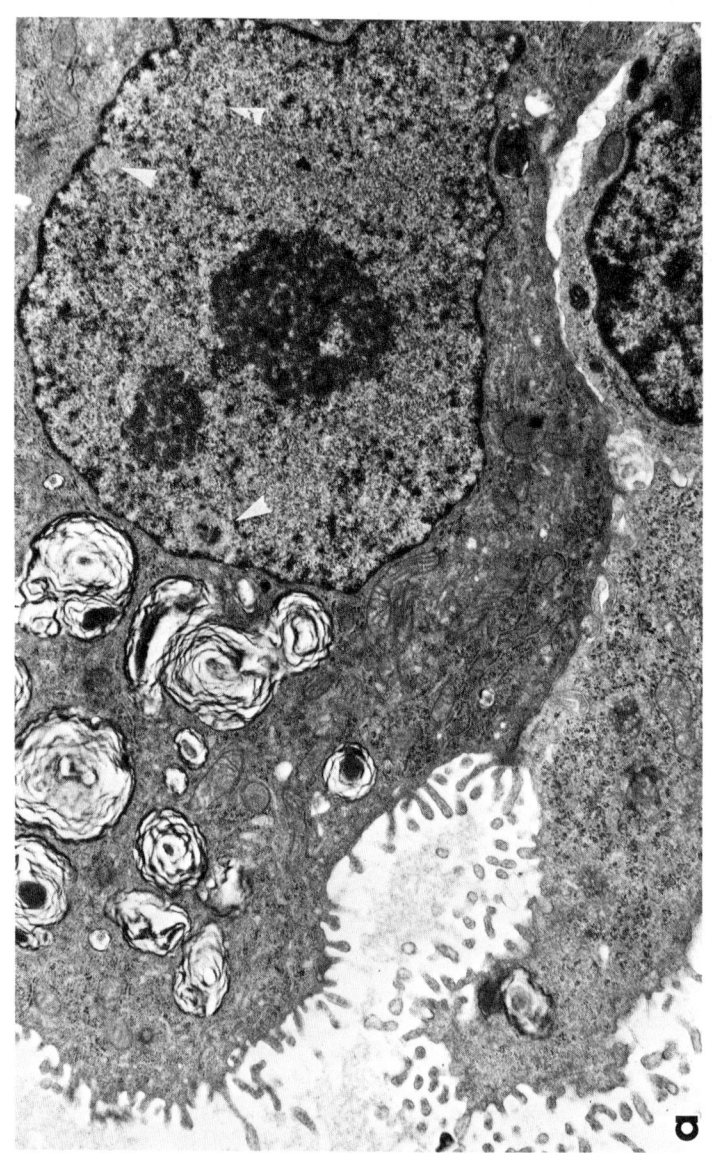

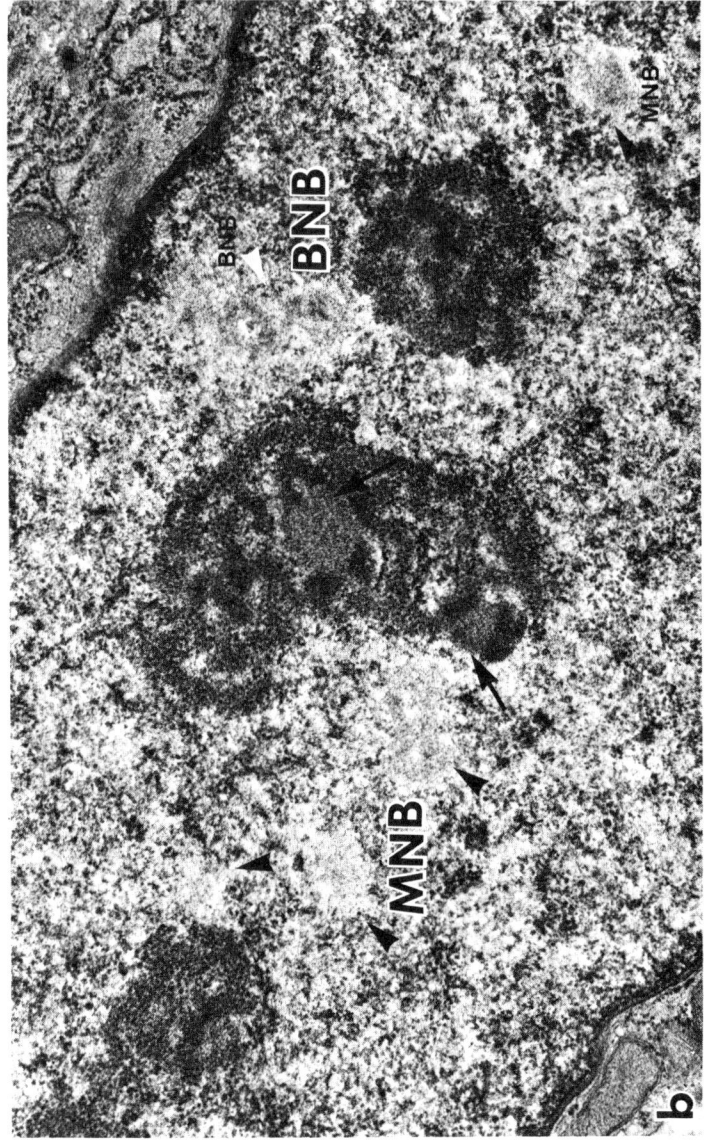

Fig. 4. (a) Type II alveolar epithelial cell from Patient B at low magnification. White pointers indicate the presence of nuclear bodies. (b) Nucleolus of an alveolar interstitial fibroblast (from Patient C) with fibrillar centers (arrow) and five nuclear bodies (pointers), most of them of the membranous variety. Lead citrate-uranyl acetate. (a) x11,284. (b) x32,725.

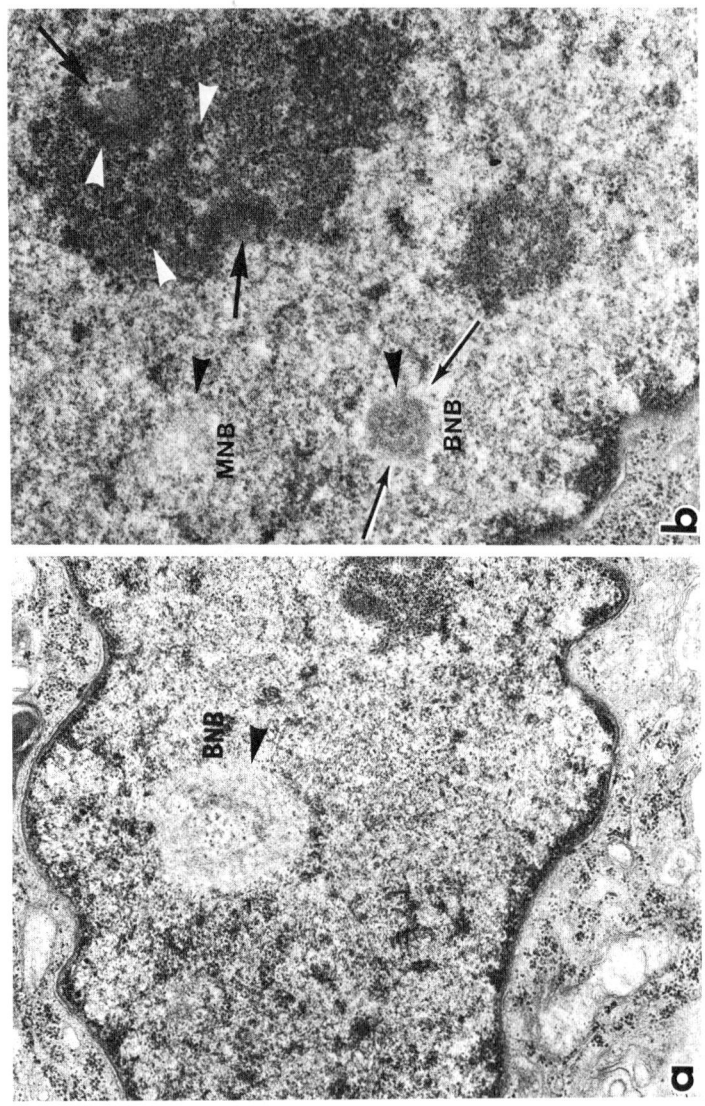

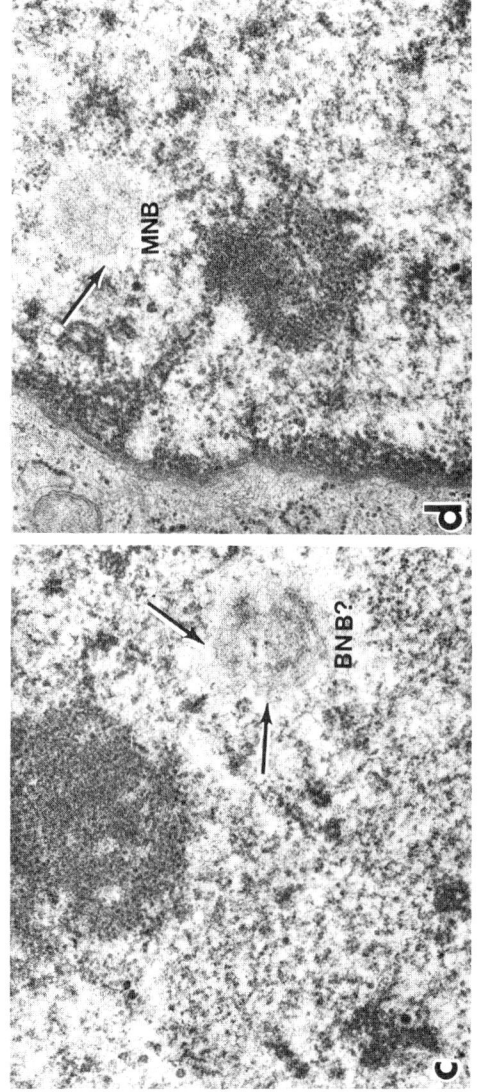

Fig. 5. Type I alveolar epithelial cells from Patient A. The BNB may be differentiated into a membranous cortex and a granular core (a, pointers). Nucleoli contain fibrillar centers (b, arrows), condensed fibrillar components, and microspherules (b, white pointers). At higher magnifications, nuclear bodies can be seen to be surrounded by a halo of low electron density (c, white arrows). In this halo, fine filaments interconnect the nuclear body and nucleoplasmic components. This particular nuclear body appears to be an intermediate between the membranous and beaded varietv. (d) Alveolar interstitial fibroblast from Patient C, with a characteristic MNB. Lead citrate-uranyl acetate. (a) x25,500; (b) x29,962; (c) x38,250; (d) x38,760.

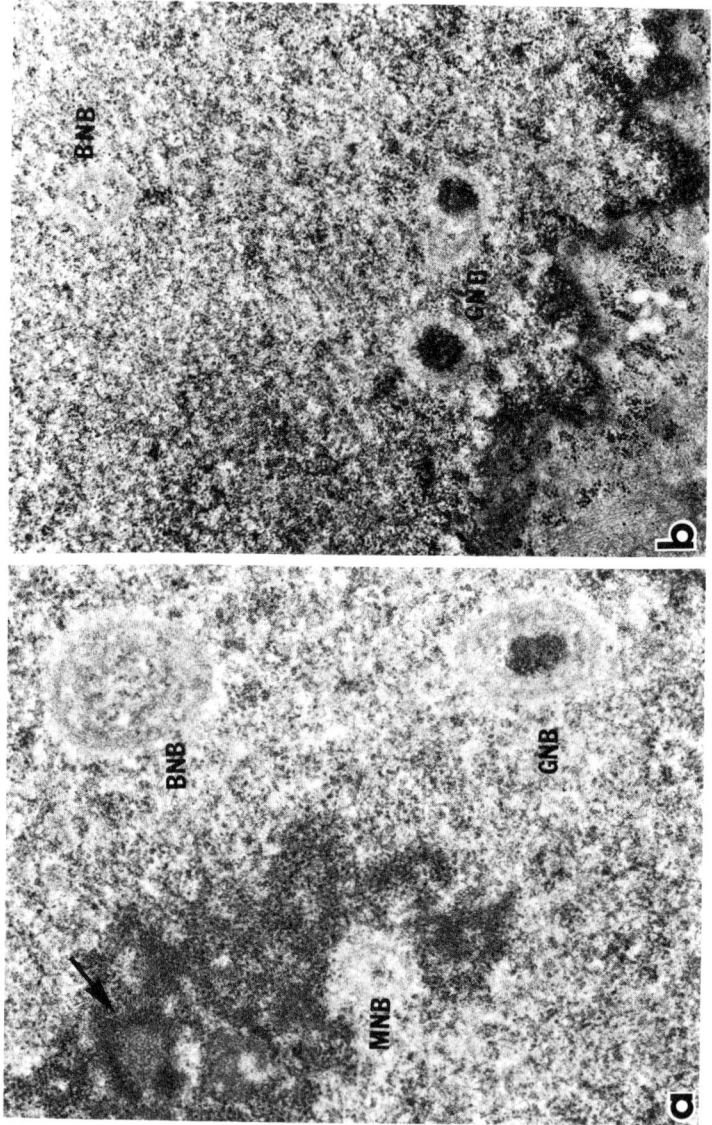

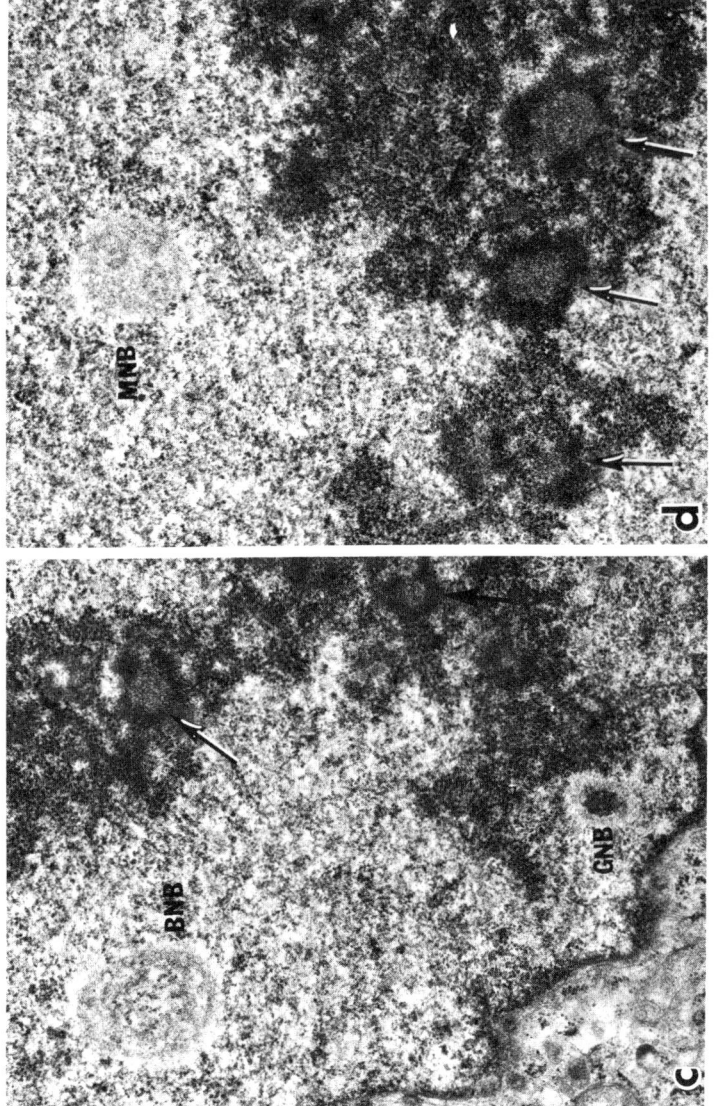

Fig. 6. Type II alveolar cell nuclei from Patient A containing characteristic nuclear bodies. In this nucleus, all three varieties of nuclear bodies are in the proximity of the nucleolus. Note the lamellated nature of the cortex of these bodies. Arrows—nucleolar fibrillar centers. Lead citrate-uranyl acetate staining. (a) x33,150; (b) x27,625; (c) x29,325; (d) x32,512.

Nuclei and nucleoli of septal fibroblasts were similar in their ultrastructure to those of Type II alveolar cells. However, the number of nuclear bodies was somewhat reduced and consisted mainly of the membranous variety (Table I). Few nuclear bodies were found in specimens obtained from untreated patients.

Type I alveolar epithelial cells were less abundant in specimens from treated patients. Their nulcei often contained two or more nucleoli. Distinct large fibrillar centers were distributed throughout the nucleolus. These fibrillar centers were surrounded by well defined fibrillar components and microspherules, as in nucleoli of Type II pneumocytes. Some localized segregation appeared between the granular and fibrillar components of the nucleolus, but it differed from the typical nucleolar segregation patterns induced by actinomycin D.

As was the case with Type II cells, the most conspicuous ultrastructural change in these nuclei was the increase in nulcear bodies which were frequently found in the proximity of the nucleolus and were of two main varieties, MNB and BNB. Frequently, these nuclear bodies were surrounded by a "halo" of nucleoplasmic matrix where fine fibers were anastomosing with the nuclear body proper and other nuclear components. Cytoplasmic fibrillar bodies or perinuclear tufts were not detected in these cells (Daskal *et al.*, 1975). The function of these nuclear bodies is unknown at present, as is their origin. Moreover, it is not clear whether these represent native nuclear components or a pathological manifestation of drug action. Additional quantitative evaluation of these specimens is needed to establish them clearly as bleomycin-induced structures. It is interesting to note that at approximately the same time these results were presented an identical observation was made by Yasuzumi *et al.* (1976); namely, they have detected the formation of nuclear bodies in human tongue carcinoma cell nuclei. Such bodies, according to the author, could not be detected prior to the onset of bleomycin therapy.

The next question to be asked was whether an ultrastructural lesion induced by bleomycin can be defined for cells *in vitro* and related to (a) the known molecular mode of action of the drug and/or (b) to the pathological manifestations at the organ level. Fujimoto (1974) studied the intracellular distribution of [^{14}C] bleomycin in mouse ascites tumor cells. He observed that within 2 hr most of the radioactivity was associated with the cell membrane, while at 4 hr bleomycin was detected on the nuclear membrane on the cytoplasmic side.

Fig. 7 is a scanning electron micrograph of an untreated Novikoff hepatoma ascites cell. The main features to be considered were cell contour and substrate interaction via numerous cellular filopodia. Vital staining of these cultures showed that viability of the normal and treated cell lines was in excess of 92%. Based on the comparison between these and other bleomycin-treated cells (Fig. 8), it must be concluded that at present it is premature to use topological markers for the evaluation of the potential drug effects on cell surface morphology. We have yet to completely define the relationship between the cell cycle and its characteristic topographical manifestations in order to interpret the effects of drugs on surface topology, since certain features may be cell-cycle-related rather than drug-induced.

Transmission electron-microscopic studies on the effects of bleomycin on cell fine structure did not appear to single out a unique lesion that could be induced by

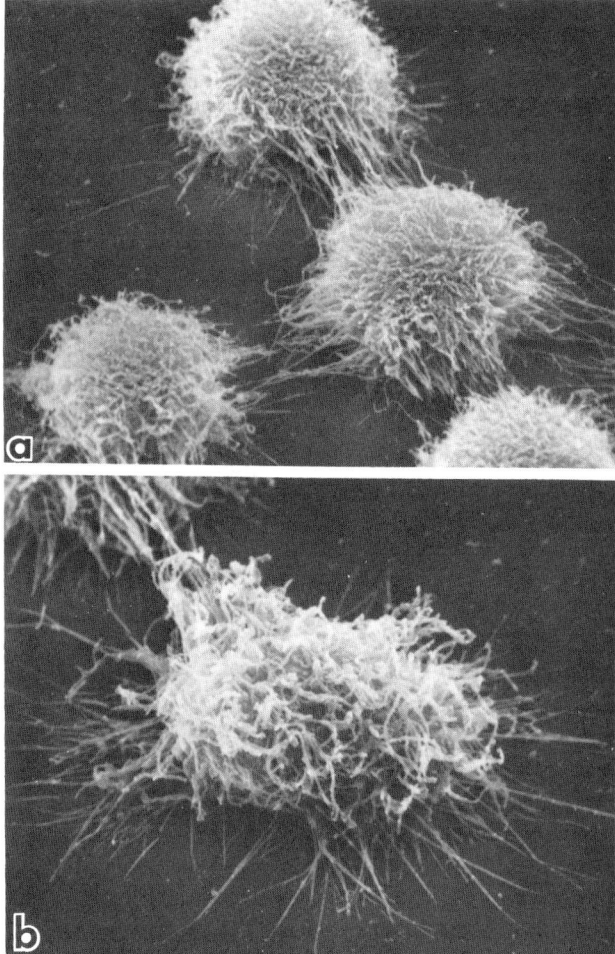

Fig. 7. Novikoff heptoma ascites cells *in vitro* for (a) 4 hr and (b) 10 hr. Note the fillopodial-substrate interactions as well as the general cell contours. (a) x1950; (b) x2925.

the drug. The wide range of effects described (Madreiter *et al.*, 1976; Mittermeyer *et al.*, 1974) were in part a universal cellular response to a noxious stimulus and in part the ultrastructural manifestation of cellular necrosis that may have been induced by bleomycin. Earlier studies by Krishan (1973) have described a wide spectrum of effects on cells treated with bleomycin. In particular, the effects on nucleolar structural segregation were mentioned. The morphological lesion known as nucleolar segregation is the ultrastructural manifestation of inhibition and cessation of rRNA synthesis. Nucleolar segregation was observed as a result of bleomycin treatment, which implies that bleomycin has a direct effect on the immediate inhibition of

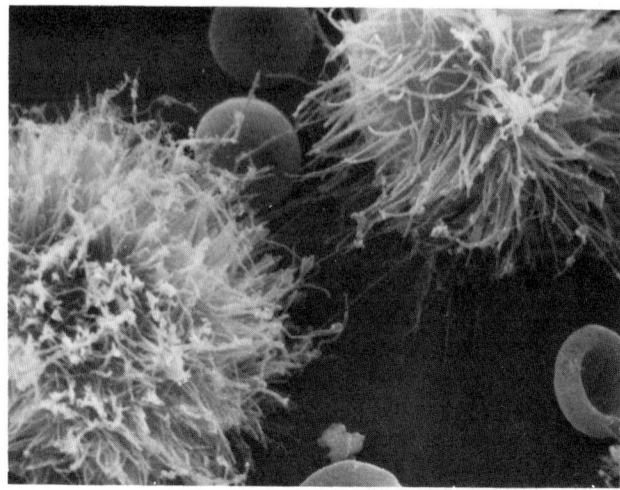

Fig. 8. Novikoff hepatoma cell treated with 100 μg/ml bleomycin for 4 hr. The only putative structural effect as a result of the bleomycin treatment may be the somewhat reduced cellular fillopodial interaction. This, however, should not be regarded as a specific response to bleomycin but rather a general response to a noxious stimulus. x2925.

rRNA synthesis. Although nucleolar segregation induced by bleomycin has been reported also by Madreiter *et al.* (1976), it appears that a better-defined lesion for nucleolar aberrations as a result of bleomycin treatment could be nucleolar fragmentation. Such nucleolar fragmentation was reported by Daskal *et al.* (1975, 1976) as well as by Yasuzumi *et al.* (1976). Figure 9a is a transmission electron micrograph of Novikoff hepatoma cells grown *in vitro* after a 2 hr incubation in the presence of bleomycin A_2 (10 μg/ml). Distinct large fibrillar centers consisting only of fibrillar components were localized in the central portion of the nucleolus. In untreated cells (Fig. 9b), small fibrillar centers were only occasionally seen. Usually, these were not well defined.

TABLE II. The Effects of Bleomycin A_2 Treatments on Novikoff Hepatoma Cells *in Vitro.*

Conditions	Cells examined	Fibrillar center/ nucleolus	Microspherules	Cytoplasmic tufts (% of total cells)	Nucleoluslike bodies (% of total cells)
10 μg/ml/2 hr	44	2.7 ± 1.2	–	–	–
50 μg/ml/2 hr	50	5.4 ± 1.1	(+)	63	24
100 μg/ml/2 hr	48	2.1 ± 1.1	+	90	87
Control	112	1 or less	–	–	< 1

With a 50 μg/ml dose of bleomycin the number of fibrillar centers increased (Table II). Concomitant nucleolar changes included an apparent loosening and fragmentation of the nucleolar fibrillar elements (Fig. 9c). In addition, this dose of bleomycin produced cytoplasmic tufts (Fig. 10) that were organized around the nuclear envelope. These structures were composed of fine fibrils 20 to 30Å in diameter. The area surrounding these tufts was devoid of ribosomes (Fig. 10).

In addition to the fibrous tufts, 25% of the cells examined at this dose (50 μg/ml) contained well defined compact cytoplasmic fibrillar bodies. These were similar to the fibrous mass of central portions of the nucleolar fibrillar centers (Fig. 9). The cytoplasmic fibrillar bodies ranged in size from 0.8 to 2.0 μm and were not surrounded by membranes.

Nucleoli of cells treated with bleomycin, 100 μg/ml, for 2 hr (Fig. 10) also contained fragmented fibrillar components around fibrillar centers. These should not be mistaken for typical nucleolar segregation. The nucleoli also contained microspherules as well as considerable granular regions. In some nucleoli that were examined the fragmented fibrillar components and their associated fibrillar centers were found on the periphery of the nucleolus or in the nucleoplasm, resulting in an overall lower count of fibrillar centers localized within the nucleolar area. In all the cells examined after treatment with bleomycin, 100 μg/ml, for 2 hr, fibrous tufts were present around the nuclear envelope (Fig. 10). Eighty-seven percent of the cells examined contained well defined cytoplasmic fibrillar bodies. These were usually observed in the proximity of lipid droplets or in the vicinity of the nuclear envelope (Figs. 10 and 11). Cross sections of the fibrillar bodies (Fig. 11) showed that they were composed of a dense fibrous cortex and a light central core. The fibrillar cortex was composed of fibrillar elements that were similar to those observed in other fibrillar bodies. The light central core consisted of fine filaments of low electron density.

Several studies have indicated that a variety of antitumor agents induce severe chromosome aberrations in treated cells. The specific effects of bleomycins on cell DNA scission will be discussed in greater detail later in these proceedings; however, the morphological manifestation of this action is in the form of chromosome aberrations reported first by Paika and Krishan (1973) and later confirmed by Hittelman and Rao (1974).

With the advent of scanning electron microscopy, such chromosomal aberrations can be easily observed and the particular lesions accurately classified.

Figure 12 represents a metaphase chromosme of CHO cells after treatment with bleomycin A$_2$ (25 μg/ml) for 30 min. Although the chromosomal lesion is not characteristic of bleomycin only, such preparations may aid in the development of specific structural marker lesions in the future.

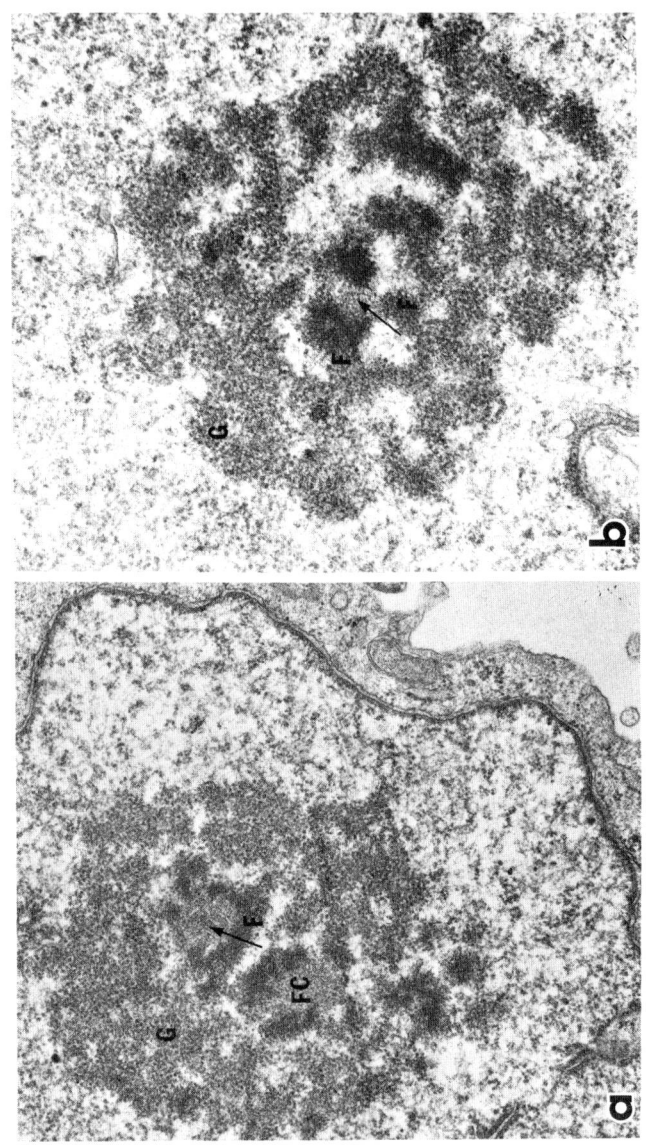

72

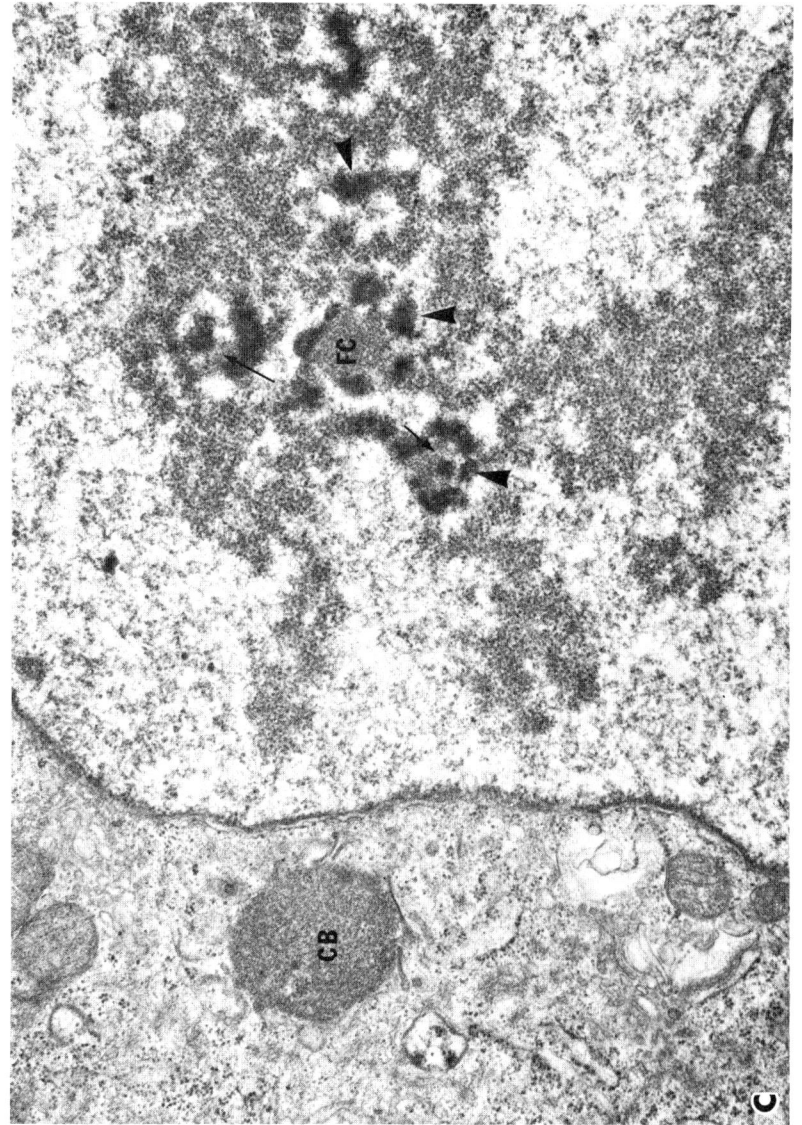

Fig. 9. Nucleolus of Novikoff hepatoma ascites cells incubated for 2 hr *in vitro* in the presence of bleomycin A$_2$, 10 μg/ml. FC, arrow, prominent fibrillar centers: F, fibrillar nucleolonemas: G, granular component. Uranyl acetate-lead citrate, x20,400.

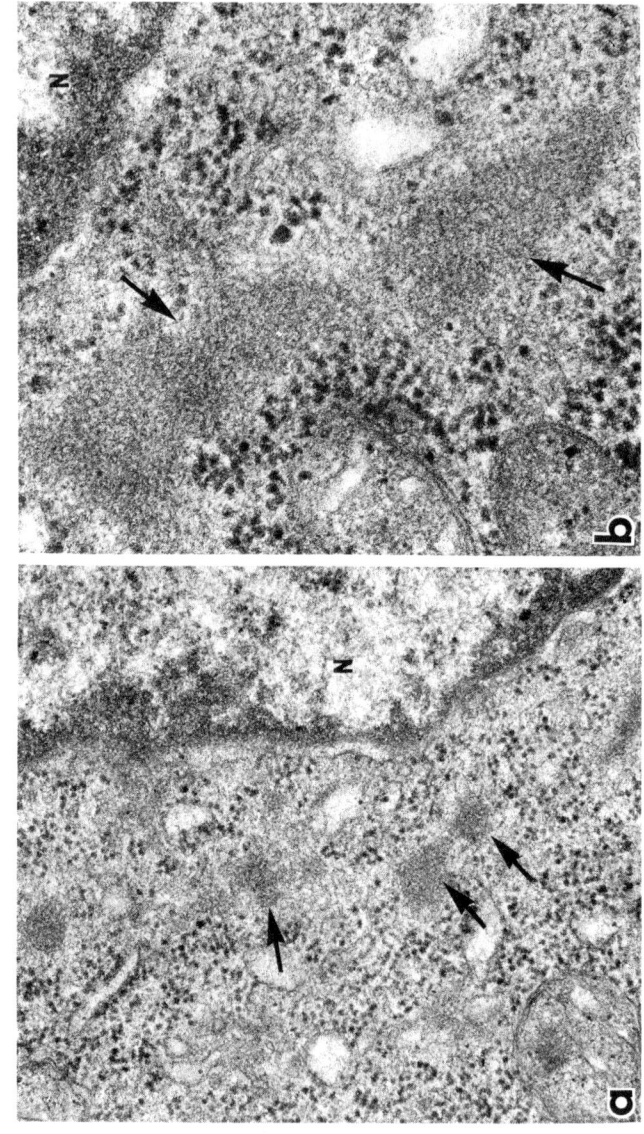

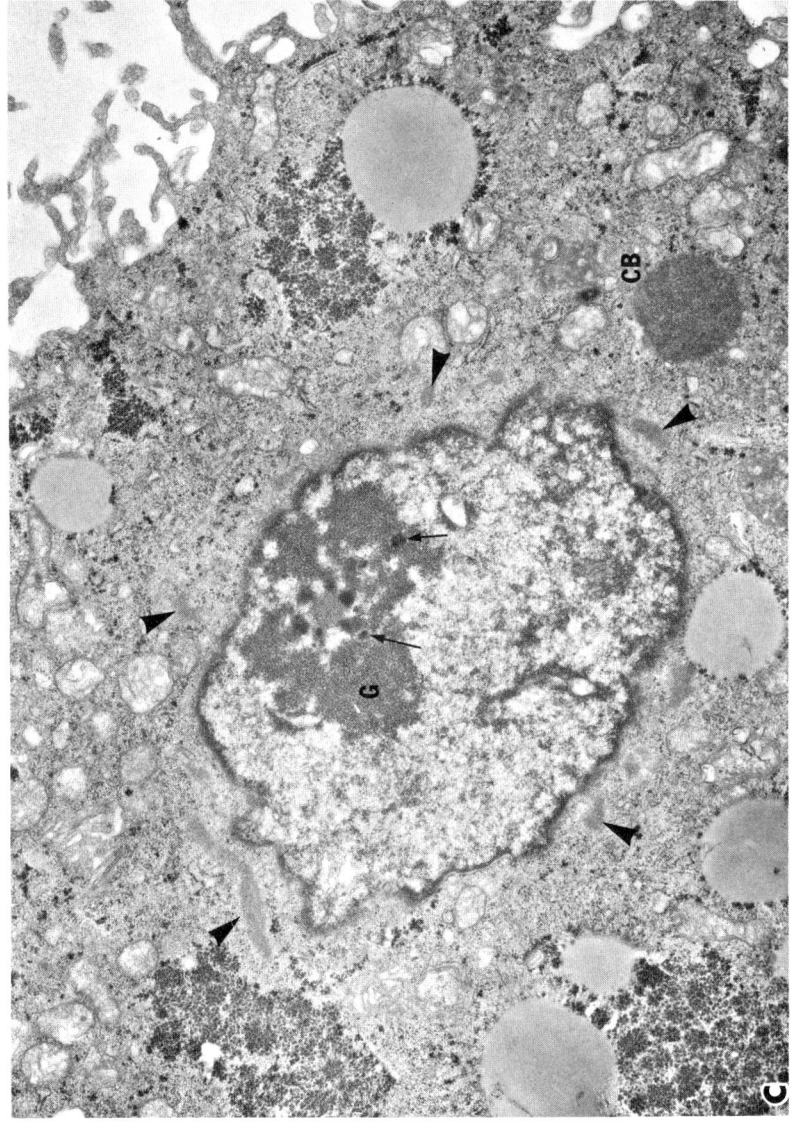

Fig. 10. Nucleolus of untreated Novikoff hepatoma ascites cells incubated for 2 hr *in vitro.* Fibrillar (F) and granular (G) elements are distributed throughout the nucleolus. Although a fibrillar center (arrow) is present, it is ill defined (compare Fig. 9). Uranyl acetate-lead citrate, x26,350.

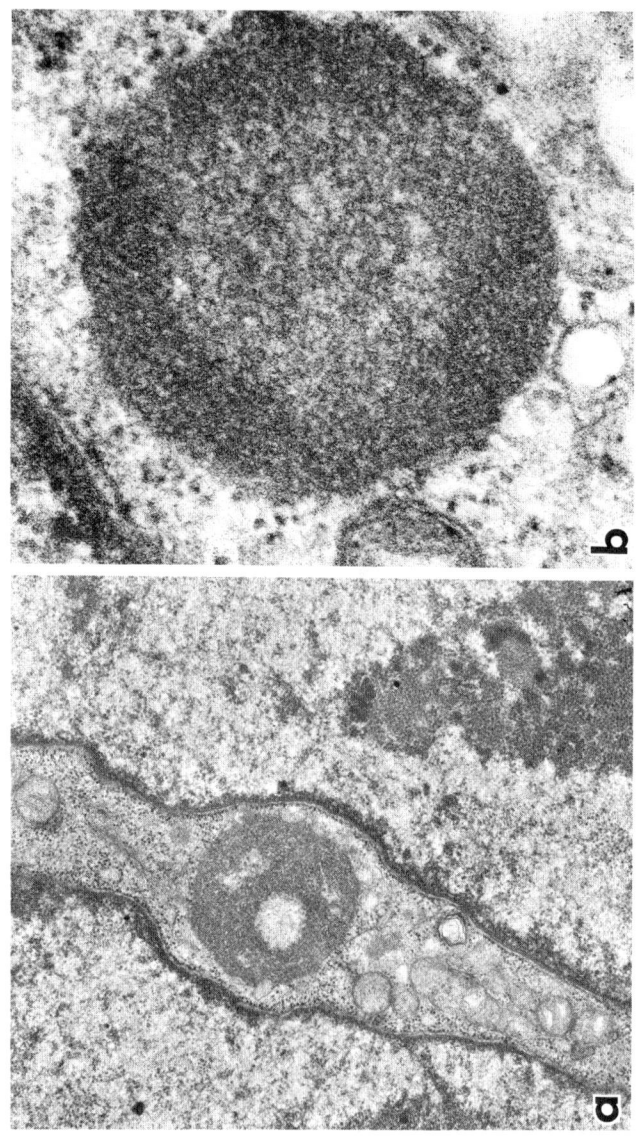

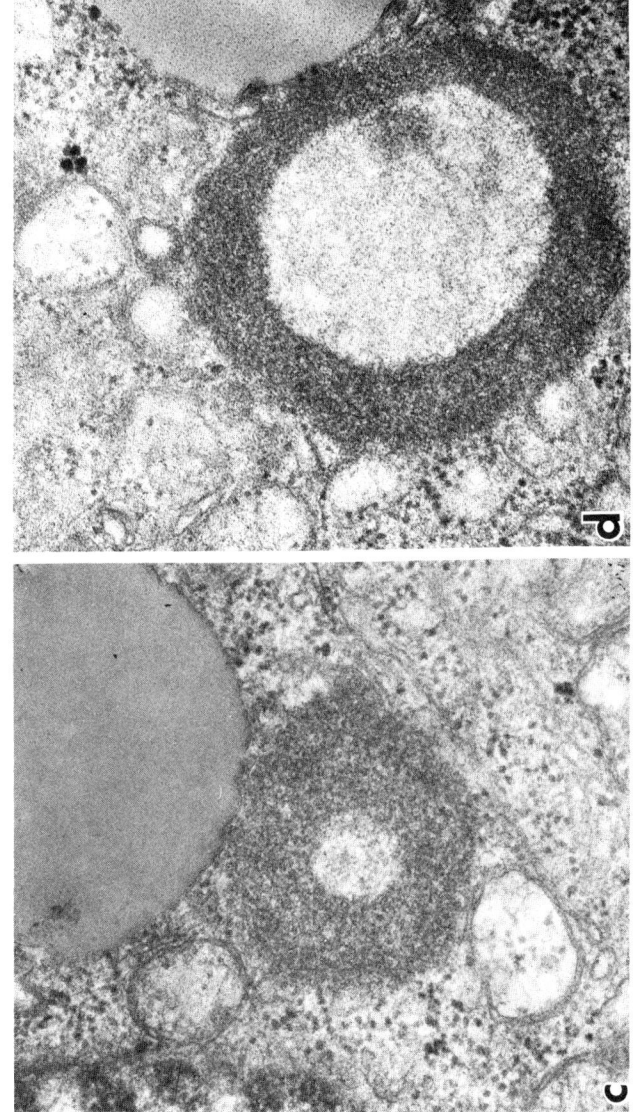

Fig. 11. Selected fibrillar bodies in the cytoplasm of bleomycin-treated Novikoff hepatoma ascites cells, showing some internal organization. (A) Cells treated for 2 hr *in vitro* with bleomycin, 100 μg/ml. (B) Cells treated for 3 days *in vivo* with bleomycin, 10 mg/kg. (C) Cells treated for 2 days *in vivo* with bleomycin, 10 mg/kg. (D) Cells treated for 2 hr *in vitro* with bleomycin, 100 μg/ml. Uranyl acetate-lead citrate. (A) x15,725; (B) x78,625; (C) x47,600; (D) x47,600.

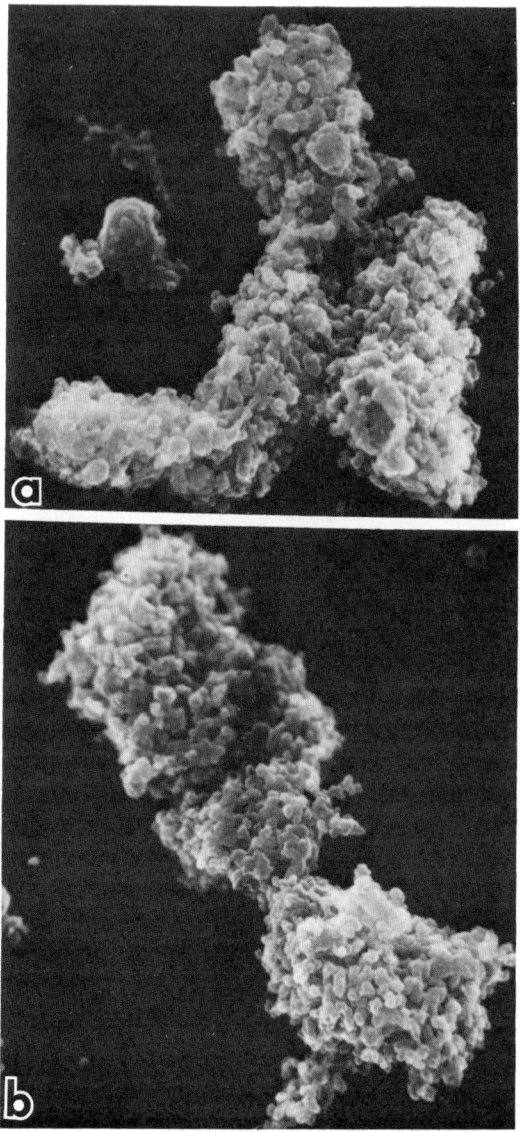

Fig. 12. Chromosomal lesions induced by bleomycin (25 μg/ml for 30 min). These isolated metaphase chromosomes exhibit lesions that are not specific for bleomycin in the form of multiple translocations and breaks (a) or specific chromatidal gaps (b). x22,100.

REFERENCES

Bedrossian, C. W. M., Luna, M. A., Mackay, G., and Lichtiger, B. (1973). *Cancer 32*, 44.

Bedrossian, C. W. M., Greenberg, S. D., Yawn, D. H., and O'Neal, R. M. (1977). *Arch. Path. Lab. Med. 101*, 248.

Bouteiile, M., Laval, M., and Dupui-Coin, A. M. (1974). In *The Cell Nucleus*, H. Busch (Ed.). Academic Press, New York, pp. 47–54.

Buttner, D. W., and Horstmann, E. (1967). *Z. Zellforsch. 77*, 589.

Daskal, Y., Crooke, S. T., Smetana, K., and Busch, H. (1975). *Cancer Res. 35*, 374.

Daskal, Y., Gyorkey, F., Gyorkey P., and Busch, H. (1976). *Cancer Res. 36*, 1267.

Fujimoto, J. (1974). *Cancer Res. 34*, 2969.

Hittelman, W. N., and Rao, P.N. (1974). *Cancer Res. 34*, 3433.

Krishan, A. (1973). *Cancer Res. 33*, 1777.

Madreiter, H., Oseika, R., Kaden, P., Rombach, A., and Mittermeyer, C. (1976). *Z. Zellforsch. 85*, 63.

Mittermeyer, C., Oseika, R., and Madreiter, H. (1974). *Arch. Derm. Forsch. 249*, 401.

Paika, K. D., and Krishan, A. (1973). *Cancer Res. 33*, 961.

Rilke, F., and Pilotti, S. (1971). *Tumori 57*, 287.

Simosato, Y., Balba, K., and Watanabe, S. (1971). *Jpn. J. Cancer Clin. 17*, 34.

Yasuzumi, F., Hyo, Y., Hoshiya, T., and Yasuzumi, F. (1976). *Cancer Res. 36*, 3574.

Chapter 7

A REVIEW OF THE SURVIVAL AND CELL-KINETICS EFFECTS OF BLEOMYCIN[1]

S. C. Barranco

I. SURVIVAL RESPONSES OF DIVIDING AND NONDIVIDING MAMMALIAN CELLS TO BLEOMYCIN

The survival responses of mammalian cells to bleomycin varies considerably, depending on whether the cells are dividing, nondividing, or synchronized into various phases of the cell cycle at the time of treatment. The bleomycin dose-response curve is biphasic (Fig. 1) suggesting the presence of sensitive and less-sensitive cells in the treated populations. The D_0 on the sensitive part of the survival curve for dividing CHO cells treated for 60 min with bleomycin is 6 $\mu g/ml$. This compared very closely to the D_{37} of 7.5 $\mu g/ml$ for mouse L5 cells originally reported by Terasima and Umezawa (1970). The D_0 for the resistant slope of the survival curve for dividing cells is 162 $\mu g/ml$. Qualitatively similar results have now been reported for EMT6 cells (Hahn et al., 1974; Twentyman and Bleehen, 1973), four strains of human melanoma cells (Barranco et al., 1973c), for a human lymphoma cell (Drewinko et al., 1972, 1973), three strains of mouse cells, a monkey kidney cell (Terasima et al., 1972), and C3H mouse mammary carcinoma in vivo (Urano et al., 1973).

[1] This work was supported in part by DHEW Grant 5R01 CA 15397.

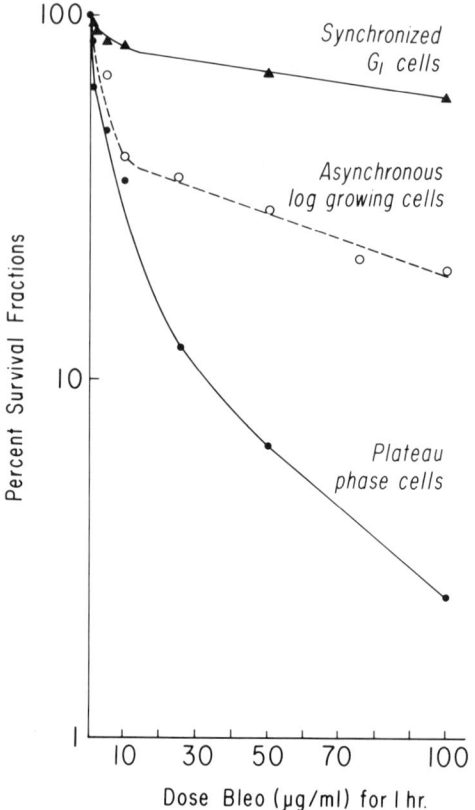

Fig. 1. Effects of bleomycin on survival of CHO cells treated while in the exponential phase of growth, or while in G_1 or plateau phase. (from Barranco *et al.*, 1973b).

The effects of bleomycin on survival of plateau phase cells are also shown in Fig. 1 (Barranco *et al.*, 1973b). Nondividing cells are several times more sensitive to bleomycin than are dividing cells. The D_0 of the sensitive slope of the survival curve is 3.4 µg/ml, and for the resistant slope is 38 µg/ml. In addition, plateau phase cells are 30 times more sensitive than are cells treated in G_1 phase (Fig. 1). These data point out that although plateau phase cells have a G_1 complement of DNA, they have widely different sensitivities to bleomycin and may not be chemically related to the normal G_1 cell. Since our initial work, Ray *et al.* (1973), using CHO cells in plateau phase, have reported similar plateau phase sensitivities to bleomycin. These findings have potential clinical significance. On the basis of our data we suggested that if a relationship existed between nondividing cells *in vitro* (plateau phase cells) and a nondividing compartment of a tumor (G_0 cells), then bleomycin would be an effective agent for killing those nondividing cells that have the potential to divide and repopulate a tumor. Hahn *et al.* (1973) have found a very close qualitative correlation between the results on *in vitro* CHO plateau phase cells and *in vivo* EMT6 tumor system. This has led to the classification of bleomycin as an agent which preferentially kills noncycling cells.

The pattern of bleomycin response during the cell cycle was first described by Terasima and Umezawa (1970). Using HeLa S3 cells, they reported that cells in mitosis and those at the G_1-S boundary were very sensitive to bleomycin. We used synchronized CHO cells to generate a family of survival curves for cells treated during different phases of the cell cycle (Barranco and Humphrey, 1971). From Fig. 2 it can be seen that the order of sensitivity is: mitotic cells (most sensitive), G_2, early S phase, late S phase, and G_1 phase (least sensitive). Since bleomycin kills dividing cells most effectively in M and G_2 phases, and because vincristine blocks cells in mitosis, the two drugs have been combined in an effective protocol for the treatment of testicular, lung, and head and neck tumors. Usually, vincristine is administered first to accumulate cells in mitosis and 6 hr later bleomycin is given. This combination was better than bleomycin given alone (Livingston et al., 1973; Spigel and Coltman, 1974).

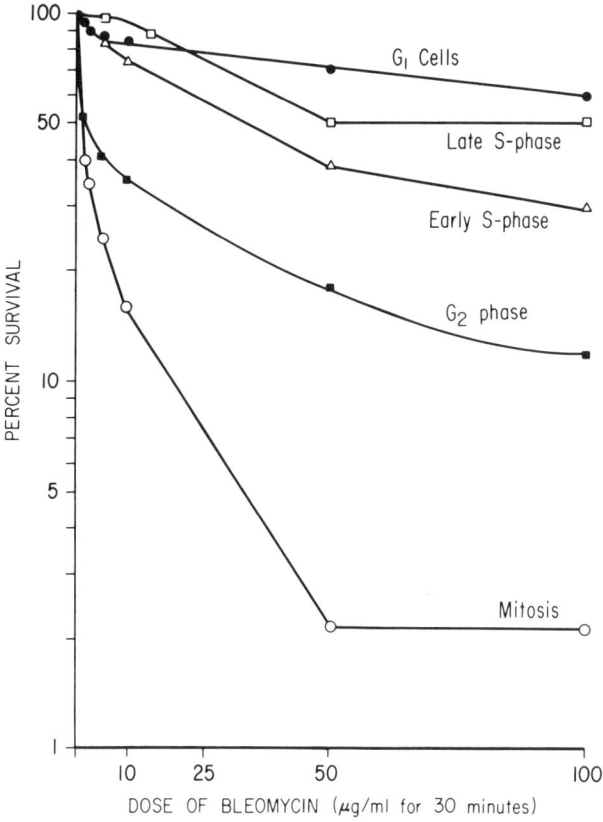

Fig. 2. Effects of increasing doses of bleomycin on survival of synchronized cells treated in G_1, S, G_2, or mitosis (from Barranco and Humphrey, 1971).

Note that the biphasic survival responses are also observed for synchronized cells (Fig. 2). Drewinko *et al.* (1973) have also reported biphasic survival curves for synchronized human lymphoma cells. Terasima *et al.* (1972), on the basis of their survival kinetics data, have suggested that the biphasic survival curve fits a model in which the drug kills cells exponentially and then induces a resistant fraction at higher doses. Following removal of the drug, the resistance is reduced and repeated doses exert a further lethal effect on the remaining viable cells.

II.   EFFECTS OF BLEOMYCIN ON CELL-CYCLE KINETICS

Kunimoto *et al.* (1967) have reported that bleomycin causes cell division delay in HeLa S3 cells. Cell progression experiments on synchronized CHO cells performed in our laboratory (Barranco and Humphrey, 1971) have shown that cells treated with bleomycin in mitosis, G_1 and S phases are not inhibited in their progression through the cell cycle. However, cells treated during G_2 phase do exhibit progression delay.

For determination of the effect of bleomycin on cells progressing from G_2 phase into mitosis, asynchronous populations of cells were pulse-labeled with $[^3H]$–TdR and then treated with 100 μg of bleomycin per milliliter. Unlabeled metaphases (accumulated in Colcemid) scored in the following 2–4 hr would have been in G_2 at the time of treatment. Labeled metaphases would have been in S phase. Thus, by differentiating between labeled and unlabeled metaphases it was possible to determine whether the delay occurred in cells treated in S or G_2 phase. Figure 3 shows that the percentage of unlabeled metaphases in untreated control cells increased linearly with time for 4 hr. Cells treated with bleomycin progressed

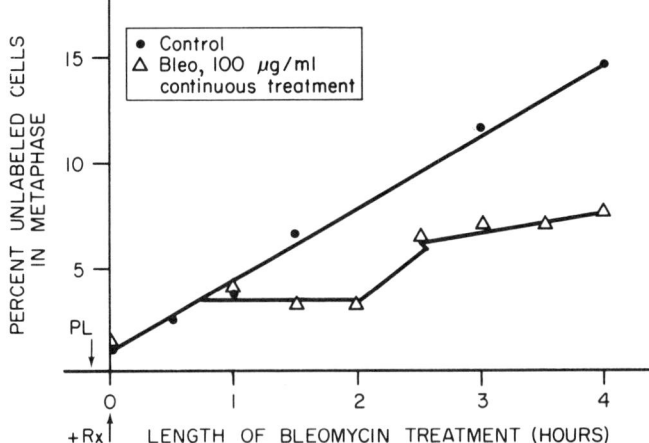

Fig. 3.   Effects on cell progression from G_2 to mitosis after bleomycin treatment of asynchronous cells in G_2 phase (from Barranco and Humphrey, 1971).

at control rates for 60 min, but then the number of unlabeled metaphases in the treated population plateaued, meaning that cells were being delayed in early G_2 phase and were not progressing into mitosis. After 2.5 hr the fraction of unlabeled metaphase cells increased again in the treated population, suggesting either that the G_2 cells could overcome the progression delay or that bleomycin was being degraded. Tobey (1972) reported a G_2 block in CHO cells at a time very similar to that reported in our laboratory, and found that the bleomycin effects were not readily reversible at high doses. Further studies by Tobey and Crissman (1972) have shown that the effects of bleomycin on G_2 traverse cannot be correlated with gross inhibition of macromolecular synthesis. Nagatsu et al. (1972) have reported that Ehrlich ascites carcinoma cells were blocked by bleomycin and accumulated in G_2. Some of these cells progressed into the next S phase without undergoing cytokinesis. Cohen et al. (1972) have presented evidence on the mouse small intestine that indicates that the bleomycin-induced delay occurs at the S-G_2 boundary. Thus the in vitro and in vivo results are in good agreement.

Because bleomycin blocks cell progression at only one place in the cell cycle, it qualifies as a potential synchronizing agent. Studies are under way (Barranco et al., 1973a) to evaluate bleomycin for this capacity in human solid tumors in vivo.

III.   RECOVERY FROM BLEOMYCIN DAMAGE BY DIVIDING AND NONDIVIDING CELLS

Irradiation studies on mammalian cells in vitro have led to the description and testing of current ideas on repair of DNA in higher organisms related to irradiation sensitivity, carcinogenesis, and mutagenesis. It is equally important that such recovery studies be carried out in detail on mammalian cells following exposure to various chemical agents. Such recovery studies may help to explain the differences in drug sensitivities of dividing and nondividing cells. The clinical implications of such studies are important since cells that recover from chemical change and survive will contribute to the regrowth of a tumor.

Hahn et al. (1973) have recently reported that potentially lethal damage (PLD) induced by bleomycin in vivo can be repaired in mice bearing EMT6 mammary sarcomas. Ray et al. (1973) have shown similar results in vitro for bleomycin. Recovery from PLD, originally described by Phillips and Tolmach (1966), is measured by the increase in survival observed when cells are exposed to various growth conditions after single-drug or irradiation treatments. Conversely, PLD is measured by a decrease in survival. Such factors as inhibition of protein synthesis, incubation in medium suboptimal for growth (nutritionally deficient), or lower temperature may influence the survival of cells after treatment with drugs or x-rays.

From Fig. 4 it can be seen that when plateau cells were treated with increasing doses of bleomycin and then held for 2-6 hr in depleted plateau phase medium (suboptimal for growth) survival was sevenfold higher than for cells treated and plated immediately for colony formation. The D_0 of the resistant part of the

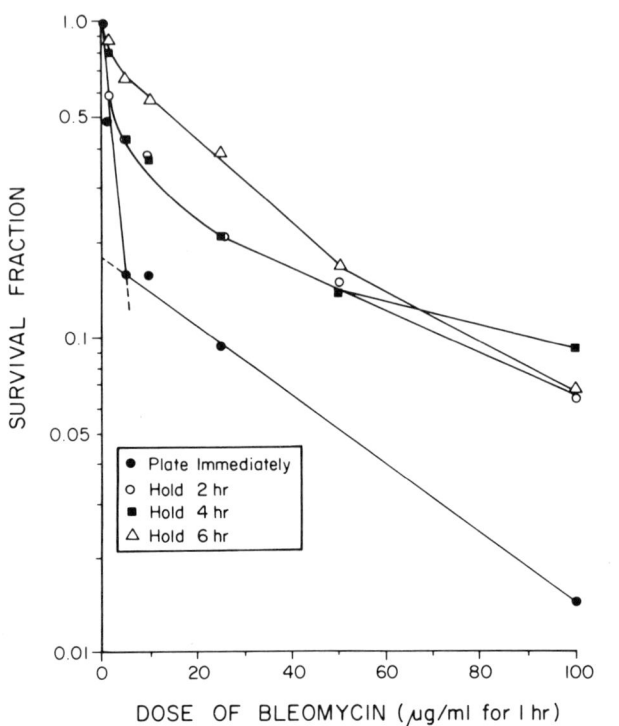

Fig. 4.   Recovery of nondividing CHO cells from PLD after being held in depleted plateau medium for 2, 4, or 6 hr (from Barranco *et al.*, 1975).

survival curve of cells plated immediately after treatment was 38 μg/ml, while cells held in suboptimal growth conditions for 2-6 hr demonstrated recovery and had higher D_0 values of 63-83 μg/ml. Identical recovery experiments performed on dividing cells resulted in survival fractions that were two- to threefold higher.

Recovery studies were extended to synchronized cell populations to determine whether the cell cycle phase-specific effects of bleomycin were related to the degree of recovery from PLD (Barranco and Bolton, 1977). It can be seen in Fig. 5 that cells treated with 100 μg/ml bleomycin for 1 hr in early G_1 or S phase can recover from bleomycin-induced PLD. G_1 cells plated for colony formation immediately after treatment had a survival fraction of 0.12 but showed fourfold increase in the survival fraction (to 0.5) within 3 hr. S-phase cells plated for colony formation immediately after treatment exhibited a survival fraction of 0.01. Within 1 hr, however, the survival fraction had increased by a factor of 40 (to 0.4).

CHO cells treated in mitosis (M) did not recover from bleomycin-induced PLD. The survival fraction immediately following the bleomycin treatment was 0.00045, and survival did not increase over the next 10 hr period of incubation. These data suggest, therefore, that the greater sensitivity of mitotic cells may be related to their inability to recover from bleomycin-induced PLD.

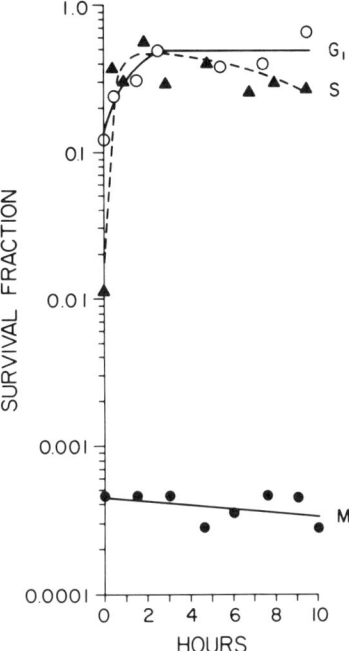

Fig. 5. Recovery from bleomycin-induced PLD by cells treated during the mitotic (M), G_1, or S phases of the cell cycle (Barranco and Bolton, 1977).

IV. INHIBITION OF RECOVERY

The inhibition of this recovery process would greatly enhance the cytotoxic effect of bleomycin. We have shown (Barranco *et al.*, 1975) that though the use of fractionated doses of bleomycin the recovery from PLD can be reduced significantly. However, PLD recovery can be completely inhibited by administering actinomycin D immediately after the bleomycin treatment (△, Fig. 6).

In CHO cells a 0.25 μg/ml dose of actinomycin D inhibited only RNA synthesis; and it can be seen in Fig. 6 (X) to reduce the survival fraction to 0.8 with a 1 hr treatment and to 0.5 after a 2-3 hr exposure. Cells which are treated first with actinomycin D for 1 hr (○) or 2 hr (□), then washed and treated for 1 hr with bleomycin, recover from PLD during further incubation.

Cells incubated in actinomycin D *after* 1 hr treatment with bleomycin showed no increase in survival. It can be seen in Fig. 6 (△) that recovery is inhibited within 30 min of the time that the cells are exposed to actinomycin D. Since a 30 min exposure to 0.25 μg actinomycin D/ml produces no cell kill by itself, these data strongly suggest that actinomycin D inhibits recovery from bleomycin-induced PLD, and illustrate that the optimal treatment schedule is bleomycin first, followed immediately by actinomycin D.

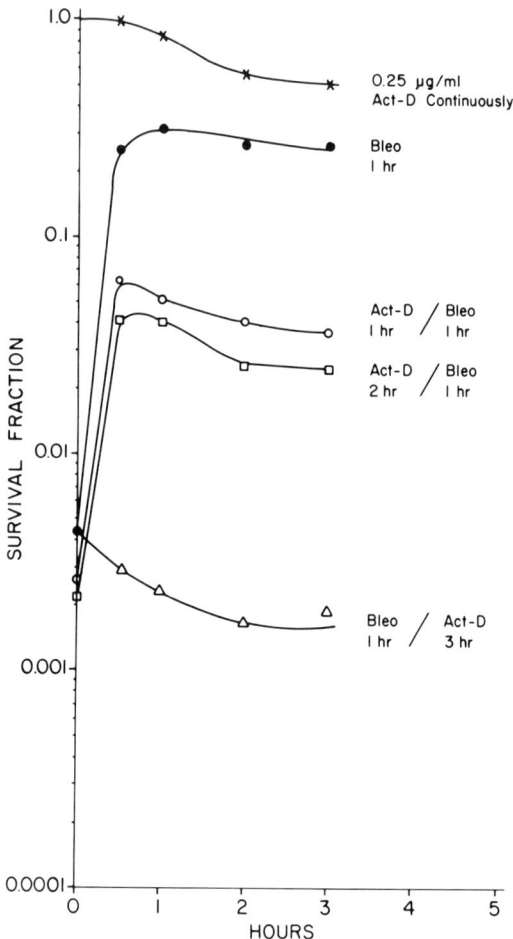

Fig. 6. The inhibition of recovery from bleomycin-induced PLD by actinomycin D

Since the dose of actinomycin D used in these studies depressed only RNA synthesis and caused only minimal cell killing (30 min and 1 hr treatments), the results in Fig. 6 suggest that RNA synthesis is required for recovery from bleomycin-induced PLD. However, it is known that actinomycin D binds selectively to DNA, and reduces the cell's ability to sustain and recover from sublethal x-ray damage (Elkind *et al.,* 1968). Its interaction with chromatin results in the inhibition of repair of x-ray damage to a DNA complex (Elkind and Chang-Liu, 1972). It might be concluded from such data that it is the binding of actinomycin D to DNA and not a specific interference with RNA synthesis that causes the inhibition of recovery. One cannot easily correlate data from DNA repair studies with the recovery experiments described in this paper. Although the possibility does exist that actinomycin inhibits recovery from bleomycin damage by its ability to complex with DNA, the requirements of RNA synthesis for such recovery cannot be ruled out.

V. CONCLUSIONS

The data presented in this paper have shown the similarities in the effects of bleomycin on a variety of *in vitro* and *in vivo* model systems. Bleomycin blocks cell progression in early G_2 phase near the S-G_2 boundary. Within the cell cycle, mitotic and G_2 phase cells are killed most effectively by bleomycin; however, non-dividing cells are the most sensitive of all. Cells in G_1 and S phase can recover from bleomycin-induced damage. That recovery can be reduced significantly through the use of dose fractionation, and can be inhibited completely by a combination treatment with actinomycin D. If such data are to be used to their greatest potential, the types of experiments presented here should be performed on all new drugs, reported, and made available to clinicians before the introduction of the agent into clinical trials. Basically we are presenting the argument for early *in vitro* testing of cancer chemotherapy agents simultaneously with the assays performed in animal tumor systems and subsequent interaction of the basic scientist with the clinician. The purpose of this interaction would be to have data available from these predictive systems at the time when they would be most valuable to the clinician in constructing effective protocols.

ACKNOWLEDGMENTS

The author wishes to acknowledge the excellent technical assistance of Mrs. J. K. Novak, Mrs. E. Gee, Miss B. Haenelt, and Mr. W. Bolton; and thanks to Mrs. R. Kenworthy for assistance in preparing the manuscript.

REFERENCES

Barranco, S. C., and Bolton, W. E. (1977). *Cancer Res. 37*, 2589-2591.
Barranco, S. C., and Humphrey, R. M. (1971). *Cancer Res. 31*, 1218-1223.
Barranco, S. C., Luce, J. K., Romsdahl, M. M., and Humphrey, R. M. (1973a). *Cancer Res. 33*, 882-887.
Barranco, S. C., Novak, J. K., and Humphrey, R. M. (1973b). *Cancer Res. 33*, 691-694.
Barranco, S. C., Romsdahl, M. M., Drewinko, B., and Humphrey, R. M. (1973c). *Mutat. Res. 19*, 277-280.
Barranco, S. C., Novak, J. K., and Humphrey, R. M. (1975). *Cancer Res. 35*, 1194-1204.
Cohen, A. M., Philips, F. S., and Sternberg, S. S. (1972). *Cancer Res. 32*, 1293-1300.
Drewinko, B., Novak, J. K., and Barranco, S. C. (1972). *Cancer Res. 32*, 1206-1208.
Drewinko, B., Brown, B. W., and Gottlieb, J. A. (1973). *Cancer Res. 33*, 2732-2736.
Elkind, M. M., and Chang-Liu, C. M. (1972). *Intern. J. Rad. Biol. 22*, 75-90.
Elkind, M. M., Sakamoto, K., and Kamper C. (1968). *Cell Tissue Kinet. 1* 209-224.

Hahn, G. M., Ray, G. R., Gordon, L. F., and Kallman, R. F. (1973). *J. Natl. Cancer Inst. 50,* 529–533.

Hahn, G. M., Gordon, L. F., and Kurkjian, S. C. (1974). *Cancer Res. 34,* 2373–2377.

Kunimoto, T., Hori, M. and Umezawa, H. (1967). *J. Antibiot., Ser. A 20,* 277–281.

Livingston, R. B., Bodey, G. P., Gottlieb, J. A., and Frei, E., III. (1973). *Cancer Chemother. Rep., Part 1 57,* 219–224.

Nagatsu, M., Richart, R. M., and Lambert, A. (1972). *Cancer Res. 32,* 1966–1970.

Phillips, R. A., and Tolmach, L. J. (1966). *Radiat. Res. 29,* 413–432.

Ray, G. R., Hahn, G. M., Bagshaw, M. A., and Kurkjian, S. (1973). *Cancer Chemother. Rep., Part 1 57,* 473–475.

Spigel, S. C., and Coltman, C. A., Jr. (1974). *Cancer Chemother. Rep., Part 1 58,* 213–216.

Terasima, T., and Umezawa, H. (1970). *J. Antibiot. 23,* 300–304.

Terasima, T., Takabe, Y., Katsumata, T., Watanabe, M., and Umezawa, H. (1972). *J. Natl. Cancer Inst. 49,* 1093–1100.

Tobey, R. A. (1972). *J. Cell. Physiol. 79,* 259–265.

Tobey, R. A., and Crissman, H. A. (1972). *Cancer Res. 32,* 2726–2732.

Twentyman, P. R., and Bleehen, N. M. (1973). *Br. J. Cancer 28,* 500–507.

Urano, M., Fukuda, N., and Koike, S. (1973). *Cancer. Res. 33,* 2849–2855.

Chapter 8

THE BLEOMYCINS:
EXPERIMENTAL TUMOR ACTIVITY

Abraham Goldin
Ira Kline

I.   INTRODUCTION

Bleomycin, a mixture of antibiotics produced by a strain of *Streptomyces verti-cillus*, was discovered by Umezawa *et al.* (1966a). These authors (Umezawa *et al.*, 1966b) separated bleomycin into fractions bleomycin A_2, the main component, and B_2 by Sephadex chromatography. A number of early reports from Japan summarized the antitumor efficacy of this chemical agent against a wide spectrum of animal tumors (Personal communication, Nippon Kayaku Co., Ltd.; Takeuchi and Yamamoto, 1968; Umezawa *et al.*, 1968).

The current report summarizes the experimental animal antitumor data for bleomycin, bleomycin fractions and analogs, and the results of combination chemotherapy with bleomycin plus other selected antitumor agents. These studies were carried out in the program of the Division of Cancer Treatment, National Cancer Institute, Bethesda, Maryland.

II. MATERIALS AND METHODS

A. Animals

All mice and rats used in these studies were obtained from the production colonies of the Developmental Therapeutics Program (DTP), Division of Cancer Treatment (DCT), National Cancer Institute (NCI). The animals were bred under the animal husbandry criteria of this group.

B. Drugs

Bleomycin, bleomycin fractions and analogs, and the other chemical agents employed in these studies were obtained from the DTP, DCT, NCI.

C. Tumors

Mouse L1210 and P-388 leukemias, B-16 melanoma, Lewis lung carcinoma, ependymoblastoma, Madison lung carcinoma, Ridgway osteogenic sarcoma, and the rat Walker carcinosarcoma were maintained by continuous passage and implanted into test animals according to protocols of the DTP, DCT, NCI (Geran *et al.*, 1972).

D. Therapeutic Studies

The drugs, given singly or in combination, were administered via the routes and on the treatment schedules indicated in the tables. The test agents were injected over a wide range of logarithmically spaced dosage levels in the constant volume of 0.01 ml/g of body weight. Each treated group consisted of 6 to 10 animals, and the untreated control groups consisted of about 16 or more animals. Antitumor activity was assessed by the median percent increase in lifespan (ILS%) relative to the untreated controls. In instances where tumor weight was used as the parameter of effect, percent tumor inhibition of the treated groups relative to the untreated controls (T/C%) was employed.

III. RESULTS

A. Single-Drug Therapy with Bleomycin versus
Various Animal Tumors *in vivo*

1. Leukemia L1210

Bleomycin was only marginally active against leukemia L1210 when the tumor was inoculated intraperitoneally (IP) or subcutaneously (SC) and the drug was given IP or SC (Table I). The best response with this drug was with daily IP treatment on days 1-9 against the IP implanted tumor. Intermittent treatment on days 2

TABLE I. Antitumor Effect of Bleomycin against Leukemia L1210

Site of inoculation	Route of administration	Treatment schedule	Opt. dose (mg/kg/inj.)	ILS %
IP	IP	Day 1 only	63	22
IP	IP	Daily, days 1-9	16	25
IP	IP	Days 2, 6	18	5
SC	IP	Daily, days 1-9	9	7
SC	SC	Daily, days 1-9	2	10

and 6 against the IP inoculated tumor, or daily treatment on days 1 through 9 given IP or SC were ineffective against the SC implanted L1210.

2. Leukemia P-388

Bleomycin had low but consistent antileukemic activity against leukemia P-388 when given on a variety of treatment schedules (Table II). Treatment on day 1 only, days 1-5, days 1-9, and on a number of intermittent schedules produced a range of activity from 22 to 56% ILS.

TABLE II. Antitumor Effect of Bleomycin against Leukemia P-388

Site of inoculation	Route of administration	Treatment schedule	Opt. Dose (mg/kg/inj.)	ILS %
IP	IP	Day 1 only	32	36
IP	IP	Daily, days 1-5	2	25
IP	IP	Daily, days 1-9	12	56
IP	IP	Days 1, 5, 9	32	22
IP	IP	Days 1, 9	64	29
IP	IP	Q_3h, day 1 only	16	22
IP	IP	Q_3h, days 1, 9	4	36
IP	IP	Q_4h, days 1, 5, 9	2	27

A comparison of the sensitivity of IP implanted L1210 and P-388 leukemias to 16 fermentation products is shown in Table III. It is clear that in most instances the P-388 tumor was more sensitive than leukemia L1210. This included bleomycin, which produced an ILS of 50% in the P-388 system and no signficiant activity in the L1210 system.

3. B-16 Melanoma

It is of interest to note that bleomycin showed greater effectiveness against the usually more refractory SC implanted B-16 melanoma than against intraperitoneally inoculated tumer (Table IV). Against SC implanted tumor, treatment on days 1-9 was highly effective (89% ILS). Even when the initiation of treatment was delayed

TABLE III. Comparative Sensitivity of IP-L1210 and IP-P388 to
16 Fermentation Products

Fermentation product	Percentage increase in lifespan over control (ILS, %)[a]	
	L1210	P388
Adriamycin	64	>200
Daunomycin	58	127
Bleomycin	N	50
Actinomycin D	45	>175
Mitomycin C	70	150
Mithramycin	N	122
Streptonigrin	N	36
Azotomycin	68	120
Streptozotocin	60	54
L-Asparaginase	N	36
Azaserine	50	97
Chromomycin A3	N	153
Neocarzinostatin	63	>200
Tubercidin	N	50
Sangivamycin	67	90
Streptovitacin A	55	81

[a] N = ILS less than 25%.

until the 5th or 10th day following SC inoculation of the tumor, treatment remained quite effective (71 and 62% ILS, respectively). Bleomycin was also active (54% ILS) against intramuscularly (IM) implanted B-16 melanoma. There was only a marginal effect against intracerebrally inoculated tumor (20% ILS).

TABLE IV. Antitumor Effect of Bleomycin against B-16 Melanoma

Site of inoculation	Route of administration	Treatment schedule	Opt. dose (mg/kg/inj.)	ILS %
IP	IP	Daily, days 1–9	3	53
IP	IP	Daily, days 5–13	6	43
IP	IP	Daily, days 10–18	6	19
SC	IP	Daily, days 1–9	4	89
SC	IP	Daily, days 5–13	12	71
SC	IP	Daily, days 10–18	24	62
IM	IP	Daily, days 1–9	16	54
IC	IP	Daily, days 1–9	8	20

TABLE V. Antitumor Effect of Bleomycin against Lewis Lung Carcinoma

Site of inoculation	Route of administration	Treatment schedule	Opt. dose (mg/kg/inj.)	ILS %
IM	IP	Day 1 only	36	24
IM	IP	Daily, days 1-9	7	60
IM	IP	Daily, days 1-11	10	67
IM	IP	Daily, days, 1-17	7	6
IM	IP	Daily, days 1-25	3	6
IM	IP	Days 1, 5, 9	20	60
IM	IP	Days 1, 5, 9, 13, 17	10	33
IM	IP	Days 1, 5, 9, ... 25	16	26
IM	IP	Days 1, 9	23	69
IM	IP	Q_3h, days 1, 5, 9	2	37
IM	IP	Q_6h, days 1, 5, 9	6	48
IM	IP	$Q_{12}h$, days 1, 5, 9	18	51

4. Lewis Lung Carcinoma

Bleomycin was also effective in increasing lifespan over a variety of treatment schedules in the Lewis lung solid tumor system (Table V). Repeated administration IP (days 1-9 or 1-11) was more effective (60 and 67% ILS) than single treatment (24% ILS) against IM inoculated tumor. It is evident that it is possible to overtreat with bleomycin, since treatment on days 1-17 or days 1-25 resulted in a reduction in survival time of the tumor-bearing animals. The drug was also active on intermittent schedules of administration but these did not result in further improvement of therapeutic response.

Bleomycin was also active when the site of inoculation of Lewis lung carcinoma and the route of administration of the drug were altered (Table VI). Bleomycin was active against IM tumor when it was administered via the SC route. It was also effective against intravenously (IV) inoculated Lewis lung carcinoma on daily or intermittent IP treatment. However, with IV inoculated tumor and IP treatment there was a loss in therapeutic effectiveness (15% ILS) when the treatment was on days 14, 18, and 22.

TABLE VI. Effect of Site of Inoculation and Route of Administration on the Antitumor Effect of Bleomycin Against Lewis Lung Carcinoma

Site of inoculation	Route of administration	Treatment schedule	Opt. dose (mg/kg/inj.)	ILS %
IM	SC	Daily, days 1-11	15	61
IV	IP	Daily, days 1-10	8	71
IV	IP	Days 1, 5, 9	32	50
IV	IP	Days 14, 18, 22	18	15

TABLE VII. Antitumor Effect of Bleomycin against Lewis Lung Carcinoma
(Delayed Therapy)

Site of inoculation	Route of administration	Treatment schedule	Opt. dose (mg/kg/inj.)	ILS %
IM	IP	Daily, days 5–8	14	42
IM	IP	Daily, days 5–13	23	57
IM	IP	Daily, days 5–15	4	34
IM	IP	Daily, days 5–18	10	24
IM	IP	Daily, days 6–14	8.4	46
SC	IP	Daily, days 8–16	32	28
SC	IP	Daily, days 7–15	16	59

The results of additional studies with delayed therapy against IM and SC inoculated Lewis lung tumor are shown in Table VII. On intraperitoneal injections delayed until day 5, 6, 7, or 8 after tumor implantation, definitive increases in lifespan were still observed (28–59% ILS).

5. Ridgway Osteogenic Sarcoma

The antitumor activity of bleomycin against the Ridgway osteogenic sarcoma is illustrated in Table VIII. Daily treatment on days 2–11 produced a marked increase in lifespan (67% ILS). With single treatment on day 2 a somewhat reduced effect was observed (43% ILS).

6. Walker 256 Carcinosarcoma

Bleomycin demonstrated a high degree of antitumor activity against the Walker 256 carcinosarcoma in the rat (Table IX). The activity was observed with a variety of schedules, including single treatment, daily treatment, and intermittent therapy. It was most effective against IP inoculated tumor when it was administered IP. Reduced antitumor activity was observed when bleomycin was given SC, IM, or IV (43, 50, and 62% ILS, respectively). The drug lost its effectiveness when administered orally.

TABLE VIII. Antitumor Effect of Bleomycin against the Ridgway Osteogenic Sarcoma

Site of inoculation	Route of administration	Treatment schedule	Opt. dose (mg/kg/inj.)	ILS %
SC	IP	Day 2 only	60	43
SC	IP	Daily, days 2–11	5.3	67

TABLE IX.   Antitumor Effect of Bleomycin on the Walker 256 Carcinosarcoma

Site of inoculation	Route of administration	Treatment schedule	Opt. dose (mg/kg/inj.)	ILS %
IP	IP	Day 1 only	3	156
IP	IP	Daily, days 1–5	3	600
IP	IP	Daily, days 1–9	0.8	600
IP	IP	Days 1, 5, 9	0.8	125
IP	SC	Daily, days 1–9	13	43
IP	PO	Daily, days 1–9	0.2	6 *oral (nonfasting)*
IP	PO	Daily, days 1–9	32	12 *oral (with prior fasting)*
IP	IM	Daily, days 1–9	32	50
IP	IV	Daily, days 1–9	32	62
				T/C%
IM	IP	Daily, days 3–6	100	14

7.   Madison Lung Carcinoma

Bleomycin was also active against Madison lung carcinoma (Table X). On the one schedule tested (days 1, 5, 9), the drug produced a 41% ILS.

8.   Ependymoblastoma

Bleomycin showed moderate antitumor efficacy against intracranially implanted ependymoblastoma (Table XI). Daily IP treatment on days 1-5 yielded a 34% increase in survival time in this tumor system.

B.   Single-Drug Therapy with Various Bleomycin Derivatives versus Animal Tumors

Antitumor data for various bleomycin derivatives are summarized in Table XII. Bleomycin A_2 (NSC-146842) comprises approximately 60–70% of the mixture that is designated as bleomycin (NSC-125066). Bleomycin A_2 on the schedule employed (days 1–9) was ineffective in the treatment of B-16 (IP) melanoma or leukemia L1210 (IP). On the same schedule, this fraction yielded only a 21% ILS in the

TABLE X.   Antitumor Effect of Bleomycin against Madison Lung Carcinoma

Site of inoculation	Route of administration	Treatment schedule	Opt. dose (mg/kg/inj.)	ILS %
IM	IP	Days 1, 5, 9	10	41

TABLE XI. Antitumor Effect of Bleomycin against Ependymoblastoma

Site of inoculation	Route of administration	Treatment schedule	Opt. dose (mg/kg/inj.)	ILS %
IC	IP	Daily, days 1–5	8	34

treatment of Lewis lung carcinoma (SC). However, in similarity to bleomycin, bleomycin A_2 was definitively effective on daily therapy (days 1–9) in the P-388 (IP) system (63% ILS).
daily therapy (days 1–9) in the P-388 (IP) system (63% ILS).

Bleomycin A_2HCl (NSC-146843) administered IP on a daily schedule (days 1–9) was ineffective against P-388 leukemia (IP).

Bleomycin platinum (NSC-278470) was essentially ineffective when administered IP daily on days 1–5 to mice inoculated IP with B-16 melanoma.

Bleomycin analog BU-2231A (NSC-279496) at the doses and schedule employed was essentially ineffective in the P-388 leukemia system. However, it was reported by Bradner et al. (1977) that this compound is highly active against the Walker 256 carcinosarcoma, moderately active against P-388 leukemia and B-16 melanoma, and slightly active in the Lewis lung carcinoma system. It was also reported by Bradner et al. (1977) that the effective doses for this analog were 2 to 11 times lower than seen with bleomycin.

Bleomycin PYP(-CU) (NSC-276381) and bleomycin PEP(-CU) (NSC-276382) showed marked activity in the B-16 (SC) melanoma system (70 and 59% ILS, respectively).

Bleomycin A_2 sulfate (NSC-149500), bleomycin A_5 sulfate (NSC-149501), bleomycin B_2 sulfate (NSC 149502), and the parent material, bleomycin (NSC-125066), were compared in the same experiment for their antitumor activity against the Lewis lung carcinoma (Table XIII). Each of the drugs was injected IP daily on days 1–11 into mice bearing the IM implanted tumor. All of the analogs were active (68, 52, and 70% ILS, respectively), but none was superior to bleomycin (70% ILS) in increasing the lifespan of the animals.

C. Combination Chemotherapy with Bleomycin and Other Chemotherapeutic Agents

Bleomycin was tested in combination with a variety of drugs and the results summarized in this report are for those combinations in which the increase in lifespan elicited by the combination was 25% or more than that produced by either of the drugs given alone (Table XIV).

The combination of bleomycin plus cyclophosphamide was more effective than the drugs employed individually in increasing the survival time of mice with Lewis lung carcinoma. The increase was observed at somewhat reduced dose levels for

TABLE XII. Antitumor Effect of Bleomycin Analogs against Various Mouse Tumors.

Drug	Tumor system	Route of administration	Treatment schedule	Optimal dose (mg/kg/inj.)	ILS %[a]
Bleomycin A$_2$ NSC-146842	B-16 melanoma (IP)	IP	Daily, days 1–9	3.9	07
	L1210 leukemia (IP)	IP	Daily, days 1–9	4.0	07
	Lewis lung (SC)	IP	Daily, days 1–9	1.0	21
	P-388 leukemia	IP	Daily, days 1–9	8.0	63
Bleomycin A$_2$HCl NSC-146843	P-388 leukemia (IP)	IP	Daily, days 1–9	16	08
Bleomycin platinum NSC-278470	B-16 melanoma (IP)	IP	Daily, days 1–9	16	19
Bleomycin analog (BU-2231A) NSC-279496	P-388 leukemia (IP)	IP	Daily, days 1–9	1.0	13
	P-388 leukemia (IP)	IP	Daily, days 1–9	0.8	13
Bleomycin PYP(-CU) NSC-276381	B-16 melanoma (SC)	IP	Daily, days 1–10	0.4	70
Bleomycin PEP(-CU) NSC-276382	B-16 melanoma (SC)	IP	Daily, days 1–10	0.4	59

[a] % Increase in mean or median lifespan over untreated controls.

TABLE XIII. Bleomycin Antitumor Activity in Lewis Lung Carcinoma Compared with Derivatives of Bleomycin[a]

Compound	Dose (mg/kg/inj.)	BW ± (g) (day 12)	Survivors (day 12)	Tumor wt. T/C% (day 12)	Deaths (days)	Median S.T.	S.T. %T/C
Bleomycin NSC-125066	30	-5.5	8/8	0	14-44	40	166
	18	-3.0	8/8	0	34-44	41	170
	10.8	-3.3	8/8	3	37-44	40	166
	6.5	-2.3	8/8	20	17-40	38	158
	3.9	-1.4	8/8	38	16-40	31.5	131
	2.3	-0.4	8/8	57	16-42	34.5	143
Bleomycin A2, sulfate NSC-149500	50	—	0/8	toxic	6-12	8	0
	30	-7.8	3/8	toxic	6-16	11	0
	18	-3.6	7/8	0	6-43	40	166
	10.8	-4.0	8/8	2	36-44	40.5	168
	6.5	-3.0	8/8	16	32-43	36.5	152
	3.9	-1.4	8/8	20	27-42	34	141
	2.3	-0.1	8/8	44	26-38	32	133
Bleomycin A2, sulfate NSC-149501	50	—	0/8	toxic	7-11	10	0
	30	-5.4	7/8	0	12-19	15	62
	18	-2.7	8/8	0	35-40	36.5	152
	10.8	-2.3	8/8	14	32-42	36	150
	6.5	-0.8	8/8	21	31-42	35	145
	3.9	-0.2	8/8	42	25-39	29	120
	2.3	-1.0	8/8	44	24-39	31.5	131
Bleomycin B2, sulfate NSC-149502	50	-5.6	5/8	toxic	5-38	33.5	139
	30	-5.0	6/8	0	10-44	40.5	168
	18	-4.6	8/8	47	36-44	41	171
	10.8	-3.1	8/8	7	20-43	36	150
	6.5	-3.0	8/8	19	17-31	27	112
	3.9	-0.1	8/8	41	27-37	29.5	122
	2.3	-0.8	8/8	63	23-34	32	133
Cytoxan NSC-26271 (day 1 only)	180	-1.1	8/8	10	14-22	44	183
Untreated controls: T.W. = 2714 (mg); S.D. = 840.			0/16		16-32		24

[a] Mice: BDF₁, male, 18–24 grams. Tumor weight was estimated from tumor size: W = 0.6d³. Treatment IP daily, days 1–11. IM tumor inoculation (2 × 10⁶ cells).

each drug and the ILS was 39% greater than that observed for cyclophosphamide alone.

Bleomycin in combination with the vinca alkaloid, vinblastine, extended the life-span of the mice bearing leukemia P-388 36% more than that observed with the optimal treatment of vinblastine injected alone. In the combination the enhanced effect was achieved with a daily dose of vinblastine that was optimal for the drug when employed individually plus one-half the optimal daily dose for bleomycin alone.

Treatment with bleomycin plus vinblastine also resulted in enhanced therapeutic effect against the B-16 melanoma implanted either IP or SC. Again, as observed in the treatment of P-388 leukemia with these drugs, enhanced therapy was obtained with reduced optimal daily dose levels of bleomycin plus dose levels of vinblastine near the optimal daily dose for vinblastine employed individually.

Combination chemotherapy with bleomycin plus the vinca alkaloid, vincristine, also resulted in therapeutic enhancement in the treatment of Lewis lung carcinoma. The combination produced an ILS of 118% which was 60% greater than that observed with vincristine given alone (58% ILS). This was observed with a daily dose of bleomycin higher than the optimal dose level of bleomycin when employed alone.

Bleomycin plus CCNU was also more effective than the drugs employed individually in increasing the survival time of mice with Lewis lung carcinoma. Similarly, bleomycin plus cis-Pt(II) provided therapeutic enhancement in the treatment of B-16 melanoma. In these studies the doses used for each of the drugs in the combination were lower than those used for single-drug administration.

Bleomycin plus procarbazine (NSC-77213) also provided therapeutic enhancement in the treatment of Lewis lung carcinoma. This observation is noteworthy since treatment with procarbazine alone was without effect.

A study was conducted employing the Wexler technique (1966) to determine the influence of bleomycin and procarbazine administered alone and in combination on lung metastases in mice with Lewis lung carcinoma (Table XV). In this experiment more than 25 nodules were found in the lungs of untreated mice on day 20. A marked retardation of the growth of metastatic foci in the lungs was observed with bleomycin as well as with procarbazine treatment, and more than 25 nodules were not apparent until day 34 of the study. It is noteworthy that no nodules were detected on days 14 through 34 in the lungs of mice treated with the combination of bleomycin and procarbazine.

IV. DISCUSSION AND SUMMARY

Bleomycin has broad-spectrum antitumor activity, as illustrated by its therapeutic action against the animal tumors leukemia P-388, B-16 melanoma, Lewis lung carcinoma, Ridgway osteogenic sarcoma, Walker carcinosarcoma 256, Madison lung carcinoma, and the intracranially inoculated ependymoblastoma.

TABLE XIV. Effect of Combination Chemotherapy with Bleomycin (NSC-125066) Plus Other Chemical Agents against a Variety of Animal Tumors

NSC No., Chemical Agent	Tumor System	Route and Treatment schedule[a]	Optimal dose (mg/kg/day)		%Ils[b]		Untreated control[c] (MST days)
			Single	Combination	Single	Combination	
125066 Bleomycin	Lewis Lung (SC)	IP daily, days 1-9	6.0	4.0 +	58	199	20.0
26271 Cyclophosphamide		PI, day 4 only	200	150	160		
125066 Bleomycin	P-388 Leukemia (IP)	IP daily, days 1-9	16.0	8.0 +	25	132	11.2
49842 Vinblastine		IP daily, days 1-9	0.5	0.5	96		
125066 Bleomycin	B-16 Melanoma (IP)	IP daily, days 1-9	16.0	2.0 +	13	209	19.3
49842 Vinblastine		IP daily, days 1-9	0.25	0.5	103		
125066 Bleomycin	B-16 Melanoma (SC)	IP daily, days 1-9	16.0	4.0 +	67	94	22.1
49842 Vinblastine		IP daily, days 1-9	0.5	0.25	13		

TABLE XIV –cont.

125066 Bleomycin	Lewis lung (IM)	IP daily, days 1-9	5.0	14.0	50	118	
67574 Vincristine		IP daily, days 1-9	0.14	+ 0.08	58		20.0
125066 Bleomycin	Lewis lung (IM)	IP daily, days 1-9	14.0	5.0 (days 2-9) 86		159	
79037 CCNU		IP, day 1 only	39.0	+ 23.0	29		23.0
125066 Bleomycin	B-16 Melanoma (SC)	IP daily, days 1-9	16.0	8.0	70	111	
119875 cis-Pt II		IP daily, days 1, 5, 9	8.0	+ 4.0	44		23.6
125066 *Bleomycin*	Lewis Lung (IM)	IP daily, days 1-9	23	8.4	35	68	
77213 Procarbazine		IP daily, days 1-9	108	+ 108	04		28.7

[a] Treatment was given over a wide range of logarithmically spaced doses.
[b] Percent increase in median or mean lifespan over controls.
[c] MST = median or mean survival time of untreated controls.

TABLE XV. Effect of Procarbazine and Bleomycin Treatment, Alone and in Combination, on Primary Tumor and Lung Metastases in Mice with (IM) Lewis Lung Carcinoma[a]

Agent	Dose (mg/kg)	MST	Tumor weight (g) (days after tumor inoculation)				(Average No. of nodules/lung) (days after tumor inoculation)			
			14	20	26	34	14	20	26	34
Procarbazine	108	21.5	2.4	2.5	6.0	—	0	0	0	—
	65	21	1.3	1.8	4.4	7.3	0	0	6	>25
Bleomycin	14	35.5	0.7	1.4	7.8	2.2	0	0	0	6
	8.4	30.5	1.4	2.2	—	6.8	0	0	0	>25
Procarbazine	108	29	0.08	0.2	0.4	2.7	0	0	0	0
+										
Bleomycin	8.4									
Untreated controls		28	2.6	4.9	11.6	—	9	>25	>25	—

[a]Eight BDF$_1$ mice per test group, 16 untreated controls used for survival. Additional mice were inoculated and sacrificed for evaluation of metastatic growth.

The sensitivity of P-388 leukemia to bleomycin was greater than that seen in L1210 leukemia. The high sensitivity of leukemia P-388 to most fermentation products makes it especially useful for detecting active materials present in low concentration and is the primary reason that this system is being used in the DCT,NCI program as a standard prescreen.

The antitumor activity of bleomycin against the Lewis lung carcinoma, a tumor which is relatively insensitive to most chemical agents, is noteworthy. This activity was still apparent when the initiation of therapy was delayed from 5 to 14 days after implantation of tumor, at a time when metastasis to the lungs from the local tumor site usually occurs (Karrer and Humphreys, 1967).

The effectiveness of bleomycin may be influenced by the schedule of treatment. The observation with several tumors including Lewis lung carcinoma, Ridgway osteogenic sarcoma, and Walker carcinosarcoma 256 that single treatment may be less effective than chronic therapy indicates the importance of continued treatment with this drug to a point short of limiting chronic toxicity.

Antitumor data for a number of bleomycin fractions and analogs are presented in this paper. Even though analogs, such as bleomycin A_2 sulfate (NSC-149500), bleomycin A_5 sulfate (NSC-149501), and bleomycin B_2 sulfate (NSC-149502) produced antitumor activity similar to that of the parent material, bleomycin, they should nevertheless be investigated further with respect to optimal schedules, broad-spectrum activity, and other characteristics. The comparative toxicities of these analogs relative to antitumor effectiveness should be explored with a view to finding analogs with greater antitumor selectivity or other desirable characteristics as compared with bleomycin.

Enhanced therapy with bleomycin plus several established antitumor agents is presented in this manuscript. It is noteworthy that the optimal dose for bleomycin in several of the combinations was lower than that observed when the drug was given alone. For most of the combinations presented here, the drugs also exerted significant antitumor effect when employed individually. The exception was procarbazine (Kline, 1974) which was ineffective, when employed alone, in increasing survival time in the Lewis lung system. Nevertheless, the combination of bleomycin and procarbazine elicited an enhanced therapeutic response as measured by the increase in survival time of the animals. One interpretation of this observation is suggested by the results of the metastasis experiment presented here. The improved therapy with the combination may result because both compounds appear to be active in inhibiting the metastatic process to the lungs. This effect of procarbazine may contribute to the therapeutic response when used in conjunction with bleomycin, even though procarbazine by itself is not sufficiently tumor-inhibitory to increase the lifespan of the animals.

Clinical groups have reported varying degrees of activity with bleomycin in lymphomas, reticuloses, and other tumors. These investigators (Blum et al., 1973; E.O.R.T.C., 1972; Halnan et al., 1972) uniformly recognized the almost complete lack of bone-marrow toxicity with bleomycin and recommended it for use in combination chemotherapy.

REFERENCES

Blum, R. H., Carter, S. K., and Agre, K. (1973). *Cancer 31*, 903.

Bradner, W. T., Imanishi, H., Hirth, R. S., and Wodinsky, I. (1977). *Proc. Am. Assoc. Cancer Res. 18*, 35.

E.O.R.T.C., Co-operative Group for Leukemia and Reticulocytoses (1972). *Br. Med. J. 1*, 285.

Geran, R. I., Greenberg, N. H., Macdonald, M. M., Schumacher, A. M., and Abbott, B. J. (1972). *Cancer Chemother. Rep. 3*(2), 1.

Halnan, K. E., Bleehen, N. M., Brewin, T. B., Deeley, T. J., Harrison, D. F. N., Howland, C., Kunkler, P. B., Ritchie, G. L., Wiltshaw, E., and Todd, I. D. H. (1972). *Br. Med. J. 4*, 635.

Karrer, K., and Humphreys, S. R. (1967). *Cancer Chemother. Rep. 51*(7), 439.

Kline, I. (1974). *Cancer Chemother. Rep., Pt. 2, 4*(1), 33.

Takeuchi, M., and Yamamoto, T. (1968). *J. Antibiot. 21*, 631.

Umezawa, H., Maeda, K., Takeuchi, T., and Okami, Y. (1966a). *J. Antibiot., Ser. A 19*, 200.

Umezawa, H., Suhara, Y., Takita, T., and Maeda, K. (1966b). *J. Antibiot., Ser. A 19*, 210.

Umezawa, H., Ishizuka, M., Kimura, K., Iwanaga, J. and Takeuchi, T. (1968). *J. Antibiot. 21*, 592.

Wexler, H. (1966). *J. Natl. Cancer Inst. 36*, 641.

Chapter 9

THE RADIOIMMUNOASSAY OF BLEOMYCIN
AND ITS ANALOGS [1]

Alan Broughton

I. INTRODUCTION

The classical methodologies to determine drug concentrations in biological fluids are often very time consuming, require expensive equipment and highly skilled personnel, and are in many instances insensitive and imprecise.

The development of radioimmunoassays first for insulin (Berson and Yalow, 1960), then for the cardiac glycosides (Smith et al., 1969), and more recently for antibiotics (Broughton and Strong, 1976a,b), has enabled the pharmacologist to study and analyze data from patients, which would otherwise have been impossible. The development of any radioimmunoassay requires the production of high avidity specific antisera and the development of a suitably labeled tracer compound. The bleomycins are no exception. This paper will describe the development of radioimmunoassays for bleomycin and its analogs.

[1] Supported by a grant-in-aid by Bristol Laboratories, Syracuse, New York.

107

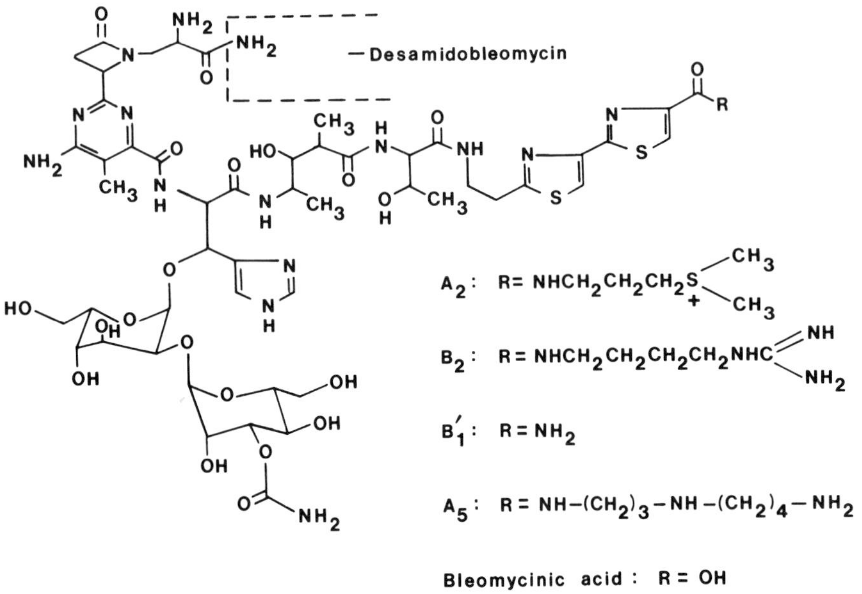

Fig. 1. Structure of bleomycin and its analogs.

II. ANTISERA PRODUCTION

The clinical preparation of bleomycin sulfate (BLM) Blexane® containing mainly bleomycin A_2 (55-70%) and B_2 (25-32%) (Fig. 1) was used to develop the assay. BLM with a molecular weight of 1500 would not be a satisfactory immunogen but when covalently linked to a macromolecule should elicit a satisfactory response. Therefore, BLM was conjugated to bovine serum albumen (BSA) using 1-ethyl 3-(dimethyl aminopropyl) carbodiimide (ECDI–Story Chemical Co., Muskegon, Michigan) to form an amide bond as described by Goodfriend et al. (1964). This conjugate was prepared as follows: 20 mg of BSA was dissolved in 1.0 ml of PBS (0.15 mole/liter NaCl in 0.01 mole/liter phosphate buffer with 1 g/liter sodium azide added as a preservative) containing 45 mg of BLM and 1.0 ml of ECDI (900 mg/ml) was added slowly to the mixture with constant stirring.

The solution was mixed at room temperature for 1 hr and then at 4°C for 3 days. It was then dialyzed for 18 hr at 4°C against PBS and purified using column chromatography (Sephadex G25). The molar incorporation of BLM to albumen was determined spectrophotometrically and found to be 28/1.

Three young New Zealand white rabbits were immunized with the conjugate by the following procedure. Each rabbit received 0.5 mg of conjugate emulsified in complete Freunds adjuvant by IM injection into all limbs. This was followed by monthly injections of 0.5 mg of conjugate to either fore or hind limbs. The animals were bled after three boosters and the resulting antisera evaluated as discussed in Section VI.

III.   IODINATION PROCEDURE

The BLM was labeled using a modified Hunter and Greenwood (1962) chlor-amine T technique. This was performed as follows: 1 mCi Na^{125}I (100 mCi/ml, in 0.1 N NaOH), 10 μl chloramine T (5 mg/ml solution in 0.1 M Borate buffer, pH 9.0), and 10 μl BLM (1 mg/ml solution in 0.1 M Borate buffer, ph 9.0) were mixed and incubated at room temperature for 1 min and then 10 μl of sodium metabi-sulfite (12 mg/ml solution in 0.1 M Borate buffer, pH 9.0) were added, followed by 10 μl of potassium iodide (20 mg/ml in 0.1 M Borate buffer, pH 9.0).

The iodination of the bleomycin probably occurred in the imidazole ring and can be compared to histamine iodination in certain polypeptides. The iodinated material was then purified by column chromatography on Sephadex C25 (30 x 0.9 cm). A linear gradient of ammonium formate (pH 6.4) from 0.1 to 1.0 M was used to elute the iodinated product.

The specific activity of the iodinated product was approximately 5 μCi/μg with an incorporation of 3.5 x 10^{-5} atoms of iodine per molecule of bleomycin.

IV.   RADIOIMMUNOASSAY PROCEDURE

A competitive protein binding assay between ^{125}I-labeled bleomycin and un-labeled bleomycin for antibody binding sites was used to quantitate unknown con-centrations of bleomycin in biological samples. The antibody bound drug was separated from the free drug by the use of a dextran-coated charcoal separation procedure. A typical system is as follows: 200 μl of 1% gelatin dissolved in phosphate-buffered saline (PBS), 100 μl sample or appropriate solution, 100 μl ^{125}I-labeled bleomycin diluted to approximately 30,000 cpm in PBS, and 100 μl of a suitable dilution of antisera, were mixed and incubated (10 min at 37°C, and 10 min at 4°C). Following this incubation, 200 μl of dextran-coated charcoal (2 g dextran T-70 and 2 g activated charcoal in 100 ml PBS) plus 400 μl PBS (4°C) were added. After incubation (5 min, 4°C) the mixture was centrifuged (2000g, 10 min, 4°C) and the supernatant counted in an automatic gamma counter.

V.   BLEOMYCIN ANALOGS

In addition to BLM, antibodies to conjugates of BU2231A (Tallysomycin A)[2] and desamido bleomycin,[2] were produced and labeled tracers to each compound prepared by the techniques described in Sections II and III.

---

[2] Provided by S. T. Crooke, Bristol Laboratories.

VI.   ANTISERA EVALUATION

The antisera to bleomycin were first evaluated for titer and avidity, then specificity. The titer, defined as that dilution of an antisera which would bind 50% of the labeled bleomycin (2 ng) was 1 in 10,000. The avidity as determined by the equilibrium technique of Odell et al. (1969) was 1.3×10^9 liters/mole. The specificity of the antisera was determined by cross-reactivity experiments using the following drugs: adriamycin, 1-(2-chloroethyl)3, cyclohexyl-1-nitrosourea, 5 fluorouracil, arabinosyl cytosine, vincristine, and prednisolone, and by determining the concentration at which 50% binding to antibody sites occurs and expressing this as a percentage related to the concentration of bleomycin. All the above drugs cross-reacted less than 1%.

The BLMs (Fig. 1) differ from each other in the terminal amine moieties and the results of the cross-reactivity studies suggest that the presence and nature of this part of the molecule determine much of its immunoreactivity. Illustrated in Table I is the percentage cross-reactivity of these analogs with the bleomycin antisera. A_2 and B_2 compete more effectively than the other analogs, although B_2 has a terminal moiety differing somewhat from A_2, there is a structural resemblance between the two side chains as shown with molecular models. BLM A_5, which has a spermidine moiety as the terminal amine, competes only 11.7% effectively against the antibody and iso BLM A_2, differing from A_2 only in the translocation of the carbamoyl group in the mannose sugar, competed with 25% the efficiency of BLM sulfate.

TABLE I. Bleomycin Analog Immunoreactivity with Rabbit Antisera [a]

Bleomycin	Mean concentration (pmole)	Standard deviation (pmole)	Percentage cross-reactivity
Sulfate	3.45	±0.11	100
A_2	2.99	±0.22	115.4
B_2	4.63	±0.17	74.5
A_5	29.50	±5.14	11.7
Iso-A_2	13.70	±0.29	25.2
Acid	>1000.00	–	<1.0
BU-2231B	>1000.00	–	<1.0
Desamido A_2	8.26	0.51	44.6
B_1^1	214.2	15.9	1.6

[a] The indicated quantity of bleomycin analog was required to produce a 50% inhibition of ^{125}I-labeled bleomycin sulfate bound to antibody. Results are expressed as the mean concentration, in picomoles, of the bleomycin analog determined in five separate analyses.

Another compound, bleomycinic acid, which is devoid of any terminal amine moiety, failed to react with the antibody, and B_1, which has an amide group in lieu of a terminal amino acid, only reacts to 1.6%.

Desamido BLM, which is a metabolite of BLM produced by the inactivating

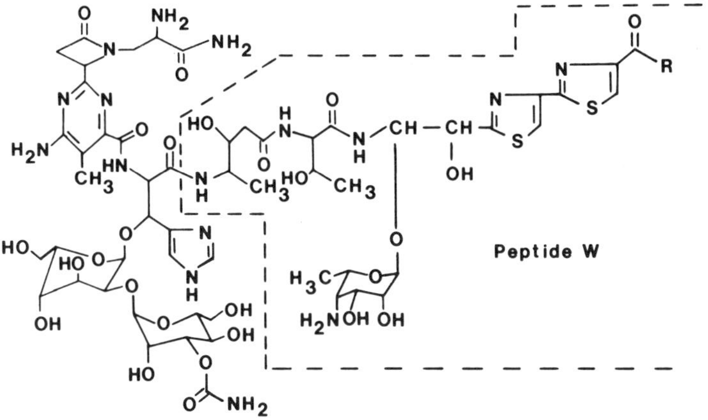

Bu 2231 A $R = -NH-(CH_2)_3-CH(NH_2)-CH_2-CO-NH-(CH_2)_3NH(CH_2)_4NH_2$

Bu 2231 B $R = -NH(CH_2)_3NH(CH_2)_4NH_2$

Bu 2231 S_2b $R = -NH-(CH_2)_3-S^{+}(CH_3)_2$

Bu 2231 E_1a $R = -NH-(CH_2)_2CH_2NH_2$

Fig. 2. Structure of the tallysomycins (BU2231) and their analogs.

enzyme described by Umezawa (1976), has intact terminal amines, but the amine group on β aminalanamide has been removed. This compound cross-reacts to 44% with the bleomycin antibody; conversely, an antibody raised against desamido bleomycin cross-reacts 100% against BLM sulfate.

Experiments using a new generation of bleomycins, the tallysomycins, give further evidence to support the immunodominance of the terminal amines. These compounds, in addition to the existing disaccharide, contain a new amino sugar and a specific terminal amine moiety. The structure of these compounds has recently been elucidated by Konishi *et al.* (1977) and is shown in Fig. 2. Tallysomycin B (BU2231B)[3] was tested against the bleomycin antibody and exhibited no cross-reactivity.

Antibodies raised in a goat against BLM sulfate exhibited different specificities (Strong *et al.*, 1977) but these were still related to the structure of bleomycin.

The compound tallysomycin A (Fig. 2) was conjugated to albumen and antibodies to this conjugate were raised in rabbits. These antibodies also produced interesting evidence concerning immunodominance. Using the criteria defined above, the bleomycins react less than 1% (Fig. 3), as do phleomycin and desamido

[3]Supplied by S. T. Crooke, M.D., Bristol Laboratories.

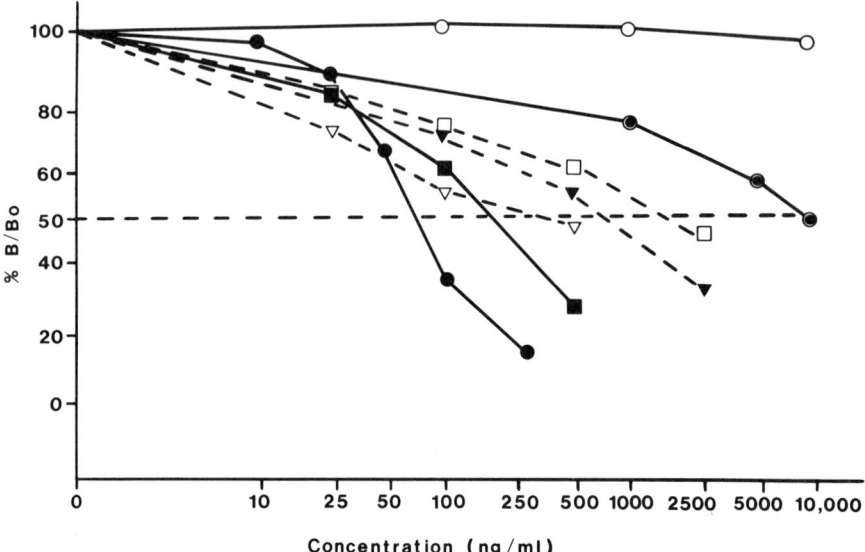

Fig. 3. Immunoreactivity studies of analogs of tallysomycin and bleomycins against rabbit antisera to tallysomycin A. (○——○) BLM, phleomycin, desamidobleomycin; (◉——◉) BU 2231 S_2B + Cu; (□ --- □) BU 2231 B - Cu; (▲--- ▲) BU 2231 WB; (△ --- △) BU 2231 B + Cu; (■ ——■) BU 2231 E_1 + Cu; (● ——●) BU 2231 A ± Cu; BU 2231 WA.

bleomycin. BU2231A, with or without copper, and BU2231 WA (Fig. 2) cross-reacted 100%, but tallysomycin B BU2231B, without copper, competes only 10% as effectively, whereas with copper in the molecule there was 40% cross-reactivity. The chelation of copper by bleomycin has been studied by Umezawa (1976) and Dabrowiak *et al.* (1977), who have produced good evidence that Cu(II), a square planar atom, ligates from nitrogen atoms situated in the β aminalanamide, imidazole ring, 4 amino pyrimidine residue, and the sugar carbamoyl function. This ligation probably produces a conformational change in the molecule, enabling antibody to bind more effectively. A similar situation may account for some loss of immunoreactivity by anti BLM against iso BLM A_2, which was also copper-free.

The analogs of BU2231, S_{2_b} and E_{1_a} (Fig. 2), both with ligated copper, exhibited interesting cross-reactivity with anti BU2231A. S_{2_b} cross-reacted less than 1%, whereas the activity of E_{1_a} was 87%. The only difference in the structure of these compounds is substitution of dimethyl thio radical in S_2B for the primary amino group of the 1–3 diaminopropane side chain of E_{1_a}.

These results reemphasize the importance of the side chain in determining immunoreactivity.

VII. EVALUATION OF THE TRACER

The four radioactive peaks from the column chromatography were evaluated for immunoreactivity, stability, and radiation damage. The first two peaks were not immunoreactive and probably represent inorganic iodide. The other two were immunoreactive and represented some form of labeled BLM. The first of these two peaks was unstable, the nonspecific radioactivity (not bound to BLM) increasing to 20% of the total radioactivity in 4 days. The second of these peaks was stable with low nonspecific activity for over 3 months. The process of iodination often results in iodination damage to the molecule being investigated. Therefore, before a product can be used it must be examined for iodination damage. This is done by two competitive binding experiments: (a) a constant amount of iodinated product and increasing amounts of noniodinated drug are mixed with antibody; and (b) increasing amounts of tracer are mixed with antibody. The results are expressed as in Fig. 4. When the two curves are superimposed there is no radiation damage, but if, as in the interrupted line, there is divergence, the product has less immunoreactivity than the native drug and should not be used as a tracer.

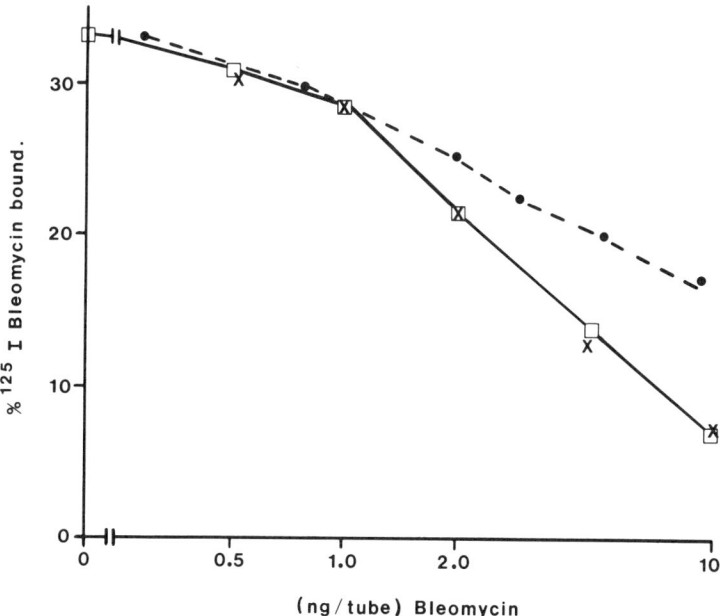

Fig. 4. Evaluation of iodinated bleomycin for radioiodination damage. (X ——X) tracer amounts of [^{125}I] BLM plus increasing amounts of unlabeled BLM; (□ —— □) increasing amounts of [^{125}I] BLM; (●----●) hypothetical curve to depict radiation damage.

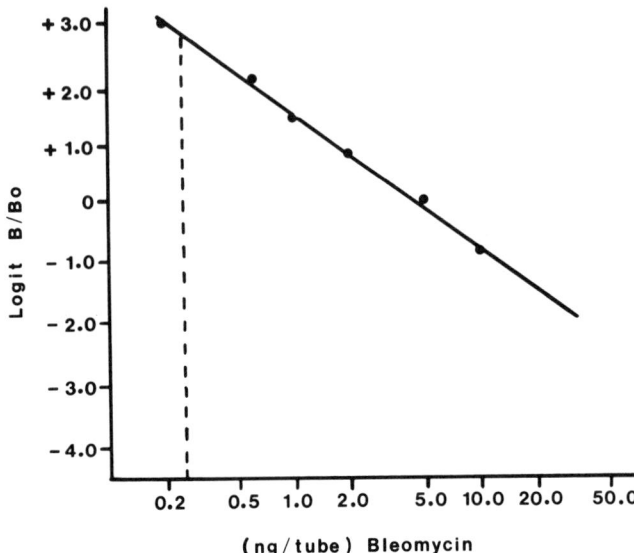

Fig. 5. Dose-response curve of bleomycin. Vertical interrupted line delineates sensitivity of the assay.

VIII. THE ASSAY SYSTEM

Figure 5 shows a logit/log transformation of the dose-response curve, with the vertical interrupted line showing the sensitivity of the assay, which was 250 pg. The precision of the assay determined from the dose-response curve using the index (Midgley *et al.*, 1969), which is defined as the ratio between the standard deviation of each Y value and the slope of the regression line between the mean values of logit Y and the corresponding log X, was 0.024 at 5 ng. This value compares favorably with those reported for polypeptide hormone assays.

Recovery experiments were performed by adding BLM in known concentrations to serum specimens and measuring these by the radioimmunoassay, and gave a mean recovery of 102.6% (±3.3% SE).

The assay system was then compared with the standard microbiological assay system using *B. subtilis* ATC 6633 as the test organism. The coefficient of correlation (r) was 0.987. Another radioimmunoassay system using [57]Co-labeled bleomycin and polyethylene glycol as a separating agent has recently been described by Elson *et al.* (1977) and compared to the same microbiological assay giving a correlation coefficient of 0.96. A comparison of the two radioimmunoassays on plasma samples showed a coefficient of correlation of 0.93. Interestingly, the coefficient of correlation between the assays performed on urine from patients receiving the drug was 0.71. Further studies are in progress to determine the reason for the fall in correlation.

IX. CLINICAL APPLICATIONS OF THE ASSAY

The radioimmunoassay of BLM has been used to study the clinical pharmacology of the drug following administration by various routes and regimes (Broughton *et al.*, 1977; Crooke *et al.*, 1977a,b). It is of interest to note that following long-term continuous intravenous infusions the elimination kinetics of BLM as determined by radioimmunoassay appear to differ from those following a bolus injection. Table II illustrates these differences and also shows that if plasma levels below 10 μu/ml of bleomycin are excluded, the kinetics are similar.

TABLE II. Averaged Pharmacokinetic Data for Bleomycin Infusions

	Group A[a]	Group B[b]	Group C[c]
Elimination half-life ($t_{1/2}$)	14.5	2.98	2.03
Volume of distribution (l/kg)	2.25	0.458	0.354
Volume of central compartment (l/kg)	0.251	0.145	0.142
Renal clearance (ml/min/1.73^2)		61.4	76.9
Total body clearance (ml/min/1.73^2)		119.0	128.0

[a] Five-day continuous infusion, all data points.
[b] Five-day continuous infusion data points <10 μ u/ml excluded.
[c] Short-term (15 min) infusion.

The data can be interpreted in different ways. There may be a deep compartment which binds bleomycin, releasing it slowly following long-term infusion. This compartment will become saturated, prolonging the elimination half-life of the drug. Another interpretation is that the assay system described here is measuring a metabolite of bleomycin, perhaps desamidobleomycin, which the antibody cross-reacts 44%. This metabolite would not be detectable following a bolus injection, but after an infusion lasting 5 days the level of the metabolite may be significant. This is currently being investigated by the development of a specific radioimmunoassay for desamidobleomycin.

The next paper will discuss in detail some of the data obtained in studies of the clinical pharmacology of bleomycin using the radioimmunoassay.

REFERENCES

Berson, S. A., and Yalow, R. S. (1960). *J. Clin. Invest.* 39, 1157.
Broughton, A., and Strong, J. E. (1976a). *Clin. Chem.* 22, 726.
Broughton, A., and Strong, J. E. (1976b). *Cancer Res. 36,* 1418.
Broughton, A., Strong, J. E., Holoyoe, P., and Bedrossian, C. W. M. (1977). *Cancer* (in press).
Crooke, S. T., Luft, F., Broughton, A., Strong, J. E., Casson, K., and Einhorn, L. (1977a). *Cancer 39,* 1430.
Crooke, S. T., Comis, R. L., Einhorn, L. H., Strong, J. E., Broughton, A., and Prestayko, A. W. (1977b). *Cancer Treatment Rep.* (in press).

Dabrowaik, S. C., Greenaway, F. T., Longo, W. E., Husen, M. V., and Crooke, S. T. (1977). *Biochem. Biophys. Acta* (in press).

Elson, M. K., Oken, M. M., and Shafer, R. B. (1977). *J. Nucl Med. 18,* 296.

Goodfriend, T. L., Levin, L., and Fasmon, G. D. (1964). *Science 144,* 1344.

Hunter, W. M., and Greenwood, F. C. (1962). *Nature 194,* 495.

Konishi, M., Saito, K., Numata, K., Tsuno, T., Asama, K. T., Sukiura, H., Naito, T., and Kawagnchi, H. (1977). *J. Antibiot.* (in press).

Midgley, A. R., Niswender, G. D., and Regar, R. W. (1969). *Acta Endocrinol. 63,* 163.

Odell, W. D., Abraham, G., Rand, H. R., Soverdioff, R. S., and Fisher, D. A. (1969). *Acta Endocrinol. Suppl. 142,* 54.

Smith, T. W., Butler, V. P., Jr., Haber, E. (1969). *N. Engl. J. Med. 281,* 1212.

Strong, J. E., Broughton, A., and Crooke, S. T. (1977). *Cancer Treatment Rep. 61,* 1509–1512.

Umezawa, H. (1974). *Fed Proc., Fed. Am. Soc. Exp. Biol. 33,* 2296.

Umezawa, H. (1976). *Gann Monogr. Cancer Res. 19,* 3–35.

Chapter 10

CLINICAL PHARMACOLOGY OF BLEOMYCIN

Archie W. Prestayko
Stanley T. Crooke

I. INTRODUCTION

Bleomycin (Blenoxane®) is excreted primarily by renal mechanisms. The pharmacokinetics of bleomycin have been reported in patients receiving the drug by a number of routes including intravenous (Fujita and Kimura, 1970; Ohnuma *et al.*, 1974; Fujita, 1971; Crooke *et al.*, 1977a, b, c; Broughton *et al.*, 1977a,b), intramuscular (Fujita and Kimura, 1970; Ohnuma *et al.*, 1974), intracavitary (Alberts *et al.*, 1977; Crooke and Bradner, 1976), intratumoral (Crooke and Bradner, 1976), intrathecal (Hayakawa *et al.*, 1976), intraarterial (Fujita and Kimura, 1970), subcutaneous (Hall *et al.*, 1977), and intravesical (Bracken *et al.*, 1977). The early reports (Fujita and Kimura, 1970; Ohnuma *et al.*, 1974; Fujita, 1971) employed a microbiologic assay in a small number of patients using *Bacillus subtilis* ATCC-6633 spore solution which was sensitive to approximately 0.2 mu/ml. The elimination of bleomycin from blood was reported to vary, with some patients demonstrating first-order kinetics and others not. The plasma half-life was reported to vary from 14 to 45 min after intravenous injection (Fujita and Kimura, 1970); however, it was unclear whether this time represented $t_{1/2}\alpha$ or $t_{1/2}\beta$.

Recently, two radioimmunoassays were developed which have greater sensitivity than the microbiologic assay (Broughton and Strong, 1976; Elson *et al.*, 1977). The pharmacokinetics of bleomycin were determined in patients after intravenous injection, intravenous continuous infusion, and intramuscular injection and will be reviewed in this report for all three methods of drug administration.

II.   MATERIALS AND METHODS

A.   Assay Procedure

The microbiologic assay was performed employing *B. subtilis* ATCC-6633 spore solution as previously described (Fujita and Kimura, 1970). The radioimmunoassays were performed as previously described (Broughton and Strong, 1976; Elson *et al.*, 1977). Replicates of each concentration were performed and the results were found to be readily reproducible.

B.   Sample Collection

Blood specimens were obtained in heparinized tubes at specified intervals up to 72 hr after a dose of bleomycin. When serum was to be assayed, blood specimens were collected in nonheparinized tubes. Specimens were refrigerated, centrifuged, and either plasma or serum obtained and stored frozen (-20 or -70°C) until analyzed. Urine specimens were collected for varying periods of time, stored refrigerated and frozen immediately at termination of the collection period.

C.   Patient Selection

1.   Intravenous Injection

Twenty patients had metastatic testicular tumors and were treated with bleomycin, 30 u/wk in combination with vinblastine and *cis*-platinum according to the regimen shown in Table I (Einhorn *et al.*, 1976). These patients were chosen for this study for several reasons; (1) they were a group of homogeneous and relatively healthy young males; (2) they were all treated with the same regimen, thereby eliminating possible effects of drugs other than vincristine and *cis*-platinum on bleomycin pharmacokinetics; (3) most of the patients had normal renal function on entry into the study and since *cis*-platinum is a nephrotoxic agent, it was possible to determine pharmacokinetics of bleomycin serially in patients with varying creatinine clearance.

Seven other patients had poorly differentiated lymphocytic lymphoma or diffuse histiocytic lymphoma and were treated with 7-10 u bleomycin as a 10 min intravenous injection.

2.   Intravenous Continuous Infusion

Patients receiving 15-30 u bleomycin per day for 4-5 days as a continuous infusion had one of the following tumors; squamous cell carcinoma of the tongue, embryonal carcinoma, squamous cell carcinoma of the scrotum, squamous cell carcinoma of the urethra, or bronchogenic adenocarcinoma.

TABLE I. Treatment Regimen for Metastatic Testicular Cancer

Bleomycin	30 u/week for 12 weeks
cis-Platinum	20 mg/m^2/day, days 1–5 q 3 weeks for 9 weeks
Vinblastine	0.2 mg/kg/day, x 2 q 3 weeks

3. Intramuscular Injection

Patients who received 2–30 u bleomycin as an intramuscular injection had various malignancies.

III. RESULTS

A. Intravenous Injection

Table II shows the characteristics of 20 patients in whom bleomycin pharmacokinetics were determined. The median age was 24 years. Ages varied from 18 to 47 years. With two exceptions, all initial performance statuses (Karnofsky) were 60 or greater. Initial creatinine clearances varied from 10.7 to 180 ml/min corrected to 1.73 m^2 body surface area. All evaluable patients achieved either a partial response (>50% decrease in the cross-sectional area of measurable lesions), or complete response. Two patients were not evaluable for response (N.E.) because of lack of measurable disease.

Table III presents the plasma $t_{1/2}\beta$ of bleomycin determined by the microbiologic and radioimmunoassays relative to creatinine clearance. In general, the data shown in Table III demonstrate that the plasma $t_{1/2}\beta$ of bleomycin determined by both methods was similar, and that the plasma clearance of bleomycin varied with creatinine clearance. The values for areas under curve (AUC) were variable and did not correlate well with the creatinine clearance or $t_{1/2}\beta$. This may be explained by slight variations in the timing of the first blood sample relative to the time of bleomycin injection. Since patient 1 received only 15 u of bleomycin, AUC data are not presented.

Figure 1 shows the semilogarithmic plot of the plasma $t_{1/2}\beta$ versus the creatinine clearance. These results demonstrate that the inflection point, i.e., the point at which the plasma $t_{1/2}\beta$ of bleomycin becomes prolonged, is at a creatinine clearance of approximately 25–35 ml/min. At creatinine clearances in excess of 25–35 ml/min the mean $t_{1/2}\beta$ was 122.7 ± 9.6 min when determined with the microbiologic assay and 115.4 ± 8.6 min when determined with the radioimmunoassay. Below a creatinine clearance of approximately 25–35 ml/min the plasma $t_{1/2}\beta$ of bleomycin increased exponentially as the creatinine clearances decreased. The mean $t_{1/2}\beta$ in patients with creatinine clearances in excess of 70 ml/min did not differ from the mean of patients with creatinine clearances in excess of 25–35 ml/min (111 or 109 min determined by the microbiologic or radioimmunoassays, respectively).

Bleomycin pharmacokinetics were evaluated sequentially in eight patients (Table IV). These studies demonstrate that, in a given patient, the plasma half-life of bleomycin varied inversely with the creatinine clearance.

TABLE II. Patient Characteristics

Patient number	Age	Body surface area (m^2)	Performance status	Initial creatinine clearance (ml/min)	Site of metastases	Tumor response
1	24	2.0	90	10.7	Pulmonary	CR
2	33	1.95	30	21.3	Pulmonary, CNS	PR
3	29	2.3	80	62	Left inguinal node	CR
4	25	1.8	80	64.6	Left cervical node, para aortic	PR
5	27	1.65	90	78	Liver	PR
6	46	1.6	80	88	Lung	PR
7	21	2.3	80	89	Bone, lung, retroperitoneal nodes	PR
8	24	1.9	60	98.6	Retroperitoneal mass	PR
9	20	1.9	90	98.7	Pelvis, mediastinum, para aortic	PR
10	47	2.1	90	107	Pulmonary, mediastinum	PR
11	22	1.5	90	108.5	Skull, shoulder, elbow	NE
12	22	2.1	90	109	Pulmonary, lymph node	CR
13	25	1.76	90	110	Adjuvant therapy	NE
14	26	2.08	90	115	Mediastinal mass	PR
15	26	1.68	90	118	Pulmonary	CR
16	26	1.88	90	123	Lung, retroperitoneal nodes	CR
17	22	2.1	90	128	Large retroperitoneal mass, lung	PR
18	18	1.84	90	140	Mediastinal mass, pulmonary	CR
19	27	1.7	100	157	Lung	PR
20	22	1.98	90	180	Pulmonary, liver nodes, para aortic	PR
Median	24	1.9				

TABLE III. Plasma $t_{1/2}\beta$ Bleomycin versus Creatinine Clearance

Patient number	Creatinine clearance (ml/min)	Microbiologic		Radioimmunoassay	
		$t_{1/2}$ (min)	AUC	$t_{1/2}$ (min)	AUC
1	10.7	1260	–	1260	–
1	15.2	660	–	660	–
2	21	375	255	341	452
11	35	276	670	178	480
7	48	119	172	–	–
3	62	157	378	114	309
4	65	171	532	177	256
7	89	158	210	117	142
15	98	129	160	150	318
8	99	92	159	68	141
9	99	114	168	133	350
12	105	123	173	103	249
10	107	100	71	106	146
11	108	41	74	25	145
12	109	121	72	86	146
13	110	85	217	74	292
14	115	94	73	117	155
15	118	173	149	129	257
7	120	63	137	79	188
20	122	134	209	209	270
16	123	114	155	103	184
14	127	115	139	98	193
18	140	112	183	98	189
18	146	121	218	98	270
20	149	114	137	124	218
20	180	95	89	140	185

Table V shows that the total apparent volume of distribution varied from 14 liters to 35 liters except for two patients who had volumes of distribution of 6.5 liters and 8.3 liters. The mean volume of distribution of bleomycin was 22.7 ± 6.02 and 19.8 ± 1.46 liters in patients with creatinine clearances greater or less than 35 ml/min, respectively (Table VI).

Table VII shows the urinary excretion of bleomycin relative to creatinine clearance. In patients with creatinine clearances approximately 50 ml/min or greater, approximately 50% (mean) of the total dose was excreted during the first 4 hr postdose. Within 24 hr postdose, approximately 70% of the total dose was excreted in the urine.

In another study (Broughton et al., 1977a,b) using a 10 min infusion in patients with non-Hodgkin's lymphoma, the mean $t_{1/2}\beta$ for bleomycin was approximately 122 min and approximately 60% of the administered dose was recovered in urine in 24 hr after injection. Six of the seven patients had a creatinine clearance > 60 ml/min. Figure 2 shows the semilogarithmic plot of the serum bleomycin concentration

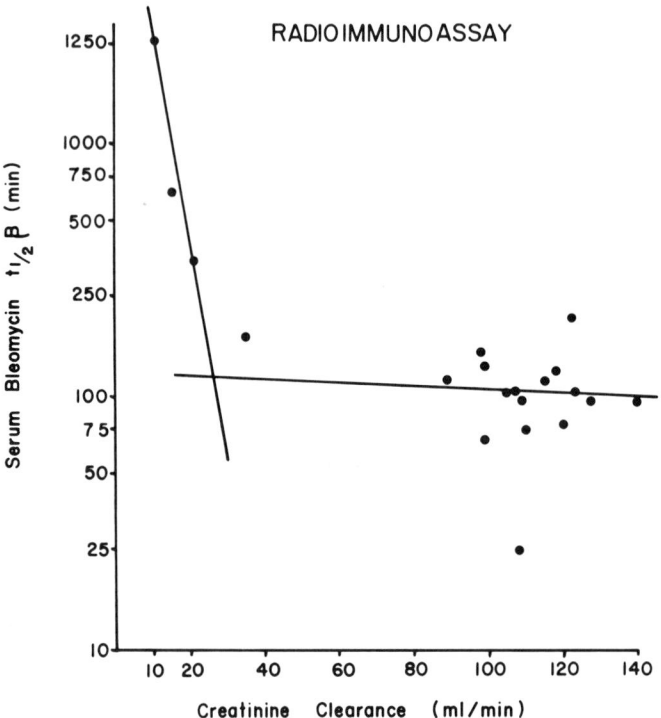

Fig. 1. Semilogarithmic plot of plasma and serum $t_{1/2}\beta$ of bleomycin versus creatinine clearance from values determined using the radioimmunoassay.

in microunits per milliliter versus time for these patients. The $t_{1/2}\beta$ and 24 hr bleomycin excretion after a 10 min infusion agree well with that determined by Crooke *et al.* (1977a) using an IV bolus bleomycin dose.

B. Continuous Infusion

Fig. 3 shows the semilogarithmic plot of serum bleomycin concentration versus time for four patients receiving a 4–5 day continuous infusion of bleomycin. Steady-state concentration was approached approximately 12 hr after initiation of infusion and ranged from 0.132 to 0.312 mu/ml. The half-life of bleomycin in the post-infusion decay period was approximately 180 min when values less than 10 μu/ml were excluded. These results compare reasonably closely to the $t_{1/2}\beta$ for a single injection. However, when all values measured were used in the determination of $t_{1/2}\beta$, the half-life of bleomycin postinfusion was approximately 10–14 hr. Approximately 63% of the dose of bleomycin administered by continuous infusion was recovered in the urine and was similar to that observed after a single injection.

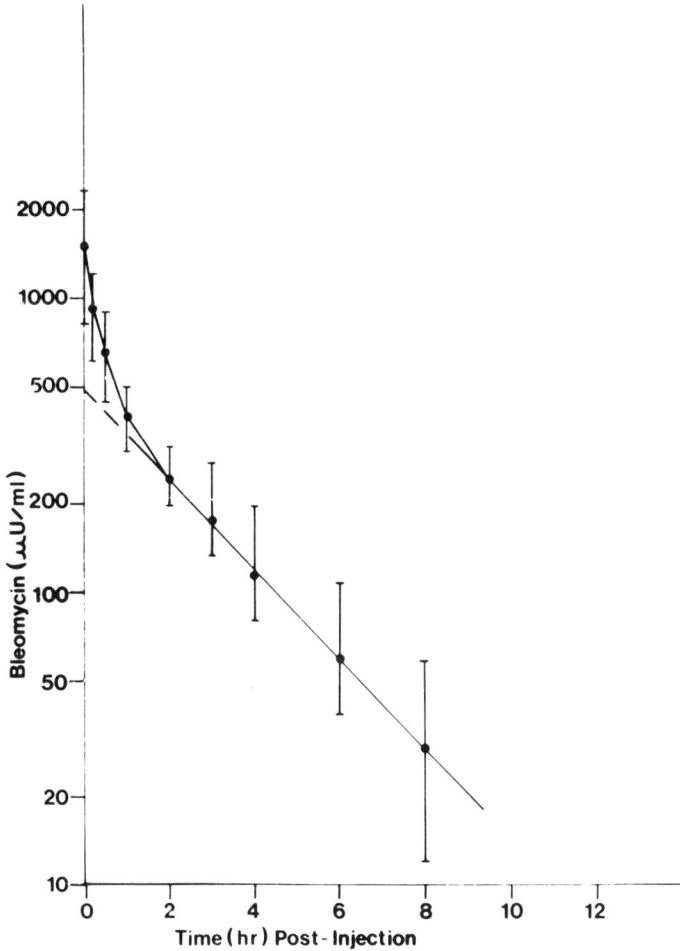

Fig. 2. Semilogarithmic plot of serum bleomycin versus time. Each point represents the average of bleomycin determinations for six patients administered 7–10 u intravenously by 10 min infusion. The standard deviation for each time point is indicated by vertical bars (from Broughton *et al.*, 1977a).

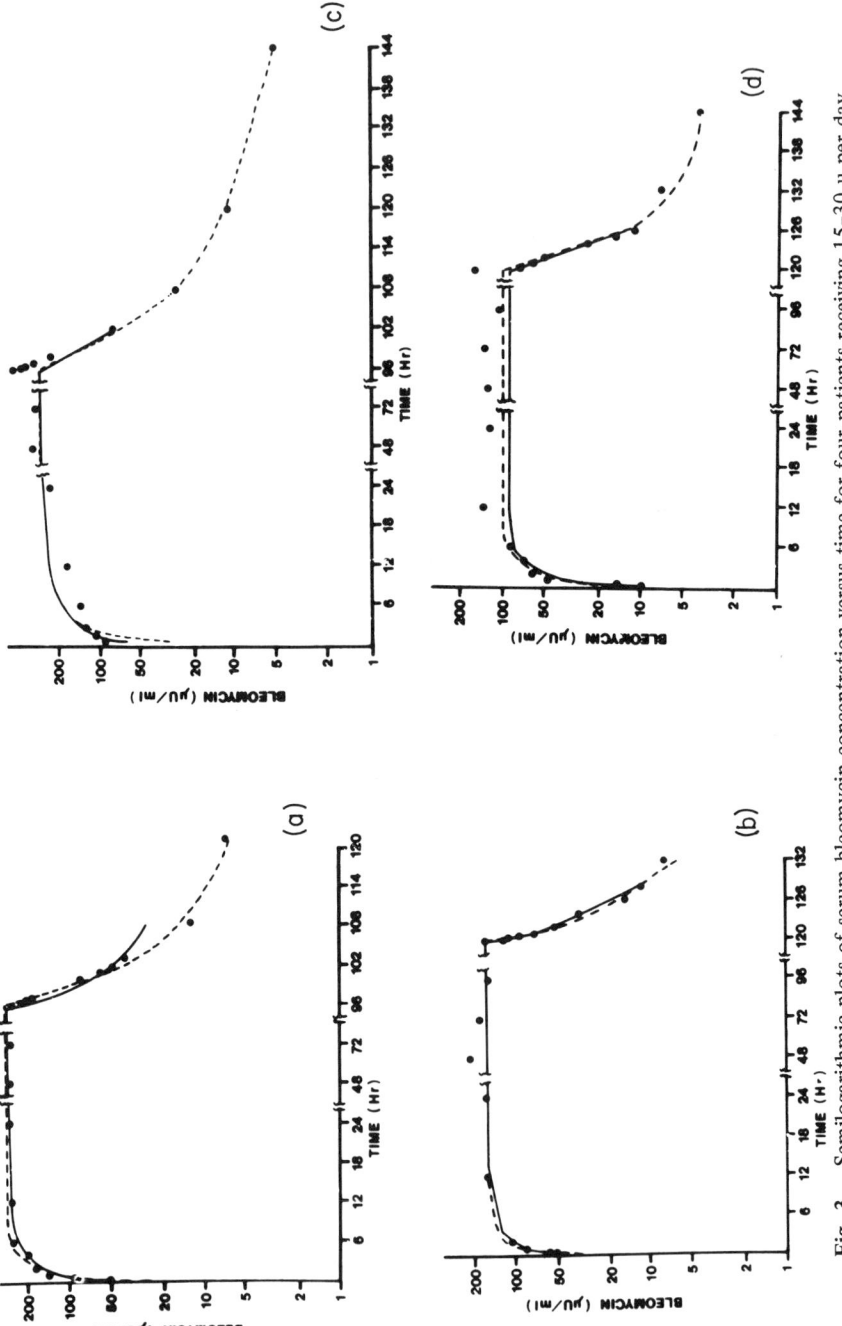

Fig. 3. Semilogarithmic plots of serum bleomycin concentration versus time for four patients receiving 15–30 u per day bleomycin as a continuous 4–5 day intravenous infusion. The experimental data are shown as (●), the curve predicted by the analysis of all the data as (---) and that predicted by excluding data less than 10 μu/ml as (——). A–D represent patients 1–4, respectively (from Broughton et al., 1977a,b).

TABLE IV. Changes in Renal Status and Plasma $t_{1/2}\beta$ Bleomycin

Patient number	Week of therapy	Creatinine clearance (ml/min)	$t_{1/2}$ (min)
15	0	118	129
15	5	98	150
14	0	115	117
14	6	127	98
18	0	140	98
18	6	146	98
12	0	109	86
12	5	105	103
20	0	180	95
20	6	149	114
20	9	122	134
11	0	108	41
11	9	35	276
7	0	89	158
7	3	120	83
7	6	48	119
1	0	10.7	1260
1	1	15.2	660

C. Intramuscular Injection

Bleomycin pharmacokinetic studies were carried out in patients receiving bleomycin by intramuscular injection. Serum concentrations of bleomycin were determined by both [57]Co and ^{125}I radioimmunoassays (Broughton and Strong, 1976; Elson et al., 1977) and by the microbiologic assay when blood levels of drug were high enough for detection. Doses ranged from 2-30 u. Maximum serum levels of bleomycin ranged from 0.13 to 0.35 mu/ml at 1 hr after injection and no bleomycin could be detected in serum at 24 hr after injection.

Table VIII compares the $t_{1/2}\beta$ of IM bleomycin determined by three methods in six patients. In only one patient was the creatinine clearance below normal (< 70 ml/min). The microbiologic assay was capable of detecting serum bleomycin only in patients who received ≥ 15 u dose. In patients with a creatinine clearance of ≥ 70 ml/min, the mean $t_{1/2}\beta$ was 158 ± 8.2 and 144 ± 9.1 as determined by the ^{125}I and [57]Co radioimmunoassays, respectively, and was independent of the dose.

Table IX shows that bleomycin elimination was predominantly via urinary excretion. Urinary bleomycin recovery was $32.2 \pm 5.0\%$ (mean) in 0-4 hr and $57.8 \pm 5.9\%$ (mean) in 0-24 hr of the administered dose. The amount of bleomycin excreted in urine did not appear to correlate with the creatinine clearance.

TABLE V. Creatinine Clearance versus Volume of Distribution

Patient	Creatinine clearance (ml/min)	Volume distribution (l)
1	15	34.8
2	21	16.3
11	35	17.2
7	48	33.1
3	62	13.9
4	65	6.5
7	89	29.4
15	98	18.8
9	99	14.5
8	99	19.1
12	105	15.8
10	107	23.6
11	108	16.3
12	109	22.9
13	110	8.3
14	115	30.1
15	118	19.8
7	120	18.1
20	122	26.7
16	123	29.4
14	127	19.7
18	140	18.8
18	146	13.6
20	149	23.4
20	180	28.6

TABLE VI. Volume of Distribution versus Creatinine Clearance

Creatinine clearance	Mean volume of distribution
≤ 35 ml/min	22.7 ± 6.02
> 35 ml/min	19.8 ± 1.46

TABLE VII. Bleomycin Excretion versus Creatinine Clearance

Patient	Creatinine clearance (ml/min)	$t_{1/2\beta}$ (min)	Cumulative % bleomycin excreted in urine			
			0–4 hr	0–8 hr	0–12 hr	0–24 hr
7	48	119	50	58.3	59.9	60.6
3	62	157	29	40.6	46.2	53.8
4	65	171	35.3	46.9	52.9	58.2
7	89	158	53	69.0	71.3	75.6
15	98	150	54	70.0	75.0	77.6
12	105	103	57.3	63.3	67.9	69.5
14	115	117	62.6	76.6	80.6	82.1
20	122	134	50	62.0	70.3	70.3
18	140	98	47.6	63.6	66.4	67.9
Mean	93.7	134	48.7	61.1	65.6	68.4
	±	±	±	±	±	±
	10.1	8.7	3.5	3.7	3.6	3.1

TABLE VIII. Comparison $t_{1/2\beta}$ Bleomycin for Microbiologic and Radioimmunoassays

Patient	Total dose (units bleomycin)	Creatinine clearance (ml/min)	RIA (^{125}I), $t_{1/2}$ (min)	RIA (^{57}Co), $t_{1/2}$ (min)	Microbiologic $t_{1/2}$ (min)
1	20	133	160	145	190
2	10	111	145	110	–
3	4	109	180	165	–
4	2	99	135	150	–
5	17	89	170	150	160
6	15	57	310	255	320
Creatinine clearance > 70 ml/min: mean			158 ± 8.2	144 ± 9.1	

TABLE IX. Bleomycin Excretion

Patient	Total dose (units bleomycin)	Creatinine clearance (ml/min)	Cumulative % urine bleomycin	
			0–4 hr	0–24 hr
1	20	133	48	69
2	10	111	46	72
3	4	109	27	58
4	2	99	32	65
5	17	89	22	33
6	15	57	19	50
Mean		99 ± 10.4	32.3 ± 5.0	57.8 ± 5.9

Table X summarizes the $t_{1/2}\beta$ for bleomycin administered by IV injection, IV prolonged infusion, or intramuscular injection and shows that the radioimmunoassays and microbiologic assay gave equivalent results.

IV. DISCUSSION

The conclusions which may be derived from the pharmacokinetic study after IV bolus injection of bleomycin are: (1) bleomycin is cleared principally by renal mechanisms; (2) at creatinine clearances >25-35 ml/min the $t_{1/2}\beta$ of bleomycin is approximately 155 min; (3) at creatinine clearances <25-35 ml/min the $t_{1/2}\beta$ increases exponentially as the creatinine clearance decreases; (4) even in frank renal failure, no bleomycin was detectable in the blood 48–72 hr after a bolus injection; (5) in patients with creatinine clearances ≥ 50 ml/min approximately 50% of a total dose of bleomycin is excreted in the urine in 4 hr, and $>70\%$ in 24 hr; (6) the mean total volume of distribution is approximately 20 liters, and does not vary with creatinine clearances; (7) bleomycin is problably not dialyzable; (8) the pharmacokinetic

TABLE X. Comparison of $t_{1/2}\beta$ Bleomycin with Route of Administration[a]

Route	$t_{1/2}\beta$, RIA ^{125}I (min)	$t_{1/2}\beta$, RIA ^{57}Co (min)	$t_{1/2}\beta$, microbiologic (min)
IV rapid injection	109	–	111
IV 10 min injection	122	–	–
IV continuous infusion	9.53 hr		–
	234 min	(< 10 μu/ml values excluded)	
IM injection	158	144	175

[a] These values are for patients with creatinine clearance ≥ 60 ml/min.

model describing bleomycin pharmacokinetics does not vary with varying renal function, i.e., a two-compartment model best explains the data in all patients; (9) the microbiologic and radioimmunoassays give comparable results in plasma or serum.

After continuous infusion of bleomycin the half-life was approximately 10-14 hr when all detectable levels of bleomycin were used in the determinations. When values <10 μu/ml were excluded the bleomycin half-life was approximately 3 hr, which approximates that for rapid IV injection of bleomycin. Possible explanations for the 10-14 hr half-life determination include interference in the radioimmunoassay by an unknown metabolite and/or strong binding of drug to tissues with release at a rate much less than the apparent half-life.

The results from the pharmacokinetic studies after intramuscular injection of bleomycin indicate that the $t_{1/2}\beta$ determined by either radioimmunoassay or microbiologic assay is similar to that after an IV injection, i.e., approximately 2 hr. Also, approximately 60-70% of bleomycin administered by this route is excreted in the urine in 24 hr.

Studies are in progress to determine whether patients who have impaired renal functions and who experience prolonged elevated blood levels of bleomycin also experience greater pulmonary toxicity. Results of these studies should provide a basis on which to make specific recommendations for dose reduction of bleomycin in patients with compromised renal function.

REFERENCES

Alberts, D., Chen, H. S., Liu, R., Himmelstein, K., Gross, J., Broughton, A., and Salmon, S. (1977). Bleomycin pharmacokinetics in man. Bleomycin Symposium, Oakland, California, October 1977.

Bracken, R., Johnson, D., Rodriguez, L., Samuels, M., and Ayala, A. (1977). *Urology 9* (2), 161-163.

Broughton, A., and Strong, J. (1976). *Cancer Res. 35,* 1418-1421.

Broughton, A., Strong, J. E., Holoye, P., Hall, S., Feldman, S., and Kramer, W. (1977b). (Submitted for publication).

Broughton, A., Strong, J. E., Holoye, P., and Bedrossian, C. (1977a). *Cancer* (in press).

Crooke, S. T., and Bradner, W. T. (1976). *J. Med. 7* (5), 333-428.

Crooke, S. T., Comis, R. L., Einhorn, L. H., Strong, J. E., Broughton, A., and Prestayko, A. W. (1977a). *Cancer Treatment Rep.* (in press).

Crooke, S. T., Comis, R. L., Einhorn, L. H., Strong, J. E., Broughton, A., and Prestayko, A. W. (1977b). In *Studies on the Clinical Pharmacology of Bleomycin: Proceedings of the U.S.-Japan Conference May 12-13, 1977,* Carter, S. K., and Umezawa, H. (Eds.). Springer-Verlag, New York (in press).

Crooke, S. T., Luft, F. T., Broughton, A. W., Strong, J. L., Casson, K., and Einhorn, L. (1977c). *Cancer 39,* 1430-1434.

Einhorn, L., Furnas, B., and Powell, N. (1976). *Am. Assoc. Clin. Oncol. 17,* 240.

Elson, M., Oken, M., and Shafer, R. (1977). *J. Nucl. Med. 18,* 296-299.

Fujita, H. (1971). *Jpn. J. Clin. Oncol. 12,* 151-162.

Fujita, H., and Kimura, K. (1970). *Proc. 6th Int. Congr. Chemother. 12,* 309-314.

Hall, S., Broughton, A., Strong, J., and Benjamin, R. (1977). *Clin. Res. 25,* 407A.

Hayakawa, T., Ushio, Y., Morimoto, K., Hasegawa, H., Mogami, H., and Horibata, K. (1976). *J. Neurol. Neurosurg. Psychiatry 39*, 341–349.

Ohnuma, T., Holland, J. F., Masuda, H., Waligunda, J. A., and Goldberg, G. A. (1974). *Cancer 33*, 1230–1238.

Chapter 11

DISPOSITION KINETICS OF INTRACAVITARY BLEOMYCIN IN MAN: A PRELIMINARY REPORT[1]

David Alberts
Hsiao-Sheng Chen
Rosa Liu
Joseph Chen
Michael Mayersohn
Donald Perrier
Thomas Moon
Joseph Gross
Alan Broughton
Sydney Salmon

I. INTRODUCTION

Intracavitary bleomycin instillation has resulted in frequent complete remissions of malignant pleural and peritoneal effusions as reported by Paladine *et al.* (1976). Intracavitary bleomycin appeared to be especially effective therapy for effusions associated with advanced breast and ovarian cancers. Although fever was the major toxicity experienced by 20% of patients and there were no cases of pulmonary toxicity, the largest individual total dose of bleomycin was only 240 u.

There are only limited data concerning the disposition kinetics of bleomycin following intracavitary administration. Paladine *et al.* (1976), using a microbiologic assay, reported that an average of 4.6% of the bleomycin remained in the intrapleural

[1] Supported in part by Grant CA-17094 from the National Cancer Institute and by Grant T32-GM07533, National Institutes of Health, Department of Health, Education and Welfare.

fluid 24 hr after instillation and 10–52% of the original dose was excreted in the urine during the first 16 hr in six patients. Using radioimmunoassay, Hall *et al.* (1977) observed a terminal plasma half-life of 8.6 hours in a patient who received 30 u of bleomycin intrapleurally.

We have studied the pharmacokinetics of bleomycin after both intrapleural (four patients) and intraperitoneal (four patients) instillation using a radioimmunoassay (Broughton and Strong, 1976). Additionally, we have compared the kinetics of bleomycin disappearance after intracavitary and intravenous administration (manuscript submitted for publication).

II. MATERIALS AND METHODS

A. Patients

Bleomycin disposition was examined in 17 patients whose characteristics are summarized in Tables I and II. All patients had advanced cancer at the time of study. The serum creatinine was normal in eight of nine patients receiving therapeutic intravenous bleomycin and seven of eight receiving intracavitary therapy. In all but one patient (K.D., Table II) there was cytologic confirmation of the cancer in the pleural and peritoneal effusions.

None of the patients received other anticancer drugs within 3 weeks of the bleomycin pharmacokinetic studies. An attempt was made to stop all routine-type drugs at least 3 days prior to the bleomycin disposition studies; however, it was necessary to continue narcotic administration in four of nine "intravenous" and three of eight "intracavitary" patients.

B. Treatment

All patients treated with an intravenous bolus injection of bleomycin received a dose of approximately 15 u/m^2 (Table I). All patients given intracavitary bleomycin received approximately 60 u/m^2 except one patient (P.E., Table II), who received only 15 u/m^2. Bleomycin in doses of 30–110 u (Table II) was diluted in 100 ml of normal saline and injected in bolus form into the thoracic or peritoneal cavity after maximal evacuation of effusion fluid.

C. Blood and Urine Sampling

Blood samples (10 ml) were obtained from a heparin lock and collected in tubes containing 100 I.U. of heparin. Samples were taken just prior to the start of therapy and, in most cases, at 5, 10, 15, 30, 45, and 60 min, 2, 3, 4, 6, 8, and 24 hr following drug administration. Fractional urine collections were taken for the first 8 hr after drug injection and then at known intervals for up to 24 hr and stored in sterile containiners at 4°C.

TABLE 1. Characteristics of Patients Receiving Intravenous Bleomycin

Patients	Tumor type	Sex	Age (yr)	BSA (m²)	Serum creatinine (mg %)	Bleomycin dose (u/m²)
S.H.	Head and neck	M	55	1.51	1.0	19.9
E.G.	Cervix	F	59	1.83	1.0	13.7
E.M.	Head and neck	F	64	1.67	0.9	15.0
H.H.	Cervix	F	61	1.60	1.2	15.0
M.M.	Head and neck	F	61	1.86	0.9	16.1
M.A.	Head and neck	M	56	2.05	1.0	14.6
S.R.	Cervix	F	42	1.57	0.9	14.6
M.R.	Head and neck	M	84	1.65	1.1	14.5
J.S.	Ovary	F	61	1.41	1.5	15.6

TABLE II. Characteristics of Patients Receiving Intracavitary Bleomycin

Patient	Tumor type	Sex	Age (yr)	BSA (M^2)	Serum creatinine (mg %)	Bleomycin dose (u/M^2)	Administration route[a]
E.L.	Ovary	F	63	1.63	1.1	61.3	IP
V.O.	Ovary	F	21	1.38	0.8	54.3	IP
J.P.	Endometrial	F	64	1.60	0.5	60.0	IP
P.E.	Hepatoma	M	50	2.00	3.9	15.0	IP
D.B.	Ovary	F	44	1.62	0.8	55.6	IPl
G.P.	Ovary	F	56	1.53	0.5	60.8	IPl
K.D.[b]	Lung	M	57	1.52	1.0	59.2	IPl
C.J.	Breast	F	54	1.80	0.8	61.1	IPl

[a] Route: IP = Intraperitoneal; IPl = intrapleural.
[b] Ccr = 42.7 ml/min.

D. Assay Procedure

Blood samples were centrifuged at 2000g for 10 min and the plasma separated and immediately frozen at -70 C. The bleomycin concentrations in plasma and urine were determined using the antiserum and radioimmunoassay technique developed by Broughton and Strong (1976).

E. Data Analysis

Bleomycin plasma concentration versus time data obtained from each patient were fitted by computer to a multiexponential equation using a nonlinear regression program NONLIN (Metzler, 1969). Preliminary parameter estimates were obtained using a recently published computer method CSTRIP (Sedman and Wagner, 1976). The equation used for intravenous injection has the form

$$C = A_1 e^{-\alpha t} + A_2 e^{-\beta t} \tag{1}$$

where C is the bleomycin plasma concentration, t is time after the injection, A_1 and A_2 are coefficients, and α and β are apparent first-order rate constants.

For intraperitoneal and intrapleural injections the bleomycin concentration data were fitted with

$$C = A[e^{\beta t} - e^{-K_a t}] \tag{2}$$

where K_a and β are the apparent first-order rate constants for absorption and elimination, respectively.

The plasma decay half-life, $t_{1/2}$, was determined from the terminal slope of the computer-fitted bleomycin plasma concentration versus time curve:

$$t_{1/2} = \frac{(\ln 2)}{\beta} \tag{3}$$

The area under the plasma concentration versus time curve (CXT) was calculated by integrating equations (1) and (2) from time zero to infinity.

The apparent volume of distribution V_d for bleomycin was determined from

$$V_d = \frac{\text{IV dose}}{(\text{CXT} \cdot \beta)} \tag{4}$$

III. RESULTS

A. Bleomycin Pharmacokinetics after Intravenous Administration

The pharmacokinetic parameters of bleomycin obtained from nonlinear regression fitting of the plasma concentration versus time data are summarized in Table III. The mean terminal plasma half-life for eight of these patients who had normal serum creatinine values was 4.0 ± 0.6 hr. The mean area under the plasma decay curve (i.e., CXT) was 300 ± 45 mu·min/ml and the volume of distribution was 17.5 ± 3.5 l/m^2. Finally, the mean 24 hr urinary bleomycin excretion was $44.8 \pm 12.6\%$

David Alberts et al.

TABLE III. Pharmacokinetic Parameters of Bleomycin after Intravenous Administration[a]

Patient	$t_{1/2}$ [b] (hr)	CXT (mu·min/ml)	CXT[c]	Vd (l/m^2)	24 hr urinary excretion (% dose)
S.H.	4.5	378	253	20.5	29.1
E.G.	3.2	263	360	14.4	27.4
E.M.	3.0	302	397	13.0	49.2
H.H.	4.3	309	286	18.2	45.5
M.M.	3.8	226	223	23.3	[d]
M.A.	4.4	351	328	15.9	46.2
S.R.	4.6	296	265	19.7	61.5
M.R.	4.4	367	342	15.2	54.8
J.S.	10.4	387	143	36.3	11.6
Mean[e]	4.0 ± 0.6	300 ± 45	307 ± 60	17.5 ± 3.5	44.8 ± 12.6

[a] Submitted separately for publication.
[b] Terminal phase plasma $t_{1/2}$.
[c] CXT normalized for $t_{1/2} = 4.0$ hr and bleomycin dose = 15 u/m^2.
[d] Urine collection incomplete.
[e] The values for Patient J.S. were not included in the calculation of the means.

for seven patients who had adequate urinary collections. Patient J.S. was excluded as she had abnormal renal function; and the urinary excretion was only 11.6% at 24 hr.

B. Bleomycin Pharmacokinetics after Intracavitary Administration

The pharmacokinetic parameters of bleomycin obtained from nonlinear regression fitting of the plasma concentration versus time data for four patients receiving intraperitoneal and four receiving intrapleural doses are summarized in Tables IV and V, respectively. Corresponding plasma decay curves are shown in Figs. 1-3. Peak bleomycin plasma concentrations after 60 u/m^2 in seven patients (excluding P.E., who received 15 u/m^2 intraperitoneally) ranged between 0.6 and 3.2 mu/ml. The mean terminal phase plasma half-life for three of four patients with normal renal function who received intrapleural bleomycin was 3.6 ± 0.8 hr. This was considerably shorter than the mean terminal half-life of 6.3 ± 2.2 hr seen in three of the four patients with normal renal function who received intraperitoneal bleomycin. Intrapleural and intravenous half-lives were essentially the same. In patients with normal renal function for which urinary collection was complete, bleomycin excretion during the first 24 hr was in most cases lower following intracavitary than after intravenous administration ($p < 0.03$).

For those patients with normal serum creatinines, the mean plasma CXT (concentration x time product normalized for $t_{1/2} = 4$ hr and bleomycin dose = 15 u/m^2) for "intrapleural" patients of 153 ± 140 was similar to that of 145 ± 82 for the "intraperitoneal" patients and significantly smaller ($p < 0.01$) than that for the "intravenous" patients. Although patient P.E. (Tables II and IV, Fig. 1) received

TABLE IV. Pharmacokinetic Parameters of Bleomycin
after Intraperitoneal Administration

Patient	$t_{1/2}$ (hr)	CXT[a] (mu·min/ml)	CXT [b]	24 hr urinary excretion (% dose)	Response to therapy
E.L.	8.8	2079	232	–	None
V.O.	4.8	571	131	33.6	CR[c]
P.E.	8.2	4230	2066	–	None
J.P.	5.3	374	70	11.3	None
Mean[d]	6.3 ± 2.2	1008 ± 933	145 ± 82	22.5 ± 15.8	

[a] CXT = concentration x time product of bleomycin in plasma.

[b] CXT normalized for $t_{1/2}$ = 4.0 hr and bleomycin dose = 15 u/m^2.

[c] CR = complete clinical remission of effusion for >30 days.

[d] The values for patient P.E. were not included in the calculation of the means.

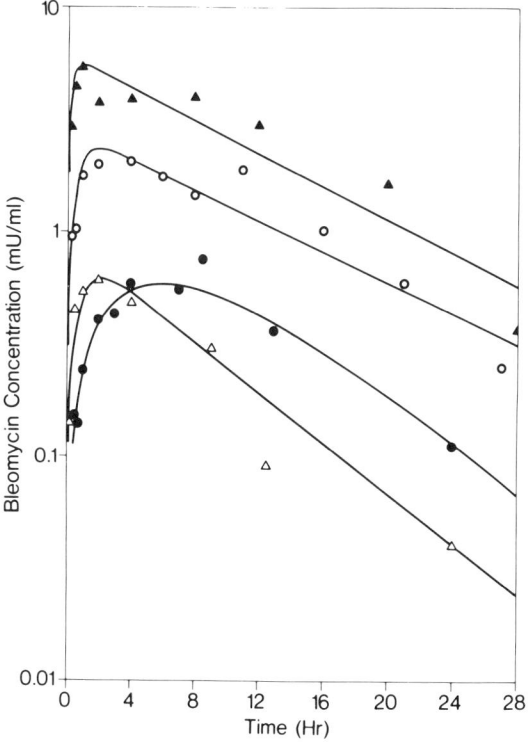

Fig. 1. Bleomycin plasma decay curves for three patients receiving 60 u/m^2 and one receiving 15 u/m^2 (patient P.E.) intraperitoneally (▲ P.E., △ J.P., ● V.O., ○ E.L.).

TABLE V. Pharmacokinetic Parameters of Bleomycin
after Intrepleural Administration

Patient	$t_{1/2}$ (hr)	CXT [a] (mu·min/ml)	CXT [b]	24 hr urinary excretion (% dose)	Response to therapy
D.B.	2.9	839	316	13.9	CR[c]
G.P.	3.5	263	75	–	None
K.D.	9.3	506	55	4.0	None
C.J.	4.5	312	68	20.6	None
Mean [d]	3.6 ± 0.8	471 ± 319	153 ± 141	17.2 ± 4.7	

[a] CXT = concentration x time product of bleomycin in plasma.
[b] CXT normalized for $t_{1/2}$ = 4.0 hr and bleomycin dose = 15 u/m^2.
[c] CR = complete clinical remission of effusion for >30 days.
[d] The values for patient K.D. were not included in the calculation of the means.

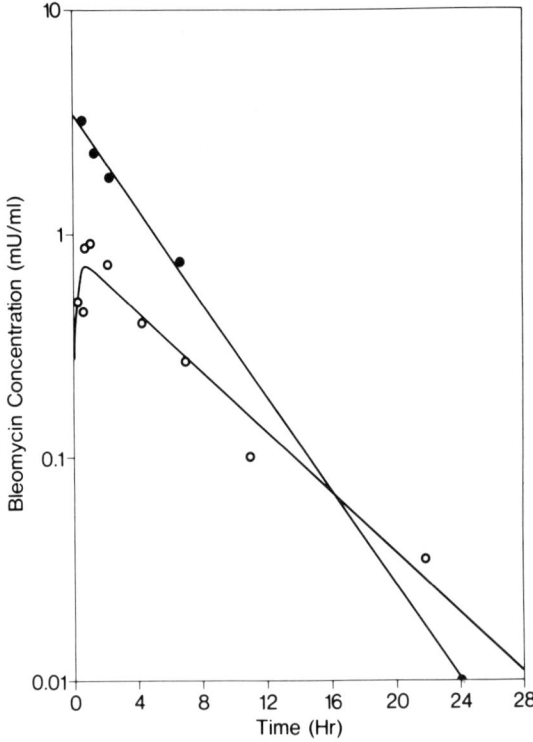

Fig. 2. Bleomycin plasma decay curves for two patients receiving 60 u/m^2 intrapleurally (● D.B., ○ C.T.).

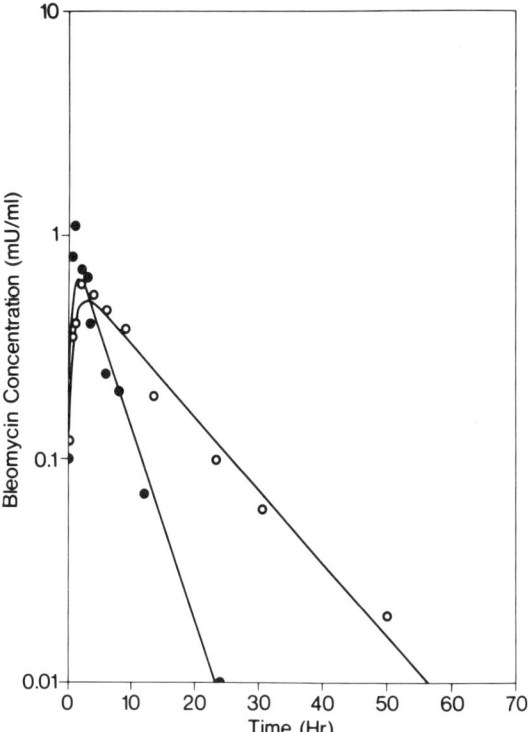

Fig. 3. Bleomycin plasma decay curves for two patients receiving 60 u/m² intrapleurally
(● G.P., ○ K.D.).

only 15 u/m² bleomycin intraperitoneally compared to the approximately 60 u/m ²
given the other seven "intracavitary" patients, his CXT was more than twice that
calculated for the high-dose patients. Patient P.E.'s serum creatinine was 3.9 mg %
(normal is 0.5-1.3 mg %) and his creatinine clearance was 10.1 ml/min on the day
of bleomycin administration.

Patient K.D. (Tables II and V, Fig. 3) had the longest plasma half-life observed
after intracavitary bleomycin. Although his serum creatinine was only 1.0 mg %,
the creatinine clearance was only 42.7 ml/min and only 4% of the total bleomycin
dose was excreted during the first 24 hr.

As seen in Table IV and V, only two of eight patients receiving intracavitary
bleomycin achieved remission from their effusions. There appeared to be no obvious
relationship between clinical response and length of bleomycin plasma half-life or
size of CXT.

IV.   DISCUSSION

In the short time since Paladine *et al.* (1976) reported clinical remissions in
response to intracavitary bleomycin for the treatment of malignant pleural and

TABLE VI. Systemic Availability of Bleomycin
after Intracavitary Administration[a]

Comparison	Plasma CXT ratio	Urinary excretion ratio
IP[b]:IV[c]	0.47	0.50
IPl[d]:IV	0.50	0.39
IP + IPl:IV	0.49	0.44

[a] Bleomycin data normalized to 15 u/m² dosage.
[b] IP = bleomycin intraperitoneal data from Table IV.
[c] IV = bleomycin intravenous data from Table III.
[d] IPl = bleomycin intrapleural data from Table V.

peritoneal effusions this new therapeutic approach has been widely applied by clinical oncologists. Unfortunately, little information has been available concerning the systemic absorption of bleomycin following intracavitary dosing.

The plasma CXT of an anticancer drug may be related to its toxicity to normal and tumor tissues. If we assume that the pharmacokinetics of bleomycin are linear at all dosage levels and that systemic absorption is complete following intracavitary drug administration, we can then compare the plasma CXT values for intravenous, intrapleural, and intraperitoneal dosing in our study patients (Table VI). We have normalized the plasma CXTs of our intracavitary patients for a bleomycin dose of 15 u/m² and a terminal phase plasma half-life of 4 hr. The "normalized" mean CXTs of the "intraperitoneal" and "intrapleural" patients with normal serum creatinines (excluding P.E., Table IV, and K.D., Table V) were 145 ± 82 and 153 ± 141 mu·min/ml, respectively. As seen in Table VI, the ratio of the normalized mean "intracavitary" plasma CXT to that of the intravenous patients is about 0.5. These data suggest that only about 50% of the intracavitary bleomycin dosage is absorbed into the systemic circulation. The mean urinary bleomycin excretion of 19.9 ± 10.0% for the four patients who had complete 24 hr urine collections following intracavitary drug administration was about 44% that observed following equivalent intravenous dosing and again suggests decreased, but important, systemic drug absorption. When calculating total bleomycin dosage for a given patient it is essential to take all routes of drug administration into consideration. We suggest using a weighting function of one-half the intracavitary dosage when calculating *total* systemic bleomycin availability.

The potential efficacy of administering bleomycin by the intracavitary route for the treatment of malignant effusions is enhanced by its incomplete systemic absorption. The approximately 50% decrease in systemic availability of bleomycin following intracavitary administration suggests the persistence of high drug concentrations in the peritoneal or pleural spaces, although Paladine *et al.* (1976) have reported that only an average of 4.6% of the initial dosage remained in intrapleural fluid 24 hr after instillation. Thus, intracavitary drug administration may result in exposure of intracavitary tumor to higher and more persistent bleomycin concentrations than that which would be achieved after intravenous dosing.

The absorption rate of bleomycin following intrapleural instillation appears more rapid than that for intraperitoneal injection. The plasma decay curves associated with intrapleural bleomycin have clearly defined peaks as compared to those seen after intraperitoneal dosing. The longer bleomycin plasma half-life for the intraperitoneal versus the intrapleural administration route is probably due to a slow but continuous absorption of the drug into the systemic circulation.

The large plasma bleomycin CXT seen after only 15 u/m^2 intraperitoneally in patient P.E. (Tables II and IV) points to the importance of renal function in the disposition of this anticancer drug. Crooke *et al.* (1977) have previously reported a prolongation of bleomycin terminal phase plasma half-life in a patient with severe renal failure (creatinine clearance of 10.7 ml/min). Although there is no evidence to document a relationship between either length of bleomycin plasma half-life or size of CXT to normal tissue toxicity, our data for patient P.E. suggest that total intracavitary dosage should be kept below 300 u in patients with decreased renal function.

ACKNOWLEDGMENTS

We wish to thank Ms. Patricia Dombrowski and Ms. Katherine Griffith for their help in patient care and sample collection and Ms. Elva Seidel for manuscript preparation.

REFERENCES

Broughton, A., and Strong, J. E. (1976). *Cancer Res. 36*, 1418.
Crooke, S. T., Luft, F., Broughton, A., Strong, J. E., Casson, K., and Einhorn, L. (1977). *Cancer 39*, 1430.
Hall, S. W., Broughton, A., Strong, J. E., and Benjamin, R. S. (1977). *Clin. Res. 25*, 407A.
Metzler, C. M. (1969). Upjohn Co., Kalamazoo, Michigan, Technical Report 7292/69/7292/005, November 25.
Paladine, W., Cunningham, T. J., Sponzo, R., Donavan, M., Olson, K., and Horton, J. (1976). *Cancer 38*, 1903.
Sedman, A. J., and Wagner, J. G. (1976). *J. Pharm. Sci. 65*, 1006.

Chapter 12

THE IMMUNOPHARMACOLOGY OF
BLEOMYCIN IN MAN [1]

Daniel E. Lehane
Montague Lane

I. INTRODUCTION

Since it has been shown by many investigators that cancer patients with good immunologic function have better survival and response to therapy than patients with poor immunocompetence, there have been innumerable clinical trials attempting to improve patients' immunocompetence by using immunostimulants and chemotherapy schedules designed to permit recovery of the immune system from immunosuppression.

Bleomycin, as one of its many unique pharmacologic properties, produces little or no myelosuppression. Therefore, the immunopharmacologic effects of bleomycin have been of great interest. Initially, Ohno et al. (1971) demonstrated that bleomycin did not affect the primary antibody response in mice Andrews (1972) studied the effects of bleomycin on graft rejection times using a non-H_2 allograft system in mice and found that there was no delay in graft rejection times except when lethal doses of bleomycin were administered. Dolgi et al. (1974) confirmed these observations by showing that bleomycin had no effect on the primary antibody response and did not alter IgM or IgG antibody production. Furthermore,

[1] Supported by USPHS Research Grants CA 10893 and CA 03392.

they showed that cell-mediated immunity in the mouse was not altered by several drug administration schedules except for lethal doses of bleomycin. However, Tisman *et al.* (1973), using an assay system dependent on DNA synthesis to measure lymphocyte blastogenesis, showed marked immunosuppression in man using bleomycin.

We have studied the immunopharmacology of bleomycin in man measuring multiple parameters of both antibody- and cell-mediated immunity both *in vivo* and *in vitro* and have concluded that bleomycin does not suppress immunocompetence in man.

II. MATERIALS AND METHODS

A. Subjects

In vivo studies of immunocompetence were conducted in six patients with advanced disseminated cancer who were being treated with bleomycin (three squamous cell carcinoma of the lung. and one each of adenocarcinoma of the colon, adenocarcinoma of unknown primary, and squamous cell carcinoma of the esophagus). Bleomycin was administered at a dose of 15 u/m^2 IM twice weekly. Prior to each dose of bleomycin patients were examined for evidence of toxicity and tumor response. If there was evidence of toxicity bleomycin was withheld until toxicity completely was resolved. No patient received greater than 300 u/m^2 cumulative dose. Two patients developed transient stomatitis and one, subsequently, pulmonary fibrosis. Informed consent was obtained from each patient prior to immunologic testing.

B. Immunological Testing

Patients were tested 2 days prior to initiating bleomycin and after 2 and 4 weeks of treatment. Six normal volunteers were used for controls for both *in vivo* and *in vitro* immunologic studies.

C. Antibody-Mediated Immunity

Three parameters of established antibody immunity were studied. Isoantibodies to human blood group antigens were measured using the saline agglutination technique. Recall virus antibody titers to polio virus Type I and herpes simplex Type I were measured by the microneutralization test. Cytomegalovirus antibody was measured by the microtiter compliment fixation test. Immunoglobulin levels and serum complement levels were measured by the radial immunodiffusion technique. The primary antibody response to vaccination with KLH was performed by administering 1 mg of KLH intradermally 2 days prior to beginning bleomycin treatment. KLH antibody was measured by the passive hemagglutination test adapted to the microtiter method. Anti KLH IgM antibody titers were determined by measuring 2 mercaptoethanol resistant antibody titers.

D. Cellular Immunity

Recall of established cell-mediated immunity was measured using delayed hypersensitivity reactions to six skin test antigens which included mumps, streptokinase, streptodornase, PPD, monilia, dermatophyton, and dermatophyton "O." Primary cell-mediated immune reaction was measured using delayed hypersensitivity reaction to KLH following vaccination with KLH as above. All skin tests were read at 48 hr and the diameter of induration was measured in two perpendicular diameters for each reaction. On the basis of these measurements the mean diameter of all skin tests with measurable induration was calculated for each patient.

Lymphocyte blastogenesis following PHA stimulation was performed using a microtiter culture system with tritiated thymidine incorporation as the indicator of blastogenesis. Lymphocytes were collected using the Ficoll Hypaque technique and were grown using RPMI 1640 supplemented with 20% calf serum. Each culture well contained 50 μl of lymphocyte suspension (4 x 10^6 ml), 50 μl of PHA M (diluted 1 to 10), and 100 μl of growth medium. Replicate cultures were incubated at 37° for 72 hr. Tritiated thymidine was added 3 hr prior to harvesting for liquid scintillation counting. The results of lymphocyte blastogenesis are expressed as a stimulation index which is the ratio of the mean counts per minute in PHA-stimulated cultures to those of unstimulated control cultures. The percentage of circulating lymphocytes which formed E rosettes was determined by mixing equal volumes of lymphocytes (1 x 10^7 ml) suspended in phosphate buffered saline pH 7.2 with 10% fetal calf serum added and sheep red blood cells (0.5%). The mixture was centrifuged to a pellet at 200g for 5 min, incubated at 4°C for 30 min, gently resuspended, and counted in a hemocytometer.

The *in vitro* effects of bleomycin on normal human lymphocytes stimulated with PHA utilizing the thymidine incorporation assay were measured for seven volunteers. Bleomycin was added to the culture medium at final concentrations of 0.15, 1.5, and 15 μg/ml. The average plasma concentration achieved in man is approximately 0.15 μg/ml and the average tissue concentration of bleomycin in sensitive tumors has been reported to be as high as 1.5 μg/ml. In an effort to stimulate the *in vivo* clearance of bleomycin, one-half of the lymphocyte cultures containing bleomycin were washed free of bleomycin while the other half were cultured with bleomycin present continuously during the 72 hr culture period.

Lymphocytes from six volunteers were also cultured *in vivo* using a protein synthesis assay for determining lymphocyte blastogenesis as described by Levy and Kaplan (1974). In this assay serial dilutions of PHA were cultured with lymphocytes for 20 hr in leucine-free RPMI 1640 to which tritiated leucine 0.5 μ Ci per well was added. Simultaneous cultures containing continuous bleomycin exposure, lymphocytes from which bleomycin had been removed following 1 hr of culture, and lymphocytes that had not been exposed to bleomycin were prepared.

TABLE I. Isoantibody Titers [a]

	Pretreatment	Week 2	Week 4	Controls
Anti A or Anti B	27	33	25	388 [b]

[a] Expressed as $1 \times 10^{-1} \times$ the last positive serum dilution.
[b] $p < 0.05$.

E. Statistical Methods

A comparison of the results from immunocompetence testing prior to chemo-therapy was made with the results obtained following 2 and 4 weeks of bleomycin treatment. The significance of the differences between the means was evaluated by the analysis of variance and by the Students t-test.

III. RESULTS

A. Antibody-Mediated Immunity

The results of established antibody immunity testing are shown in Tables I–IV. While isoantibody titers were significantly lower in the patient group as a whole compared to controls, there was no significant change in isoantibody titer during bleomycin therapy. When recall virus antibody titers are compared it is evident that patients had significantly higher antibody titers to herpes simplex Type I than controls, but again there are no significant changes in virus antibody titer for polio virus, herpes simplex virus, or cytomegalovirus in patients during treatment with bleomycin. The results of serum immunoglobulin testing showed that serum IgG titers and serum IgA titers were higher (although not significantly so) in patients compared to controls. There was again no significant change in serum immunoglob-ulin levels or serum complement levels during treatment with bleomycin. Patients were able to make a normal primary immune response to KLH while receiving bleo-mycin. Antibody titers were low in both the patient and control groups 2 weeks postvaccination and had increased by 4 weeks. The difference between patients and controls at 4 weeks was not statistically significant. Of even greater importance was the fact that both patients and controls began to make serum IgG anti-KLH anti-body at 4 weeks postvaccination. Of the measurable antibody titer at 4 weeks 54% was 2 mercaptoethanol-sensitive in the patient group and 64% in the control group, indicating a normal conversion from IgM to IgG antibody synthesis during bleomycin therapy.

TABLE II. Recall Virus Antibody Titers [a]

	Pretreatment	Week 2	Week 4	Controls
Polio	26	30	24	19 [b]
Herpes simplex	408	467	645	54
Cytomegalo-virus	43	52	64	41

[a] Expressed as 1×10^{-1} x the last positive serum dilution.
[b] $p < 0.01$.

TABLE III. Serum Immunoglobulins [a]

	Pretreatment	Week 2	Week 4	Controls
IgG	1438	1492	1635	1043
IgA	305	293	347	199
IgM	154	148	115	149
C'	138	153	148	101

[a] Expressed as mg/100 ml.

TABLE IV. KLH Antibody Titers [a]

	Pretreatment	Week 2	Week 4
Patients	0	5	79
Controls	0	8	240

[a] Titer equals 1×10^{-1} x the last positive dilution.

B. Cell-Mediated Immunity

The results of cell-mediated immunity testing are shown in Tables V and VI. As noted in prior studies, patients had a significantly lower mean diameter of delayed hypersensitivity reaction to recall antigens when compared to controls (Lehane and Lane, 1975). However, during bleomycin treatment there was no depression of existing delayed hypersensitivity reaction. Furthermore, patients were able to develop a primary delayed hypersensitivity reaction during treatment with bleomycin. The percentage of E rosettes was likewise significantly lower in patients than in controls and the percentage of E rosettes in patients remained constant during

TABLE V. Delayed Hypersensitivity

	Pretreatment	Week 2	Week 4	Controls
Recall	6.1 [a]	5.1	8.1	27.7 [b]
Primary KLH	–	28.8	15.4	55

[a] Mean diameter of induration, mm.
[b] $p < 0.001$.

TABLE VI. Lymphocyte Testing

	Pretreatment	Week 2	Week 4	Controls
E Rosettes %	24	19	33	48 [b]
Lymphocyte blastogenesis (PHA)	99 [a]	19	31	112

[a] Stimulation index.
[b] $p < 0.01$.

bleomycin treatment. The results of lymphocyte blastogenesis testing following PHA stimulation showed no difference between patients and control groups prior to bleomycin therapy, but a steady decrease in stimulation index during bleomycin therapy was observed.

C. *In Vitro* Studies

The effects of bleomycin cultured *in vitro* on normal lymphocyte PHA-induced blastogenesis are shown in Table VII. Lymphocytes exposed to bleomycin continuously through the culture period showed a significant reduction in stimulation index at concentrations of bleomycin equal to tissues levels or greater. When bleomycin was washed from the culture media after 1 hr of incubation there was no depression of stimulation index at bleomycin concentrations similar to plasma or tissue levels and only partial suppression of the stimulation index at bleomycin con centrations equivalent to 100 times the usual plasma concentration.

Lymphocyte blastogenesis was also measured by the protein synthesis assay utilizing tritiated leucine incorporation and is shown in Fig. 1. It is evident that when protein synthesis is used as an indicator for blastogenesis there is no inhibition of lymphocyte blastogenesis following PHA stimulation even at very high concentrations of bleomycin despite the fact that bleomycin was present continuously during the culture period.

TABLE VII. *In Vitro* Bleomycin–PHA Blastogenesis [a]

Bleomycin concentration	Continuous	Washed
0	144 [b]	234
1.5 μg	129	382
15 μg	30[c]	264
150 μg	6[d]	131

[a] [³H] thymidine incorporation.
[b] Stimulation index.
[c] $p < 0.05$.
[d] $p < 0.001$.

IV. DISCUSSION

Several investigators using animal models have shown that bleomycin does not suppress either antibody or cell-mediated immunologic function. None of the immunologic assays utilized in these animal studies was dependent on DNA synthesis or utilized thymidine incorporation as an indicator of immunologic response. Previous studies in man have demonstrated suppression of PHA-induced lymphocyte blastogenesis by bleomycin, but these studies used assay systems dependent on DNA synthesis as indicators of blastogenesis.

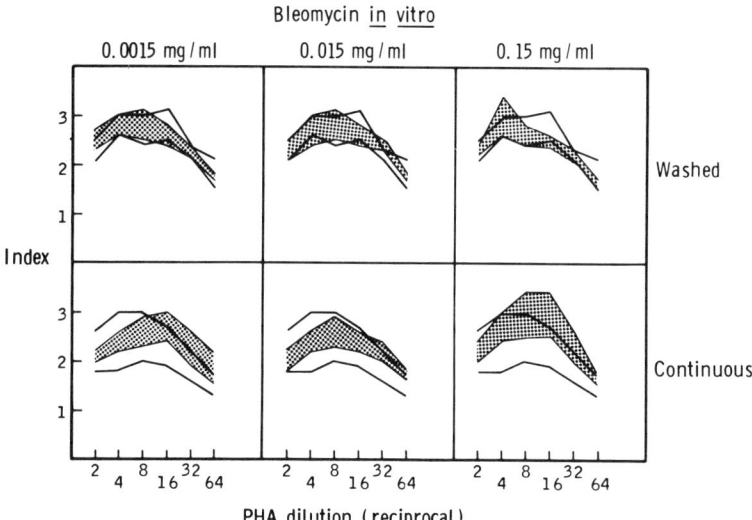

Fig. 1. *In vitro* blastogenesis as measured by [³H] leucine incorporation in bleomycin treated and control lymphocyte expressed as the mean stimulation index + 1 standard deviation of the mean at each dilution of PHA (shaded = bleomycin treated, open = controls). Reproduced with permission from *Cancer Research 35*, 2724-2728 (1975).

Our studies on the immunopharmacology of bleomycin in man examined multiple parameters of immunologic function. There was no depression of antibody-mediated immunity as measured by recall virus antibody titers, serum immunoglobulin, and serum complement levels or isoantibody titers. The primary antibody response to KLH vaccination was not suppressed during bleomycin treatment even to the extent that there was normal conversion from IgM to IgG antibody production during bleomycin therapy. Several parameters of cell-mediated immunity were likewise not depressed during bleomycin treatment, including recall delayed hypersensitivity reaction, primary delayed hypersensitivity reaction to KLH, and percent circulating E rosettes. However, using a lymphocyte blastogenesis assay dependent on tritiated thymidine incorporation there was a marked reduction in the stimulation index during bleomycin treatment. *In vitro* studies using lymphocytes from normal volunteers showed marked reduction of blastogenesis measured by thymidine incorporation if the lymphocytes were exposed to very high concentrations of bleomycin continuously during the culture period. This inhibition was reversed by washing the lymphocytes after 1 hr exposure to bleomycin simulating plasma clearance. Since bleomycin is known to interfere with DNA synthesis and thymidine incorporation as a biochemical action of the drug, we elected to study lymphocyte blastogenesis utilizing a protein synthesis indicator of blastogenesis, i.e., tritiated leucine incorporation. Levy and Kaplan (1974) have shown that this method of measuring PHA-induced blastogenesis is more sensitive than the thymidine incorporation assay for detecting small differences in lymphocyte function. As shown in Fig. 1 there was no inhibition in lymphocyte blastogenesis even in cultures continuously exposed to very high concentrations of bleomycin when the leucine incorporation assay was employed. We have therefore interpreted the observed inhibition of thymidine incorporation by PHA-stimulated lymphocytes following prolonged exposure to high concentrations of bleomycin as a specious indication of inhibited lymphocyte blastogenesis. The inhibition of thymidine incorporation by PHA-stimulated lymphocytes probably reflects the biochemical action of the drug on DNA metabolism rather than impaired blastogenesis. It occurs only after prolonged incubation of lymphocytes with high concentrations of the drug Consequently the failure of high doses of the drug to reduce leucine incorporation with PHA-stimulated lymphocytes indicates that blastogenesis is not inhibited. We have concluded that bleomycin administered by a high-dose continuous schedule for 4 weeks does not suppress either antibody- or cell-mediated immunity in man.

REFERENCES

Andrews, E. J. (1972). *Cancer Res. 32*, 1993–1994.
Dolgi, A. M., Robie, K. M., and Mitchell, M. S. (1974). *Cancer Res. 34*, 2504–2507.
Lehane, D. E., and Lane, M. (1975). *Oncology 30*, 458–466.
Levy, R., and Kaplan, H. S. (1974). *New Engl. J. Med. 290*, 181–186.
Ohno, R., Nishwaki, H., Kawashima, K., Tadaaki, U., Hirano, M., Miura, M., and Yamada, K. (1971). *Gann Monogr. Cancer Res. 62*, 267–274.
Tisman, G., Herbert, V., Go, L. T., and Brenner, L. (1973). *Blood 41*, 721–726.

Chapter 13

THE ROLE OF BLEOMYCIN IN THE TREATMENT OF ADVANCED HEAD AND NECK CANCER

Andrew T. Turrisi, III
Marcel Rozencweig
Daniel D. Von Hoff
Franco M. Muggia

I. INTRODUCTION

The management of head and neck cancer is a challenging problem for medical oncologists. This tumor occurs with relative infrequency, principally among elderly patients, and accounts for only 5% of all malignancies in the United States. Chemotherapy is employed generally for tumors beyond the control of surgery and radiotherapy. Unfortunately, at this stage of the disease the rapidly declining performance status and lack of clearly evaluable lesions often hamper the administration of cytoxic agents. Nevertheless, a number of active compounds have been identified and, among them, bleomycin is filling an increasingly important therapeutic role. This review summarizes published data on bleomycin as a single agent or in combination chemotherapy regimens in the treatment of advanced head and neck cancer. Hopefully, this information will provide some insight into areas worthy of further investigation. The combined used of bleomycin and radiotherapy is discussed elsewhere in this volume.

II. SINGLE-AGENT ACTIVITY OF BLEOMYCIN

A response rate ranging between 6 and 45% has been reported in the large series of patients receiving systemic treatment with bleomycin (Table I). Most of these data were obtained in broad phase II trials that included patients with undefined prognostic factors or with far advanced disease refractory to prior chemotherapy. The duration of responses has generally not exceeded 2-3 months. This short duration may have, in part, resulted from a selection of poor risk population, but also could be related to a limited treatment duration because of the cumulative toxicity of bleomycin.

Bonadonna *et al.* (1972, 1976) investigated a variety of dose schedules of bleomycin given by rapid IV injection in a broad phase I-II study that largely included patients with prior radiotherapy and/or chemotherapy. Of the 48 patients with epidermoid head and neck carcinomas, the largest treatment group received the drug as a daily dose of 15 mg/m² for 5 consecutive days. Courses were repeated twice at 3 week intervals and followed by weekly maintenance bleomycin until progression or definite lung toxicity was evident. Responses, including I-A responses according to Karnofsky's criteria, occurred in half of the 26 patients treated with this regimen. In another treatment group reported separately (Bonadonna *et al.*, 1976), bleomycin was administered twice weekly at a dose of 10 mg/m² and, with this dose schedule, only 2 out of 14 patients showed tumor regression.

The trial conducted by Halnan *et al.* (1972) involved various tumor types, largely in patients who were in poor general condition. Bleomycin treatment was usually initiated after recurrence on prior therapy with surgery, radiotherapy, and/or chemotherapy. The drug was usually given as a single agent at a dose of 30 mg weekly to a total of 300 mg or until toxicity became apparent. Three complete and 21 undefined partial responses were noted among the 53 patients with squamous cell carcinoma of the head and neck. Results detailed by tumor site did not suggest that site might influence the response rate, but the number of patients was small in each category.

The Southwest Oncology Group (Haas *et al.*, 1976) carried out a broad phase II trial with bleomycin in 382 patients, of whom 64 had squamous cell head and neck tumors. The drug was given at 10 mg/m² twice weekly for 12 weeks. Responding patients received a subsequent course at weekly doses of 10 mg/m² for 12 weeks, provided there was no pulmonary toxicity after 3 months without therapy. The trial was partially randomized to compare IV versus IM administration. The response rate in the head and neck cancer group was 19%, but only partial remissions were noted. These findings were not detailed according to route of administration, tumor site, or prior therapy.

The European Organization for Research on the Treatment of Cancer (E.O.R.T.C., 1970) also investigated the value of bleomycin in a large phase II trial. Patients were generally treated with an IV or IM dose of 10-20 mg/m² daily for 10 to 38 days to a total dose ranging from 150 to 820 mg; some patients received 20 mg/m² IV twice weekly. Of 54 evaluable patients with tumors of the oropharynx and nasal sinuses, one apparently complete regression and eight partial

TABLE I. Single-Agent Activity of IV or IM Bleomycin[a]

Investigator	Dose (mg/m²)	Schedule	Route	No. of evaluable patients	No. of responses (%)	Duration (mo)
Bonadonna et al. (1976)	10, 15, 30 15, 30	Twice weekly Daily x 5-8	IV	62	28 (45)	2-5
Halnan et al. (1972)	20[b]	Twice weekly	IV or IM	53	24 (45)	
Haas et al. (1976)	10	Twice weekly	IV vs. IM	64	12 (19)	
E.O.R.T.C. (1970)	10-20 20	Daily x 10-38 Twice weekly	IV or IM	54	9 (17)	
Yagoda et al. (1972)	9.25	Daily to toxicity	IV	46	6 (13)	1-11
Durkin et al. (1976)	10	Twice weekly	IV vs. IM	81	5 (6)	2-3

[a] Limited to studies including at least 25 patients with head and neck carcinoma.

[b] Actual doses were 30 mg regardless of body weight or body surface area.

regressions were noted after these systemic treatments. The population selected for this trial was not defined and no attempt was made to characterize response rate as a function of potential prognostic factors.

Yagoda *et al.* (1972) reported the overall experience with bleomycin at the Memorial Sloan-Kettering Cancer Center. The drug was administered by slow IV injection at a dose of 0.25 mg/kg given daily until the appearance of skin or mucosal ulceration or both. Nearly all patients with head and neck tumors had undergone extensive surgery, many had received high-dose radiotherapy, and some had prior chemotherapy. Of 46 evaluable patients, six achieved an objective response (I-A responses according to Karnofsky's criteria) but only one lasted longer than 2 months. In this trial, no correlation could be found between response rate and tumor site, histologic type, or prior therapy but the corresponding data were not provided.

In a study of the Western Cancer Study Group (Durkin *et al.*, 1976), 110 evaluable patients with far advanced squamous cell carcinoma of the head and neck or with metastatic testicular malignancy were randomly assigned to IV or IM bleomycin, 10 mg/m^2 twice a week, to a toal dose of 300 mg or less in the case of disease progression or development of abnormal respiratory function. Among 81 head and neck cancer patients there was one complete response and five partial responses for an overall response rate of 6%. This disappointing figure might have been due, at least partially, to selection of patients with disease refractory to or not suitable for all conventional treatment modalities, including chemotherapy. In addition, disease was often at a far advanced stage, as illustrated by the relatively high frequency (25%) of pulmonary metastases. Neither the route of administration nor the site of the tumor appeared to influence the response rate but larger series might be necessary to draw firm conclusions regarding these factors.

The broad range of response rates encountered illustrated the difficulties of accurately assessing the antitumor activity of cytotoxic agents. Patient selection, response criteria, and method of data reporting greatly modulate therapeutic results. The available data do not allow a meaningful comparison of the therapeutic effectiveness of bleomycin versus other chemotherapeutic agents in head and neck carcinoma.

An optimal mode of administering bleomycin remains to be determined. The route of administration, IV or IM, and the dose schedules investigated in the aforementioned large studies (Table I), do not seem to influence response strikingly but there is some suggestion that response rates seen with doses of 10 mg/m^2, daily or twice weekly, are likely to be improved with higher dosage levels. Experience with continuous infusions is presently limited despite a fair amount of available background information.

Barranco and Humphrey (1971) demonstrated cell-cycle specificity of bleomycin in Chinese hamster ovary cells *in vitro*. These studies showed bleomycin to be most active on cells in mitosis or in G_2 phase. The reported cell-cycle time for epidermoid tumors is between 25 and 48 hr (Frindel *et al.*, 1968). Bleomycin may be more effective on cells exposed to it for the duration of their cell cycle

(Drewinko *et al.*, 1972). One of the postulated mechanisms of bleomycin is DNA strand scission. Takabe *et al.* (1977) have recently shown that "potentially lethal damage" produced by strand scission can rapidly be repaired, but this repair mechanism is likely to be minimized by repeated drug administration at short intervals and particularly by continuous infusion therapy.

Krakoff *et al.* (1977) reported the results of a broad phase I-II trial using continuous infusions of bleomycin at a daily dose of 0.02 to 0.50 mg/kg until limiting toxicity was apparent. When the dose was increased to 0.25 mg/kg per day, mucocutaneous toxicity developed between the seventh and eleventh day of the infusion. Some of the patients in this trial had previously been treated with conventional IV push bleomycin. Eleven patients with head and neck cancer were adequately treated and two achieved partial remissions. Little information was provided concerning these patients or their treatment and, despite the relatively unfavorable results, additional studies of this mode of administration seem warranted in head and neck cancer.

Few data are available to estimate the role of intraarterial versus systemic administration of chemotherapy in head and neck cancer. No controlled trial has compared the two modalities. The IA technique has been extensively used in the past, mainly with methotrexate (Goldsmith and Carter, 1975). Overall, this procedure has produced significant morbidity and a very modest response rate in view of the relatively favorable prognosis of the patients selected for this treatment modality.

The largest published series of patients treated with IA bleomycin was reported by Richard and Sancho (1973). In this series, 27 evaluable patients received 30 mg of bleomycin over 10-12 hr daily for 6 to 10 days. Disappointingly, a response rate of only 18% was achieved in these patients.

The E.O.R.T.C. has recently completed a randomized trial comparing IA methotrexate + systemic citrovorum rescue versus IA bleomycin. A total of 93 evaluable patients with T_3-T_4 squamous cell carcinoma of the oral cavity were included in the trial. A definite conclusion must await publication of the final report.

III. BLEOMYCIN IN COMBINATION CHEMOTHERAPY REGIMENS

A. Two Drug Combinations

The combination of methotrexate and bleomycin has been the two-drug regimen most frequently investigated in head and neck carcinoma (Tables II and III). Several combinations of these two compounds have been developed, but superiority of any of these treatments over each drug given alone has not been established.

As might be expected, mucocutaneous toxicity is dose-limiting. In addition, the severe myelosuppression encountered (Broquet *et al.*, 1974; Lokich and Frei, 1974; Medenica *et al.*, 1976; Mosher *et al.*, 1972) suggests a synergistic effect of bleomycin and methotrexate on the bone marrow stem cells. A possible potentiation of bleomycin-induced pulmonary toxicity has also been suggested (Lokich and Frei,

1974). perhaps as a result of either agent impairing the excretion of the other agent or as a result of an additive effect of each of these drugs on the lung.

The largest experience with this combination has been reported by Swiss investigators. In their first study (Broquet et al., 1974), the twice weekly administration of bleomycin at 30 mg and methotrexate at 0.4 mg/kg produced impressive toxicities, especially myelosuppression. The total dose of bleomycin was limited to 300 mg and no pulmonary toxicity was encountered. The treatment elicited nine partial responses for 7 to 15 weeks among the 15 patients entered in the study. In the subsequent study (Medenica et al., 1976), much lower doses were given (Table II). This combination was well tolerated and achieved a response rate similar to that of the former trial but with noticeably more prolonged response duration. Nine patients who failed to respond to this low-dose program were treated with the initial higher dose regimen and four additional patients responded for a median duration of 7 weeks.

cis-Diamminedichloraplatinum (II) (DDP) is a new anticancer agent that has recently introduced in the treatment of head and neck cancer (Rozencweig et al., 1977a, b). The potential of DDP in the chemotherapy of this malignancy has been suggested by data obtained at Memorial Sloan-Kettering Cancer Center. First detected in an early clinical trial (Lippman et al., 1973), the activity of the drug was subsequently documented in a pilot study using high doses of the drug with hyperhydration and mannitol diuresis (Hayes et al., 1977). Twenty-six patients with far-advanced epidermoid head and neck cancer were entered in their most recent study (Wittes et al., 1977a). All patients had previous radiotherapy and a majority of them also had surgery and/or chemotherapy. Two complete remissions for 2+ and 6+ months and six partial remissions for periods ranging from 1 to 8+ months were achieved.

Two regimens combining DDP and bleomycin have been successively investigated. The potential for these combinations to enhance toxicity by impairing renal excretion, as in methotrexate-bleomycin combinations, is certainly reasonable; however, these interactions have not yet been observed with DDP-bleomycin combinations. The first study included 28 patients previously treated with surgery and/or radiotherapy (Wittes et al., 1975); 11 patients had received prior chemotherapy. DDP was administered at 2 mg/kg every 3 weeks without particular attention to hydration; bleomycin was given at 0.25 mg/kg daily until mucocutaneous toxicity developed. Disappointingly, this treatment yielded only 3 partial remissions and considerable toxicity was encountered. In the next study (Randolph et al., 1977), DDP was given at higher doses (3 mg/kg) with forced diuresis as in their most successful single-agent study. Bleomycin (0.25 mg/kg) was administered by rapid injection on day 3, followed by continuous infusion of 0.25 mg/kg/day from day 3 through day 10. This regimen was given prior to radiotherapy in patients with unresectable disease not previously treated. Of 18 evaluable patients on day 22, five achieved complete and seven achieved partial remissions.

Other two-drug combinations including bleomycin have been tested, but these trials have been generally limited to a small number of patients and have sometimes

TABLE II. Activity of Bleomycin (BLM) and Methotrexate (MTX) Combinations

Investigator	IV Dose		Schedule	No. of responses/ No. of evaluable patients	Response duration (mo.)
	BLM	MTX			
Medenica et al. (1976)	15 mg	0.6 mg/kg	Weekly	13/26	6
Bonadonna et al. (1976)	Unspecified	40 mg/m^2	Weekly	2/16	—
Broquet et al. (1974)	30 mg	0.4 mg/kg	Twice Weekly	9/15	2–3.5
Yagoda et al. (1975)	15 units	15 mg/m^2	4–14 day intervals	8/15	1–8+
Lokich and Frei (1974)	10–15 mg/m^2	15–25 mg/m^2	Twice Weekly	4/5	—
Mosher et al. (1972)	105 mg [a]	480 mg/m^2 [b]	Sequential	2/4	—

[a] BLM given IM over 5 days every 12 days.

[b] MTX given over 36 hrs. followed by citrovorum factor between BLM courses.

used agents apparently endowed with only weak effectiveness against head and neck carcinoma, such as adriamycin (Knight *et al.*, 1972; Benjamin *et al.*, 1974; Bonadonna *et al.*, 1975; Dowell *et al.*, 1975; Krakoff, 1975) and CCNU (Rozencweig *et al.*, 1977b) (Table III). Of particular interest was the sequential combination of vincristine-bleomycin initially investigated by Livingston *et al.* (1973). The rationale of this regimen was based on the ability of vincristine to increase the percentage of cells in mitosis (Frei *et al.*, 1964) and on the maximum cell-killing effect observed with bleomycin during the mitotic phase of the cell cycle. However, interpretation of the data is obscured by the intrinsic antitumor activity of vincristine in head and neck tumors (Livingston *et al.*, 1975a, b). Whether this approach actually results in improving the therapeutic effect of bleomycin remains entirely speculative but the concept is attractive and is being widely used.

TABLE III. Activity of Two-Drug Combinations Including Bleomycin

Treatment and References[a]	No. of evaluable patients	No. of responses (%)
BLM-MTX (from Table II)	81	38 (47)
BLM-DDP (Wittes *et al.*, 1975; Randolph *et al.*, 1977)	42	15 (36)
BLM-DBD (Ohnuma *et al.*, 1972)	20	5 (25)
BLM-ADM (Cortes *et al.*, 1972 Tormey *et al.*, 1973)	15	7 (47)
BLM-VCR (Livingston *et al.*, 1973)	9	3 (33)
BLM-CCNU (Mosley *et al.*, 1976)	7	3 (43)
BLM-MMC (Van Dyk *et al.*, 1972)	3	0 (0)

[a] BLM = bleomycin; MTX = methotrexate; DDP = *cis*-diamminedichloroplatinum (II); DBD = dibromodulcitol; VCR = vincristine; MMC = mitomycin C.

B. Multiple Drug Combinations

Most of the multiple drug combinations that have been tested in head and neck cancer have included bleomycin. As yet, none of these combinations has proven to be more active than single agents. The median response duration has not exceeded 6 months in any of these studies (Table IV).

The highest response rate was reported by Price *et al.* (1975) using a seven-drug regimen given sequentially in 36 hr per course repeated every 3 weeks. However, all patients who did not receive at least three courses of therapy (12/36) were excluded from the final analysis.

Costanzi *et al.* (1976) employed 48 hr bleomycin infusion at a daily dose of 7.5

TABLE IV. Multiple Drug Combinations Employing Bleomycin [a]

Treatment [b]	No. of evaluable patients	No. of responses (%)	Duration (mo)	Investigators
VCR-ADM-BLM-MTX-5FU HYD-6MP	24	19 (79)	—	Price et al. (1975)
BLM-MTX/BLM-HYD	17	10 (59)	1–8	Constanzi et al. (1976)
BACON[c] ± BCG	34	15 (44)	3–4.5	Richman et al. (1976)
CTX-VCR-BLM/MTX/ADM MeCCNU	28	12 (43)	6	Livingston et al. (1976)
BLM-CTX-MTX-5FU	25	9 (36)	—	Stathopoulos et al. (1976)
CTX-ADM-MTX-BLM	26	9 (35)	2.5	Wittes et al. (1977b)
COMB[d]	32	11 (34)	3	Livingston et al. (1975, 1976)
CTX-ADM-VCR-BLM/MTX-CTX-ADM	19	5 (26)	—	Murphy et al. (1977)

[a] Systemic administration.

[b] ADM = adriamycin; BLM = bleomycin; CTX = cytoxan; 5FU = 5-fluorouracil; HYD = hydroxyurea; 6 MP = 6-mercaptopurine; MTX = methotrexate; HN_2 = nitrogen mustard; VCR = vincristine.

[c] BACON = BLM + ADM + CCNU + VCR + HN_2.

[d] COMB = CTX + VCR + MeCCNU + BLM.

mg/m² followed, after a 24 hr rest period, by either methotrexate, 30 mg/m² IV push, on odd-numbered courses, or hydroxyurea, 2000 mg/m² orally, on even-numbered courses. Courses were repeated every 10-14 days for the first three courses, and then every 2 to 3 weeks if a response was noted. This treatment was extremely well tolerated. Of the 17 patients with epidermoid head and neck carcinoma, 10 responded for an overall response rate of 59% and a response duration in the range of 1 to 8 months.

At M. D. Anderson Hospital, the BACON regiment was investigated in a randomized study with or without BCG (Richman et al., 1976). This regimen induced noticeable toxicity; there were five drug-related deaths, four of infection and one of bleomycin pulmonary toxicity. Response rate and response duration were similar in both treatment groups, but survival was significantly prolonged in the BCG group with median values of 30.5 versus 13.5 weeks.

In the study carried out by Livingston et al. (1976), 28 patients who had not received prior chemotherapy were treated with a sequential program in an attempt to delay the development of drug resistance. Treatment consisted of a cyclophosphamide–vincristine–bleomycin combination for 6 weeks followed by alternated cycles of methotrexate and adriamycin-MeCCNU. This treatment elicited five complete and seven partial remissions for an overall response rate of 43%. The median response duration was 25 weeks but the median survival time for all patients entered in the study was 24 weeks from the start of chemotherapy.

Various other combination chemotherapy regimens have been investigated in the systemic treatment of head and neck squamous cell carcinoma (Table IV). Overall, results have been disappointing with response rates and duration in the range reported with bleomycin alone. These results have often been achieved at the expense of higher toxicity.

Combination chemotherapy has also been used intraarterially but, again, data are difficult to interpret since this treatment can be applied only in a favorable selection of patients. The most promising results were reported by Donegan and Harris (1976) with a combination of methotrexate, 5-fluorouracil, and bleomycin. An 87% response rate (13/15) was reported but this dropped to the more usual figure of 60% when only tumor shrinkage of more than 50% was considered.

IV. DISCUSSION

The difficulties in evaluating efficacy of chemotherapeutic agents have led to an increasing emphasis on knowledge of prognostic factors and continuous attempts to improve and standarize the design of clinical trials. General parameters predictive for the response to chemotherapy have been identified in various malignancies. They include primarily the performance status and extent of prior cytotoxic therapy. The former roughly reflects the stage and aggressiveness of the disease whereas the latter, besides the possibility of remnant or cumulative toxicity, may be indicative of a more advanced disease and also the emergence of "more malignant" cancer cells resistant to conventional treatment. The problem is further complicated in head and neck cancer because these tumors include malignancies arising from different sites and occasionally with different histological types. Presumably, location and pathology might be variables of strong prognostic significance, but limited data are available to assess their predictive value on responsiveness to chemotherapy.

Clinical trials must consider all these prognostic factors and should be designed to the questions addressed in these trials. The very fact that these questions are usually not clearly defined may generate endless controversies in this type of study. In the analysis of phase II data, establishing the ineffectiveness of a regimen with certainty is a major problem. When single agents are found active, accurate determination of their degree of activity becomes a somewhat secondary practical problem in view of the usual integration of these agents into combination chemotherapy regimens. Furthermore, degree of activity is truly pertinent only to homogeneous populations and, even then, requires a large number of patients to be accurately determined. Finally, the trial design itself may be responsible for considerable elasticity in response rates.

Bleomycin has shown definite activity as a single agent in head and neck tumors, but its precise role in the treatment of these malignancies remains unsettled. Inconsistent findings have been reported and the available information does not allow estimation of the efficacy of bleomycin (i. e., response rate and duration) relative, for example, to methotrexate, which is usually referred to as a standard chemotherapeutic treatment. The antitumor activity of bleomycin has often been tested in patients who failed on prior methotrexate treatment. Moreover, most of the published methotrexate data were obtained in older studies and should perhaps be reevaluated according to current criteria of drug assessment.

The data under the scope of this review do not provide much information relative to an optimal method of bleomycin treatment, if indeed there is one. A dose-response relationship has been suggested but remains to be ascertained. The effect of schedule and route of administration should be further explored.

Combination chemotherapy has been introduced relatively recently in head and neck cancer and most regimens have included bleomycin. These combinations have generally achieved response rates in the range of those reported with single agents and conclusions are difficult to reach in view of the breadth of this range. However, results have not been too promising with combination chemotherapy if one considers response duration, which remains a matter of weeks. These combinations have often proven more toxic and less manageable than single agents and, in many instances, have included drugs with borderline intrinsic antitumor activity in head and neck cancer.

Of the currently ongoing trials sponsored by the National Cancer Institute, there is only one random comparison of a single agent versus combination chemotherapy. This trial, conducted by the Southwest Oncology Group, is testing methotrexate alone versus a combination of methotrexate, bleomycin, and methyl CCNU. Unfortunately, MeCCNU is highly myelosuppressive and probably inactive in head and neck carcinoma (Rozencweig *et al.*, 1977b). None of the other ongoing trials of bleomycin in advanced disease is randomized. The most recent studies are investigating the high-dose DDP in combination with bleomycin, usually given as a continuous infusion. The sequential administration of this regimen and high-dose methotrexate is being explored at the Memorial Sloan-Kettering Cancer Center and at the Baltimore Research Center.

While this paper has not discussed treatment other than chemotherapy, establishment of the final role for chemotherapeutic agents will most likely involve combined modality studies. Diligent investigation of this therapeutic approach will hopefully lead to significant improvements in the prognosis of head and neck cancer.

REFERENCES

Barranco, S. C., and Humphrey, R. M. (1971). *Cancer Res. 31,* 1218–1223.

Benjamin, R. S., Wiernik, P. H., and Bachur, N. R. (1974). *Cancer 33,* 19–27.

Bonadonna, G., DeLena, M., Monfardini, S., Bartoli, C., Bajetta, E., Beretta, G., and Fossati-Bellani, F. (1972). *Eur. J. Cancer 8,* 205–215.

Bonadonna, G., Beretta, G., Tancini, G., Brambilla, C., Bajetta, E., DePalo, G. M., DeLena, M., Fossati-Bellani, F., Gasparini, M., Valagussa, P. and Veronesi, U. (1975). *Cancer Chemother. Rep., part 3 6,* 231–245.

Bonadonna, G., Tancini, G., and Bajetta, E. (1976). *Prog. Biochem. Pharmacol. II,* 172–184.

Broquet, M. A., Jacot-Descombe, E., Montandon, A., and Alberto, P. (1974). *Schweiz. Med. Wochenschr. 104,* 18–22.

Cortes, E. P., Shedd D., Albert, D. J., Ohnuma, T., and Hreshchyshyn, M. (1972). *Proc. Am. Assoc. Cancer Res. 13,* 86.

Costanzi, J. J., Loukas, D., Gagliano, R. G., Griffiths, C., and Barranco, S. (1976). *Cancer 38,* 1503–1506.

Donegan, W. L., and Harris, P. (1976). *Cancer 38,* 1479–1483.

Dowell, K. E., Armstrong, D. M., Aust, J. B., and Cruz, A. B., Jr. (1975). *Cancer 35,* 1116–1120.

Drewinko, B., Novak, J. K., and Barranco, S. C. (1972). *Cancer Res. 32,* 1206–1208.

Durkin, W. J., Pugh, R. P., Jacobs, E., Sadoff, L., Pajak, T., and Bateman, J. R. (1976). *Oncology 33,* 260–264.

E.O.R.T.C. Clinical Screening Group (1970). *Br. Med. J. 2,* 643–645.

Frei, E., III, Whang, J., Scoggins, R. B., Van Scott, E. J., Rall, D. P., and Ben, M. (1964). *Cancer Res. 24,* 1918–1925.

Frindel, E., Malaise, E., and Tubiana, M. (1968). *Cancer 22,* 611–620.

Goldsmith, M. A., and Carter, S. K. (1975). *Cancer Treatment Rev. 2.* 137–158.

Haas, C. D., Coltman, C. A., Jr., Gottlieb, J. A., Haut, A., Luce, J. K., Talley, R. W., Samal, B., Wilson, H. E., and Hoogstraten, B. (1976). *Cancer 38,* 8–12.

Halnan, K. E., Bleehen, N. M., Brewin, T. B., Deeley, T. J., Harrison, D. F. N., Howland, C., Kunkler, P. B., Ritchie, G. L., Wiltshaw, E., and Todd, I. D. H. (1972). *Br. Med. J. 4,* 635–638.

Hayes, D. M., Cvitkovic, E., Golbey, R. B., Scheiner, E., Helson, L., and Kradoff, I. H. (1977). *Cancer 39,* 1372–1381.

Huntington, M. C., DuPriest, R. W., and Fletcher, W. S. (1973). *Cancer 31,* 153–158.

Knight, E. W., Horton, J., Reilly, C., and Olson, K. B. (1972). *Proc. Am. Assoc. Cancer Res. 13,* 92.

Krakoff, I. (1975). *Cancer Chemother. Rep., Part 3 6,* 253–257.

Krakoff, I. H., Cvitkovic, E., Currie, V., Yeh, S., and LaMonte, C. (1977). *Cancer 40,* 2027–2037.

Lippman, A. J., Helson, C., Helson, L., and Krakoff, I. H. (1973). *Cancer Chemother. Rep. 57,* 191–200.

Livingston, R. B., Bodey, G. P., Gottlieb, J. A., and Frei, E., III. (1973). *Cancer Chemother. Rep. 57,* 219–224.

Livingston, R. B., Einhorn, L. H., Bodey, G. P., Burgess, M. A., Freireich, E. J., and Gottlieb, J. A. (1975a). *Cancer 36,* 327–332.

Livingston, R. B., Einhorn, L. H., Burgess, M. A., Gottlieb, J. A., and Freireich, E. J. (1975). In *Cancer Chemotherapy,* Yearbook Medical Publishers, Chicago, pp. 233–249.

Livingston, R. B., Einhorn, L. H., Burgess, M. A., and Gottlieb, J. A. (1976). *Cancer Treat. Rep. 60,* 103–105.

Lokich, J. J., and Frei, E., III. (1974). *Cancer Res. 34,* 2240–2242.

Medenica, R., Alberto, P., and Lehman, W. (1976). *Schweiz. Med. Wochenschr. 106,* 799–802.

Mosher, M. B., DeConti, R. C., and Bertino, J. R. (1972). *Cancer 30,* 56–60.

Mosley, H. S., Sasaki, T., McConnel, D. B., Merhoff, G. C., Wilson, W. L., Grage, T. B., Weiss, A. J., and Fletcher, W. S. (1976). *J. Surg. Oncol. 8,* 35–42.

Murphy, W. K., Livingston, R. B., Gehan, E., and Bodey, G. P. (1977). *Proc. Am. Assoc. Cancer Res. 18,* 190.

Ohnuma, T., Holland, J. F., Sako, K., and Shedd, D. P. (1972). *Cancer Chemother. Rep. 56.* 625–633.

Price, L. A., Hill, B. T., Calvert, A. H., Shaw, H. J. and Hughes, K. B. (1975). *Br. Med. J. 3,* 10–11.

Randolph, V. L., Vallejo, A., Strong, E. W., and Wittes, R. E. (1977). *Proc. Am. Assoc. Cancer Res. and A.S.C.O. 18,* 336.

Richard, J. M., and Sancho, H. (1973). *Biomedicine 18,* 429–435.

Richman, S. P., Livingston, R. B., Gutterman, J. U., Suen, J. Y., and Hersh, E. M. (1976). *Cancer Treatment Rep. 60.* 535–539.

Rozencweig, M., Von Hoff, D. D., Slavik, M., and Muggia, F. M. (1977a). *Ann. Intern. Med. 86,* 803–812.

Rozencweig, M., Von Hoff, D. D., and Muggia, F. M. (1977b). *Sem. Oncol. 4,* 425–429.

Stathopoulos, G., Wiltshaw, E., and Price, L. A. (1976). *Br. J. Clin. Prac. 30,* 188–189.

Takabe, Y., Miyamoto, T., Watanabe, M., and Terasima, T. (1977). *J. Natl. Cancer Inst. 59,* 1251–1255.

Tormey, D. C., Bergevin, P., Blom, J., and Petty, W. (1973). *Cancer Chemother. Rep. 57,* 413–418.

Van Dyk, J. J., Falkson, G., and Falkson, H. C. (1972). *S. Afr. Med. J. 46,* 1921–1926.

Wittes, R. E., Brescia, F., Young, C. W., Magill, G. B., Golbey, R. B., and Krakoff, I. H. (1975). *Oncology 32,* 202–207.

Wittes, R. E., Cvitkovic, E., Shah, J., Gerold, F. P., and Strong, E. W. (1977a). *Cancer Treat. Rep. 61,* 359–366.

Wittes, R. E., Spiro, R. H., Shah, J., Gerold, F. P., Koven, B., and Strong, E. W. (1977b). *Med. Ped. Oncol. 3,* 301–309.

Yagoda, A., Mukherji, B., Young, C., Etcubanas, E., Lamonte, C., Smith, J. R., Tan, C. T. C., and Krakoff, I. H. (1972). *Ann. Intern. Med. 77,* 861–880.

Yagoda, A., Lippman, A. J., Winn, R. J., Schulman, P., and Cohen, F. B. (1975). *Proc. Am. Assoc. Cancer Res. and A.S.C.O. 16,* 245.

Chapter 14

BLEOMYCIN IN THE TREATMENT OF LUNG CANCER

Robert B. Livingston

I. USE IN EXTENSIVE DISEASE

The high tissue concentrations of bleomycin achieved in lung tissue and its efficacy in squamous carcinoma of other sites, as originally reported by Japanese investigators, led to clinical trials of the drug as a single agent in patients with advanced inoperable lung cancer. The results of giving bleomycin primarily on schedules of once or twice weekly administration were uniformly disappointing (Blum *et al.*, 1973).

However, the apparent cell-cycle specificity of bleomycin for G_2 and M in both tissue culture (Barranco and Humphrey, 1971) and *in vivo* systems (Nagatsu *et al.*, 1972), coupled with the ability of vincristine to produce reversible mitotic arrest 6 to 24 hr after its administration (Frei *et al.*, 1964), led to trials of these agents as a sequential two-drug combination. We found encouraging evidence of activity in patients with lung cancer when vincristine at 0.75–1.0 mg was administered 6 hr before bleomycin in a dose of 30 u: 4/15 patients responded, included 1/5 squamous, 1/1 with small cell, and 2/9 with adenocarcinoma (Livingston *et al.*, 1973). No myelosuppression was observed, nor was toxicity seen which appeared to be unique to the combination. This led to its incorporation into a four-drug program with methyl CCNU and cyclophosphamide (COMB) (Livingston *et al.*, 1975).

Three sequential COMB programs were developed. The first involved methyl CCNU at 100 mg/m² and cyclophosphamide at 1000 mg/m² every 6 weeks, coupled with vincristine 0.75–1.0 mg in the morning and bleomycin 30 u in the afternoon, twice weekly for a total of 6 weeks (total bleomycin dose, 360 u). In the second program the dose of cyclophosphamide was reduced to 800 mg/m² and the frequency of administration of methyl CCNU and cyclophosphamide was changed to every 4 weeks; the doses of vincristine and methyl CCNU were unchanged; and the dose of bleomycin was halved, to 15 u twice weekly for a total of 12 weeks. In the final COMB regimen the other drugs were kept the same but bleomycin was again reduced, to a dose of 7.5 u twice weekly. Overall, the COMB programs led to response in 11/33 squamous, 13/15 small cell, and 3/28 adenocarcinoma patients with lung cancer. However, only in small cell patients was there evidence of an impact on overall survival: The median was 30 weeks. There appeared to be a relationship between the dose rate of bleomycin and the response rate in squamous lung carcinoma: 9/20 patients responded at weekly total doses of 30 u or more, while only 1/11 responded at the weekly total dose of 15 u. Besides the myelosuppression and gastrointestinal toxicity associated with methyl CCNU and cyclophosphamide, there were substantial side effects attributable to vincristine and bleomycin in these programs. The incidence of definite or probable bleomycin-related pulmonary fibrosis was 4%. Vincristine neuropathy was observed in practically all patients. With the administration of the vincristine–bleomycin combination for periods longer than 6 weeks there was in addition a striking 'debilitation syndrome,' characterized by lethargy, anorexia, weight loss, and apathy. This was reversible when vincristine and bleomycin were discontinued.

Other investigators have reported on COMB combinations subsequently. The Working Party for Lung Cancer, using a program identical to the third COMB combination, observed only one response in 20 patients with extensive squamous lung cancer, while one of 27 patients treated with cyclophosphamide alone responded, in a prospective, randomized trial (Wilson et al., 1976). The Western Cancer Study Group administered a somewhat different regimen: either methyl CCNU or CCNU at 50 mg/m² was given with cyclophosphamide at 400 mg/m² on day 1; vincristine 0.75 mg/m² was given 6 hr before bleomycin on day 2; and courses of the four agents were repeated only at 4 to 6 week intervals. Overall, 9/15 small cell and 5/28 squamous lung patients showed objective response, while 2/6 large cell and 1/5 adenocarcinoma patients had tumor regression. Responders lived longer than nonresponders (Armentrout et al., 1975). McMahon et al. (1975) reported their experience with a somewhat different COMB regimen in which methotrexate was added and doses of the other drugs were modified: 2/14 squamous and 0/11 adenocarcinoma patients responded, with a median survival of 13 weeks. Finally, Samson et al. (1977) recently reported their results with three different COMB combinations: The first involved twice weekly vincristine and bleomycin, the second a change to weekly, and the last, deletion of cyclophosphamide. The bleomycin dose was 15 u. Overall, responses were seen in 5/54 squamous, 2/11 adenocarcinoma, and 0/12 large cell patients, with no evidence of survival impact. There was no apparent difference among the three regimens.

The next bleomycin-containing combination, confined to patients with squamous histology, which we employed at M. D. Anderson Hospital was built on the COMB experience. Because adriamycin had now been demonstrated to have real activity as a single agent in extensive nonsmall cell carcinoma of the lung, it was incorporated into the new regimen. Vincristine and bleomycin were retained, but because of the debilitation syndrome associated with prolonged, twice weekly administration, they were given only once weekly, using the 'total' weekly dose of bleomycin which we believed necessary for therapeutic effect. CCNU was substituted for methyl CCNU, based on reports of its possible superiority over other nitrosoureas. Lastly, nitrogen mustard was substituted for cyclophosphamide because of the experience of the VA Lung Group which suggested its superiority in squamous lung cancer (Green et al., 1969). The resulting regimen (BACON) is shown in Table I. The total dose of bleomycin in this regimen was limited to 180 u. In our pilot study at M. D. Anderson Hospital and the University of Indiana, it had striking reported activity: 42% of 50 patients with squamous carcinoma of the lung, including 45% of 42 patients with extensive disease (Livingston et al., 1976). Early in the study, we observed that CCNU administration every 4 weeks was associated with cumulative myelosuppression; changing it to every 8 weeks had no unfavorable effects on response rate and eliminated this problem. The median survival of all patients was 20 weeks (16 weeks for extensive and 32 weeks for limited disease). When we analyzed survival in extensive disease patients by performance status, obtained in a retrospective fashion, we found that the median survival of patients with a Karnofsky rating of 5-7 was 20 weeks and that of patients with a rating of 1-4 was 8 weeks from the start of treatment. Both appeared to be superior to historical control results from the VA Lung Study Group of 10 and 2.5 weeks, respectively, for patients on no specific therapy.

TABLE I. BACON Regimen

Adriamycin	40 mg/m^2 every 4 weeks
Nitrogen mustard	8 mg/m^2 every 4 weeks
CCNU	65 mg/m^2 every 8 weeks [a]
Vincristine	0.75-1.0 mg in A.M., weekly x 12
Bleomycin	15 u 6 hr later, weekly x 12

[a] Initially every 4 weeks: See text.

The reported activity of the BACON regimen led to its incorporation in a large-scale, randomized trial by the Southwest Oncology Group (SWOG). This study compared BACON (as shown in Table I) to a simpler three-drug regimen (NAC) in which nitrogen mustard, adriamycin, and CCNU were given on exactly the same dose and schedule, but vincristine and bleomycin were deleted. The intent was a direct test of the hypothesis that the vincristine–bleomycin combination added to therapeutic efficacy in extensive squamous lung cancer. The results were disappointing (Livingston et al., 1977). Of 116 patients randomized to BACON and 115 to NAC, only 21 and 16%, respectively, had >50% regression of measurable tumor. If only fully evaluable patients were considered (those receiving at least 2 weeks of therapy), the response rates rose to 28% for BACON and 20% for NAC. There was no statistically significant difference between BACON and NAC response rates. There was, however, a significantly higher response rate (26 versus 13%, p < 0.05) among fully ambulatory patients versus those who were partially confined to bed (Karnofsky 5-7) or bedfast (Karnofsky 1-4) at the start of treatment.

To try to understand the discrepancy between the response rate in the BACON pilot and that reported in the SWOG study, several factors were analyzed. There did not appear to be an imbalance in known prognostic factors other than performance status (advanced age, liver or brain metastases) between the BACON and NAC groups. When compared to the pilot study, the SWOG study involved a much higher proportion of patients with prior radiation therapy to the primary tumor (51 versus 26%), although there was no difference in the proportion of such patients on the two regimens (53% for BACON, 49% for NAC). There was however, an apparent effect of prior radiation therapy on the response rate to BACON in the group-wide study: 31% for those without prior radiation versus 15% for those who had received it. No such difference in response rates was apparent for the NAC group (17 versus 18%). The fraction of patients who had life-threatening toxicity or drug-related fatality was comparable between the group study and the pilot study (11 to 18%). The response rate at M. D. Anderson Hospital to BACON was also comparable (31 versus 27%).

Although prior exposure to radiation may have adversely affected the response rate to BACON in the group-wide study, it had no overall impact on survival: The survival curves of patients with and without prior radiation to the primary tumor were superimposable. Median survival was comparable between BACON and NAC for patients in performance status 8-10 and 1-4; in the 5-7 category NAC appeared superior. Only for fully ambulatory patients (PS 8-10) was there a suggestion of superiority over historical controls, with a median survival of 26-28 weeks. The only difference favoring BACON over NAC at a statistically significant level was in the survival of fully ambulatory responders (median, 52 versus 40 weeks, respectively).

While the BACON pilot study was in progress, Lanzotti *et al.* (1976) at M. D. Anderson Hospital were studying another bleomycin-containing regimen (Bleo-COMF). In this program bleomycin was administered as a continuous infusion at either 30 or 15 u per day (depending on pulmonary status and prior radiation) for 4 days; after a 24 hr rest period, cyclophosphamide (200 mg/m^2, days 6-10), vincristine (2 mg, days 6 and 9), methotrexate (20 mg/m^2, days 6 and 9) and 5-fluorouracil (450 mg/m^2, days 6-10) were given. It was hoped that continuous infusion of bleomycin would synchronize tumor cells reversibly at the S-G$_2$ boundary, which would then enter the sensitive S phase 24 hr later. Chemotherapy was repeated at monthly intervals. Among 38 patients with extensive non-small-cell lung cancer, 15 responded (39%) including 5/14 squamous, 6/17 adenocarcinoma, and 4/7 large-cell carcinoma. Of interest is the fact that there were 8/17 responders in the group who received 15 u per day, implying no dose-response relationship to bleomycin (at these two levels) on a continuous infusion schedule. Experience by other investigators with the COMF regimen used alone (Bearden *et al.*, 1977) suggests, but does not prove, that bleomycin addition resulted in an increased response rate. The median survival in this study was 19 weeks, not substantially better than that of a historical control group from M. D. Anderson Hospital. As in the BACON studies, the median survival for responders was significantly longer than that of non-responders (36 versus 12 weeks, $p < 0.0001$). The bleomycin–COMF combination is currently being used in a study which randomizes between intravenous hyperalimentation and no intravenous hyperalimentation. No information is yet available concerning the results of this study.

In a small series who received bleomycin as a continuous infusion at 7.5 u/m²/day followed by 'S-phase' active therapy with hydroxyurea or methotrexate, Costanzi et al. (1976) observed no responses in five patients with extensive squamous lung cancer.

In summary, bleomycin has been employed widely in combination chemotherapy programs for extensive non-small-cell carcinoma of the lung. Although both the BACON and bleomycin-COMF combinations offer a response rate which seems to be higher than that of single-agent treatment programs, neither has been translated into improved survival for the majority of patients. Furthermore, BACON was not superior overall to a simpler combination in which bleomycin and vincristine were deleted. The only place for further investigation of bleomycin in these patients would seem to be on a continuous infusion schedule, probably in combination with adriamycin or other drugs.

II. USE IN REGIONAL DISEASE WITH RADIATION THERAPY

Samuels et al. (1975) were the first to carry out a study of bleomycin in combination with other drugs and radiation, among patients with non-oat-cell carcinoma of the lung which was locally advanced and inoperable (regional or limited disease). Bleomycin was given intramuscularly in a fixed dose of 15 u twice weekly for 3 weeks; vincristine was given intravenously in a fixed dose of 2.0 mg once weekly for 3 weeks; and methotrexate was given orally at 25–30 mg twice weekly for 3 weeks. After a 2 week rest period, split-course radiation therapy was started, with 3000 rads in 10 fractions over 2 weeks delivered as a first course. The patient was then reevaluated after a 4 week rest period. If no evidence of distant metastases had developed, a second course of 3000 rads in 2 weeks was delivered, shielding the spinal cord for the final 1500 rads. Chemotherapy in the same dose and schedule was resumed after recovery from radiation, usually within 2–4 weeks. It was given for one additional course. Objective regression of measurable tumor >50% was noted in nine of 21 patients with squamous histology and in 0/6 with adenocarcinoma. Nearly complete responses to chemotherapy alone were seen in two patients, and five of the squamous patients went on to complete responses with the addition of radiation. No survival benefit was apparent in adenocarcinoma, but the median survival for the 21 patients with squamous histology was 52+ weeks; all were fully ambulatory at the start of treatment. There was no significant difference in median survival of the entire group, compared to historical controls from M. D. Anderson Hospital who received only split-course radiation therapy (42 versus 39 weeks), nor were the overall survival curves significantly different. However, survival beyond 18 months was projected for 30% of the combined treatment group, and was observed in only 15% on radiation alone. Only one patient in this series developed clinical interstitial pneumonitis after bleomycin, in a total dose of 300 u. This was reversible. Ten patients on the combined drug program had severe stomatitis, usually after four doses of bleomycin and methotrexate (at 2 weeks). Seven patients had severe radiation esophagitis, without unusual sequelae.

Other studies of bleomycin and radiation therapy have involved its simultaneous administration with radiation. The rationale for this lies in the ability of bleomycin, in tissue culture (Bleehen *et al.*, 1974) and in some *in vivo* systems (Jorgensen, 1972), to potentiate the cytotoxic local effects of radiation. This appears to occur through prevention of repair of what would otherwise be sublethal injury to DNA, with loss of the 'shoulder' characteristic of radiation survival curves. Chan *et al.* (1976) reported a small, randomized study in which patients with unresectable squamous carcinoma of the lung were treated with either radiation alone (2000 rads in 5 days–rest 3 weeks–repeat 2000 rads in 5 days, with shielding of cord and esophagus) or the same radiation with added bleomycin, 10 u/m^2 twice weekly for 6 weeks. There were 15 patients in each treatment group and almost all were fully ambulatory. Tumor regression >50% was observed in 4/15 patients with radiation alone and 7/15 on combined treatment. More impressively, median survival was more than twice as long in the combined treatment group, 13 versus 6 months. At 2 years of follow-up, 0/15 in the radiation along and 4/15 in the combined treatment group were alive. Local control also appeared to be superior in the group on combined therapy: There were eight local failures in the control group and three in the combined therapy group. Toxicity of the two regiments appeared comparable, except that one patient in the combined treatment group developed bilateral, diffuse pulmonary fibrosis (at a total bleomycin dose of 274 mg).

Subsequently, Chan *et al.* (1977) have extended their studies of simultaneous radiation and chemotherapy to include adriamycin as well as bleomycin. Radiation therapy was delivered as in the previous study by the rapid split-course technique: 2000 rads in 5 days, repeated after 3 weeks with shielding of the spinal cord. Adriamycin and bleomycin were given during each course of radiation, with the former at 40 mg/m^2 on the first day and the latter at 10 units/m^2 (15 u) on day 1 and 4. After a 3 week rest period, adriamycin was given at 50 mg/m^2 and bleomycin at 15 u. These were repeated every 3 weeks to tumor progression or a cumulative adriamycin dose of 450 mg/m^2. Of 40 patients treated with this combined program, 33 had regional, inoperable non-oat-cell carcinoma: 19 squamous, seven adenocarcinoma, and seven large-cell carcinoma. Approximately one-fourth achieved complete regression of measurable tumor and two-thirds had > 50% regression. Long-term survival in this group appears at least comparable to that in the earlier study of radiation plus bleomycin alone, and both are suggestively superior to that of historical controls treated with similar radiation alone (Abramson and Cavanaugh, 1973; Scruggs *et al.*, 1974).

Large-scale controlled studies will be necessary to answer the question of whether bleomycin really provides useful potentiation of radiation in the setting of regional lung cancer. These should probably be confined to patients with non-oat-cell histologies, since results reported by Einhorn *et al.* (1976) suggest a dangerous interaction of simultaneous bleomycin and radiation. The reasons for this remain obscure but there seems to be real potentiation of the risk of bleomycin lung damage, which is apparently unique to the oat-cell situation.

REFERENCES

Abramson, M., and Cavanaugh, P. (1973). *Radiology 108,* 685–687.

Armentrout, S., Bateman, J., and Pajak, T. (1975). *Proc. Am. Assoc. Cancer Res. and A.S.C.O. 16,* 242.

Barranco, S., and Humphrey, R. (1971). *Cancer Res. 31,* 1218–1223.

Bearden, J., Coltman, C., Moon, T., Costanzi, J., Saiki, J., Balcerzak, S., Rivkin, S., Morrison, F., Lane, M., and Spigel, S. (1977). *Cancer 39,* 21–26.

Bleehen, N., Gillies, N., and Twentyman, P. (1974). *Br. J. Radiol. 47,* 346–351.

Blum, R., Carter, S., and Agre, K. (1973). *Cancer 31,* 903.

Chan, P., Byfield, J., Kagan, A., and Aronstam, E. (1976). *Cancer 37,* 2671–2676.

Chan, P., Byfield, J., Aronstam, E., and Kagan, A. (1977). *Proc. Am. Assoc. Cancer Res. and A.S.C.O. 17,* 347.

Costanzi, J., Loukas, D., Gagliano, R., Griffiths, C., and Barranco, S. (1976). *Cancer 38,* 1503–1506.

Einhorn, L., Krause, M., Hornback, N., and Furnas, B. (1976). *Cancer 37,* 2414–2416.

Frei, E., III, Whang, J., and Scoggins, R. (1964). *Cancer Res. 24,* 1918–1925.

Green, R., Humphrey, E., Close, H., and Patno, M. (1969). *Am J. Med. 46,* 516–525.

Jorgensen, S. (1972). *Eu. J. Cancer 8,* 531–534.

Lanzotti, V., Thomas, D., Holoye, P., Boyle, L., Smith, T., and Samuels, M. (1976). *Cancer Treatment Rep. 60,* 61–68.

Livingston, R., Bodey, G., Gottlieb, J., and Frei, E., III. (1973). *Cancer Chemother. Rep. 57,* 219–224.

Livingston, R., Einhorn, L., Gottlieb, J., and Freireich, E. (1975). *Cancer 36,* 327–332.

Livingston, R., Fee, W., Einhorn, L., Burgess, M., Freireich, E., Gottlieb, J., and Farber, M. (1976). *Cancer 37,* 1237–1242.

Livingston, R., Heilbrun, L., Lehane, D., Costanzi, J., Bottomley, R., Palmer R., Stuckey, W., and Hoogstraten, B. (1977). *Cancer Treatment Rep. 61* (in press).

McMahon, L., Jones, S., Durie, B., and Salmon, S. (1975). *Cancer Lett. 1,* 97–102.

Nagatsu, M., Richart, R., and Lambert, A. (1972). *Cancer Res. 32,* 1966–1970.

Samson, M., Baker, L., Fraile, R., Izbicki, R., and Vaitkevicuis, V. (1977). *Cancer Treatment Rep. 61,* 59–64.

Samuels, M., Barkley, H., Holoye, P., Rosenberg, P., and Smith, T. (1975). *Cancer Chemother. Rep. 59,* 377–383.

Scruggs, H., El-Mahdi, A., Marks, R., and Constable, W. (1974). *Am. J. Roentgen Radiat. Ther. 121,* 754–760.

Wilson, H., Lagakos, S., Bodey, G., Gutieruz, A., Selawry, O., Sealy, R., and Ryall, R. (1976). *Proc. Am. Assoc. Cancer Res. and A.S.C.O. 17,* 294.

Chapter 15

A BLEOMYCIN COMBINATION FOR DISSEMINATED CERVICAL CANCER

Laurence H. Baker

I. INTRODUCTION

Despite the fact that cervical carcinoma is the sixth most lethal variety of cancer in American women there have been relatively few formal chemotherapeutic studies of this disease (Kaufman, 1970; Talley, 1970). Following the encouraging pilot experience at Wayne State University (Baker et al., 1976) using a combination of mitomycin C, vincristine, and bleomycin in patients with disseminated or far-advanced cervical carcinoma, the Southwest Oncology Group (Baker et al., 1977b) studied an additional 130 patients with this disease. This cooperative group study represents the largest chemotherapy study of cervical cancer to date. This pilot study and cooperative group study form the basis of this report.

Over a 5 year period prior to the pilot study, our institution observed 17 responses (18%) out of 92 patients treated with a variety of single chemotherapeutic agents. Eleven of those responses resulted from porfiromycin therapy (38 patients treated) and have been reported by our group (Izbicki et al., 1972). We had previously shown that little difference exists in clinical efficacy between mitomycin C and its N-methyl analog, porfiromycin (Baker et al., 1977).

Wasserman and Carter (1977) recently reviewed the status of chemotherapy studies of cervical carcinoma based on the literature and studies reported to the Division of Cancer Treatment of the National Cancer Institute. They concluded that there are 12 drugs with evidence of clinical activity including mitomycin C, vincristine, and bleomycin. Seven of the drugs have significant alkylating activity and include cyclophosphamide, chlorambucil, melphalan, methyl CCNU, hexamethylmelamine, mitomycin C, and porfiromycin. Ochoa *et al.* (1977) reported the benefits of bleomycin infusion in cervical cancer.

Vincristine has been shown to produce a marked increase in the mitotic index (Frei *et al.,* 1964; Meyer and Donaldson, 1969; Shepstone *et al.*, 1973) in normal, as well as tumor cells in 6-12 hours, whereas bleomycin has been shown to exert its cytotoxic effect on cells in G_2 and M (Barranco and Humphrey, 1971; Nagatsu *et al.*, 1972).

Livingston *et al.* (1973) have shown that the combination of vincristine and bleomycin given 6 hours apart has produced modest clinical benefit in squamous cell carcinomas.

Combination chemotherapy has produced higher remission rates and, more importantly, more complete responses than single-agent therapy in several malignant diseases (Moore *et al.*, 1968; Masterson and Nelson, 1965; DePalo *et al.*, 1973; Suzuki *et al.*, 1970; Papadimitriou *et al.*, 1974; Barlow *et al.*, 1973; Blum *et al.,* 1973; Halnan *et al.*, 1972; Ansfield *et al.,* 1972; Cooper, 1969; DeVita *et al.*, 1970; Freireich *et al.*, 1964; Hoogstraten *et al.*, 1969; Li *et al.*, 1960; Luce *et al.,* 1971). One of the advantages of combining agents of dissimilar toxicities is that the individual agents can often be employed in full therapeutic doses. An additional advantage is that such agents often have different sites of action as well as different mechanisms of action. The combination of mitomycin C, vincristine, and bleomycin fulfills the above criteria of differing limiting toxicities, sites of action, and mechanisms of action (Barranco and Humphrey, 1971; Frei *et al.*, 1964; Livingston *et al.*, 1973; Meyer and Donaldson, 1969; Nagatsu *et al.*, 1972; Shepstone *et al.*, 1973).

II. MATERIALS AND METHODS

In both studies all patients had incurable carcinomas of the uterine cervix and were no longer considered candidates for further surgery or radiotherapy. All patients had histologic proof of their malignancy as well as documented evidence of dissemination or recurrence. No patient was to have had an uncontrolled active site of infection, evidence of renal impairment (serum creatinine >1.5 mg%), or to have received prior treatment with any of the drugs in the study.

The initial pilot series consisted of 30 patients seen on our service who were eligible for this study and were entered between May 1973 and November 1974. The mean age of these women was 49.1 years (range 26-74 years).

Prior radiotherapy had been given to 25 of these patients. Sixteen patients received both radium insertion and external ^{60}Co radiotherapy. Nine patients received only ^{60}Co radiotherapy to the entire pelvis (4000-5600 rads). Major prior surgery had been done in nine patients of the study group. Hysterectomy was performed in eight patients, whereas one patient had a previous segmental resection of the lung for metastatic disease. Biopsy was the only surgical procedure in the remaining 21 patients. Only one patient had received any prior chemotherapy (cyclophosphamide). This patient did not benefit from the prior chemotherapy.

All patients had extensive metastatic disease. Lesions recorded for evidence of dissemination were located in: lung (11 patients); pelvis (nine patients); lymph node (seven patients); genitourinary tract (four patients); liver (three patients); skeleton (two patients); brain (two patients); and skin (one patient).

Patients were considered to have received an adequate trial of this therapy if one complete course was administered (6 weeks). Complete response was defined as total disappearance of observable tumor and partial response defined as 50% or more decrease in the product of the perpendicular diameters of all measurable tumor.

Treatment consisted of vincristine 0.5 mg/m² twice weekly for 12 weeks beginning on day 1, bleomycin 6 mg/m² intramuscularly (IM) 6 hours following vincristine administration for 12 weeks, and mitomycin 20 mg/m² IV every 6 weeks beginning on day 2. Subsequent mitomycin doses were adjusted to the previous white blood cell and platelet nadir. Vincristine and bleomycin were discontinued if significant toxicity resulted from either agent.

The group study was conducted from October 1974 until October 1976, and 130 patients were entered into the protocol. The first 58 patients received vincristine 0.5 mg/m² twice weekly for 12 weeks beginning on day 1, bleomycin 6 u/m² IM or IV 6 hours following the vincristine administration for 12 weeks and mitomycin C 20 mg/m² IV every 6 weeks beginning on day 2 (identical schedule to pilot experience). Beginning in October 1975, patients were randomly allocated to vincristine 0.5 mg/m² IV on days 1 and 4 for two cycles, bleomycin 30 u per day as a continuous 96 hour infusion for two cycles (total dose 240 u), and mitomycin C 20 mg/m² on day 2 of each cycle, then 10 mg/m² every 6-8 weeks thereafter, or vincristine 0.5 mg/m² once weekly for 24 weeks beginning on day 1, bleomycin 6 u/m² IM or IV 6 hours following vincristine administration and mitomycin C, 20 mg/m² IV every 6 weeks. These later two schedules were devised in an attempt to reduce drug toxicity. Twenty-five patients received the once weekly schedule while 47 patients received the bleomycin infusion schedule. Subsequent mitomycin doses were adjusted to the previous white blood cell and platelet count nadirs. Vincristine doses were omitted or permanently discontinued if the patient developed evidence of severe vincristine toxicity such as severe constipation, muscle weakness, or foot drop. The administration of laxatives, particularly in the elderly, was recommended. The second course of bleomycin infusion was given only if repeat pulmonary function studies permitted continuation of the drug in the judgment of the managing physician.

Of the 130 patients entered into this study, four were not eligible. Seven patients were not evaluable for response or toxicity because of major protocol violations (four patients); insufficient data (two patients); and lost to follow-up (one patient).

Four patients were evaluable for toxicity but not response (early death, lost to follow-up, or refused further treatment). Thus, 50 evaluable patients were treated with the twice weekly bleomycin schedule; 24 patients with the once weekly bleomycin schedule, and 41 with the infusion bleomycin schedule.

All but nine of the patients received prior radiotherapy. Six patients received internal radiation alone; and 61 received both internal and external radiation. No significant differences existed between the three treatment arms concerning prior irradiation.

Surgery with a curative intent was previously performed on 36 patients. Surgery to relieve a complication of the cervical cancer (bowel obstruction, urinary obstruction, etc.) was performed on additional 14 patients. In 56 patients the only surgical procedure was that of a biopsy. Again, no significant statistical differences existed between the three treatment arms regarding prior surgeries.

The most common metastatic site followed was the pelvis (40%). Other sites in decreasing order of frequency were the lung, lymph nodes, liver, abdomen, and skeleton (see Table I).

The median age of the women studied was 50 years (range 23-83 years).

TABLE I. Frequency and Response of Metastatic Signal Lesion (SWOG Series)

	Twice weekly schedule (N=50)	Once weekly schedule (N=24)	Infusion schedule (N=41)	All patients (N=115)
Abdomen				
Occurrence	1	1	5	7(6.1%)
Response	1	0	2	3(42.9%)
Liver				
Occurrence	5	1	3	9(7.8%)
Response	3	1	1	5(55.6%)
Lung				
Occurrence	19	5	8	32(27.8%)
Response	10	2	4	16(50.0%)
Lymph nodes				
Occurrence	6	4	7	17(14.9%)
Response	6	1	4	11(64.7%)
Pelvis				
Occurrence	16	11	18	45(39.1%)
Response	10	2	5	17(37.8%)
Skeleton				
Occurrence	3	2	0	5(4.3%)
Response	0	0	0	0

III. RESULTS

In the initial pilot series 30 patients all with disseminated or recurrent squamous cell carcinoma of the cervix were entered.

Table II describes the clinical effect of this therapy. Three patients died before 6 weeks of therapy had elapsed. In two of the 13 responders, clinical disease totally disappeared. Median duration of response was 4 months (range 1-11 months).

TABLE II. Therapeutic Effect in Pilot Study

Total entered	Objective response	Increasing disease	No change	Inadequate trial
30	13	10	4	3
				95% confidence limits
Responders/patients evaluable = 13/27 = 48%				30–68%
Responders/patients entered = 13/30 = 43%				26–61%

Table III shows the lesions measured as documentation of response. In only two patients did disease regress in a previously irradiated area. The majority of patients had tumor regression in soft tissue of visceral metastases not previously irradiated.

Toxicity from this combination was considerable, since the drugs all had a different primary toxicity pattern when used as single agents. The toxic reactions encountered as a result of the combination of drugs appeared to be accumulation of the expected toxicities when these drugs were used as single agents.

In the Southwest Oncology Group study, of the 50 evaluable patients receiving twice weekly, eight patients (16%) achieved complete clinical remission and 22 (44%) experienced partial response. Of patients who received once weekly vincristine and bleomycin, 24 were fully evaluable. One patient (4%) had a complete response while five (21%) had partial response. Forty-one patients were fully evaluable in the bleomycin infusion group. Six patients (15%) had complete responses and 10 (24%) had partial remissions. The twice weekly schedule appeared significantly superior in terms of response rate ($p < 0.01$). Lymph node metastases (usually inguinal or supraclavicular), hepatic metastases, and pulmonary metastasis responded more frequently to the drug regimens than intraabdominal pelvic or skeletal

TABLE III. Measurable Lesions in Responders (Pilot Series)

Site	No. of patients
Lymph nodes	6
Lung	6
Pelvis	3
Liver	2
Bone	1
Skin	1

lesions (Table I). Responses were generally longer-lasting in the infusion treated group (16 weeks versus 9 for the twice weekly and 11 weeks for the once weekly schedule); however, the differences were not of statistical significance. The major toxicities encountered were leukopenia, thrombocytopenia, peripheral neuropathy, mucositis, weakness, dermatitis, fever and chills, nausea and vomiting, pulmonary fibrosis, and alopecia. In essence, the toxicities were a function of the drugs and their doses and resembled closely the toxicity reported for each of the drugs individually. Peripheral neuropathy, muscle weakness, and alopecia were much more frequent and severe in the twice weekly schedule. Both the once weekly and infusion schedules significantly reduced the toxicity. Indeed, the infusion schedule produced significantly less leukopenia ($p = < 0.025$) than either of the bolus bleomycin schedules (Median nadir of WBD 3.25×10^3 cells versus 2.40×10^3 and 2.68×10^3, respectively). Of patients receiving the twice weekly schedules, 38% had white blood cell nadirs less than 2000 compared to 27% for the once weekly schedule and 12% for the infusion schedule. A ridit analysis of the toxicities confirms the superiority of the infusion schedule in terms of producing less toxicity.

As would be anticipated, the twice weekly schedule produced much more peripheral neuropathy, muscle weakness, dermatitis, and alopecia than the other two schedules. Tabulation of the toxicity data is shown in Tables IV and V.

Survival data of all patients treated are shown (Fig. 1). Both the twice weekly and infusion schedules produced significantly longer survival than the once weekly

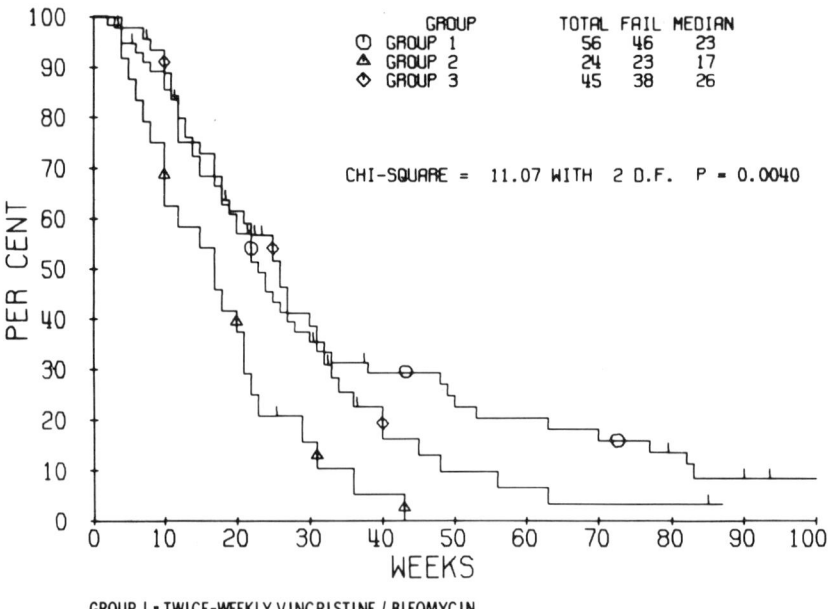

GROUP	TOTAL	FAIL	MEDIAN
GROUP 1	56	46	23
GROUP 2	24	23	17
GROUP 3	45	38	26

CHI-SQUARE = 11.07 WITH 2 D.F. P = 0.0040

GROUP 1 - TWICE-WEEKLY VINCRISTINE / BLEOMYCIN
GROUP 2 - ONCE-WEEKLY VINCRISTINE / BLEOMYCIN
GROUP 3 - BLEOMYCIN INFUSION

Fig. 1. SWOG 7412 MOB survival (all pts).

TABLE IV. Toxicity — Myelosuppression (SWOG Study)

	Leukopenia (lowest WBC x 10^3 cells)					
	0 – .99	1.0 – 1.99	2.0 – 2.99	3.0 – 3.99	≥ 4.0
Twice weekly (N=53)	6	14	17	5	11
Once weekly (N=22)	1	5	7	2	7
Infusion (N=42)	0	5	12	13	12
Total (N=117)	7	24	36	20	30

	Thrombocytopenia (lowest platelet count x 10^3)					
	0 – 25	25 – 49	50 – 74	75 – 99	≥100
Twice weekly	9	9	9	3	23
Once weekly	2	3	3	2	12
Infusion	3	6	6	7	20
Total	14	18	18	12	55

TABLE V. Toxicity (SWOG Study)

	Twice weekly [a] (53)				Once weekly [a] (22)				Infusion [a] (42)			
	1	2	3	Total	1	2	3	Total	1	2	3	Total
Peripheral neuropathy	6	13	15	34 (64%)	1	2	–	3 (13%)	1	3	0	4 (10%)
Muscle weakness	5	5	5	15 (28%)	–	1	3	4 (17%)	0	1	2	3 (7%)
Stomatitis	2	5	4	11 (21%)	1	–	1	2 (8%)	1	–	5	6 (14%)
Nausea	8	9	1	18 (34%)	6	1	1	8 (33%)	6	8	1	15 (36%)
Vomiting	3	7	1	11 (21%)	5	1	1	7 (29%)	4	2	1	7 (17%)
Fever and chills	5	4	–	9 (17%)	1	2	1	4 (18%)	–	3	–	3 (7%)
Dermatitis	3	4	6	13 (25%)	1	1	–	2 (8%)	2	2	1	5 (12%)
Pulmonary toxicity	3	5	6	14 (26%)	1	1	–	2 (8%)	4	2	–	6 (14%)
Alopecia	5	8	6	19 (36%)	1	2	–	3 (13%)	1	2	3	6 (14%)

[a] 1 = mild; 2 = moderate; 3 = severe.

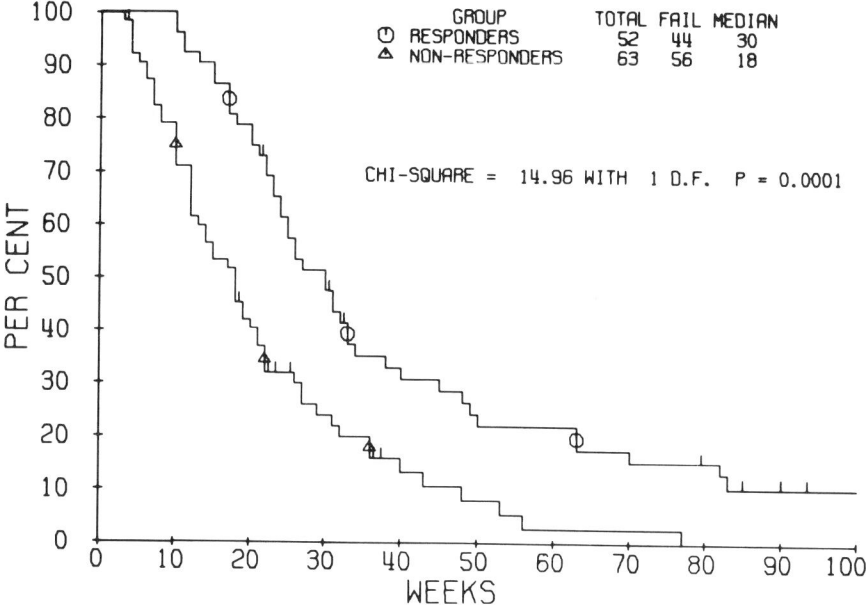

Fig. 2. SWOG 7412 MOB survival by response.

schedule (*p* = <0.0l). Median survival for the infusion group was 26 weeks versus 23 weeks for the twice weekly group and 17 weeks for the once weekly group. Responding patients lived longer than nonresponding patients (*p*<0.01). The median survival time of the responders was 30 weeks versus 14 weeks for the nonresponders (Fig. 2).

IV. DISCUSSION

Despite the relative lack of basic pharmacokinetic data of any of the three agents used in this study, it appears that tumor response and patient survival correlate with the dose of bleomycin. The once weekly schedule of bleomycin was clearly inferior to the twice weekly and continuous infusion schedules both in the response rate and survival. Compared to those who received bleomycin by continuous infusion patients receiving the twice weekly schedule of bleomycin experienced significantly more of a debilitating form of drug toxicity. Profound weakness was a serious and frequent side effect of the twice weekly schedule. This side effect is probably a function of the vincristine dosage as much as the bleomycin.

It should also be noted that the dose and schedule of administration of bleomycin affects the leukopenic toxicity of other agents and/or is myelosuppressive by itself. Significantly less leukopenia was observed in the once weekly and infusion schedules than the twice weekly schedule.

The responses to this combination were relatively short-lived, raising the possibility that it might best be viewed as an induction regime. In order to maintain the remission, other therapies may be necessary. Furthermore, this therapy may be of benefit in conjunction with radiation therapy as the initial treatment for patients with Stage III and Stage IV lesions.

Recently, Miyamoto (1977) reported that the combination of mitomycin and bleomycin produced dramatic response rates in Japanese women, raising the question of the necessity of vincristine. Yet Holland *et al.* (1973) and later Hreshchyshyn (1963) reported that vincristine is indeed an effective single agent in cervical carcinoma patients.

V. CONCLUSIONS

We tried to explore some of the known pharmacokinetic data available to date to improve the therapy of a traditionally refractory human cancer. Whether the administration of these agents in this fashion accounted for the improved response data cannot be stated at this time. Empiric reasoning was also used to develop this combination. These drugs have different sites of action, different mechanisms of action, and, perhaps most important to the chemotherapist, different toxicities. These different toxicities allowed the drugs to be combined in nearly full doses. Nonetheless, some progress has been made in the treatment of disseminated cervical cancer.

REFERENCES

Ansfield, F. J., Ramierez, G., Korbitz, B. C., and Davis, H. L., Jr. (1972). *Cancer Chemother. Rep. V, 55*, 183–187.

Baker, L. H., Opipari, M. I., and Izbicki, R. M. (1976) *Cancer 38*, 2222–2224.

Baker, L. H., Izbicki, R. M., and Vaitkevicius, V. K. (1977a). *Med. Pediatr. Oncol. 2*, 207–213.

Baker, L. H., Opipari, M. I., Wilson, H., Bottomley, R., and Coltman, C. A., Jr. (1978). *Obstet. Gynecol. 52*, 146–150.

Barlow, J. J., Piver, M. S., Chuang, J. J., Cortes, E. P., Ohnuma, T., and Holland, J. F. (1973). *Cancer 32*, 735–743.

Barranco, S. C., and Humphrey, R. M. (1971). *Cancer Res. 31*, 1218–1233.

Blum, R. H., Carter, S. K., and Agre, K. (1973). *Cancer 31*, 903–914.

Cooper, R. G. (1969). *Proc. Am. Assoc. Cancer Res. 10*, 15.

DePalo, G. M., Bajetta, E., Luciani, L., Musumaeci, R., Di Re, F., and Bonnadonna, G. (1973). *Cancer Chemother. Rep. 57*, 429–435.

DeVita, V. T., Serpick, A. A., and Carbone, P. P. (1970). *Ann. Intern. Med. 73*, 881–895.

Frei, E., III, Hang, J. W., Scoggins, R. B., Van Scott, E. J., Rall, D. P., and Ben, M. (1964). *Cancer Res. 24*, 1918–1925.

Freireich, E., Karon, M., and Frei, E., III (1964). *Proc. Am. Assoc. Cancer Res. 50*, 20 (abstr.).

Halnan, K. E., Bleaham, N. M., Brewin, T. B., Deeley, T. J., Harrison, D. F. N., Holland, C., Kunkler, P. B., Ritchie, G. L., Wittshaw, E., and Todd, I. D. H. (1972). *B. Med. J. 4*, 635.

Holland, J. F., Scharlou, C., Gailani, G., Krant, M. J., Olson, K. B., Horton, J., Shnider, B. I., Lynch, J. J., Owens, A., Carbone, P. P., Colsky, J., Grob, D., Miller, S. P., and Hall, T. C. (1973). *Cancer Res. 33*, 1258–1264.

Hoogstraten, B., Owens, A. H., Lenhard, R. E., Glidewell, O. J., Leone, L. A., Olson, K. B., Harley, J. B., Towsend, S. R., Miller, S. P., Spurr, C. L. (1969). *Blood 33*, 370-378.

Hreshchyshyn, M. (1963). *Proc. Am. Assoc. Cancer Res. 4*, 29.

Izbicki, R. M., Al-Sarraf, M., Reed, M. L., Vaughn, C. B., and Vaitkevicus, V. K. (1972). *Cancer Chemother. Rep.* (Part 1) *56*, 5.

Kaufman, R. J. (1970). *Acad. Med. NJ B-11 16*, 123-130.

Li, M. C., Whitmore, W. F., Golbey, R., and Grabstald, H. (1960). *J. Am. Med. Assoc. 174*, 1291-1299.

Livingston, R., Bodey, G. P., Gottleib, J. A., and Frei, E., III. (1973). *Cancer Chemother. Rep. 57*, 219-224.

Luce, J. K., Gamble, J. F., Wilson, H. E., Monto, R. W., Isaacs, B. L., Palmer, R. L., Coltman, C. A., Hewlett, J. S., Gehan, E. A., and Frei, E., III. (1971). *Cancer 28*, 306-317.

Masterson, J. G., and Nelson, J. H. (1965). *Am. J. Obstet. Gynecol. 93*, 1102-1111.

Meyer, J., and Donaldson, R. (1969). *Arch. Pathol. 87*, 479-490.

Miyamoto, T. (1977). *Gan To Kagaku Ryoho 4*, 273-291.

Moore, G. E., Bross, I. D. J., Ausman, R., Nakler, S., Jones, R., Slack, N., and Rimm, A. A. (1968). *Cancer Chemother. Rep. 52*, 675-684.

Nagatsu, M., Richart, R. M., and Lambert, A. (1972). *Cancer Res. 32*, 1966-1970.

Ochoa, M., Beattie, E. J., Tamimi, H., Watson, R. C., Woodruff, J. M., and Lewis, J. L. (1977). *Cancer Ther. Abstr. 18 3*, 461.

Papadimitriou, G. Razis, D., Panopoulos, C., and Gnafakis, N. (1974). *Int. Surg. 59*, 472-475.

Shepstone, B. J., Sealy, R., Greenstein, A., and Rapley, L. F. (1973). *S. Afr. Med. J. 47*, 1603-1605.

Suzuki, M., Murai, A., Watanabe, T., and Nundkawa, O. (1970). *Acta Med. Biol. Niigata 17*, 259-275.

Talley, R. W. (1970). *Geriatrics 25*, 113-125.

Wasserman, T. H., and Carter, S. T. (1977). *Cancer Treatment Rev. 4*, 25-46.

Chapter 16

A SEQUENTIAL COMBINATION OF BLEOMYCIN AND MITOMYCIN C (B-M) IN THE TREATMENT OF METASTATIC CERVICAL CANCER

Tadaaki Miyamoto

I. INTRODUCTION

For the last two decades a number of chemotherapeutic drugs such as vincristine, actinomycin D, 5-fluorouracil, 6-mercaptopurine, chlorambucil, methotrexate, and adriamycin in single and systemic use have been tested in the treatment of an advanced cervical cancer (Clasysse et al., 1976). However, no favorable results have as yet been reported. There were exceptions to this finding with bleomycin (BLM) and mitomycin-C (MMC) (Blum et al., 1973; Moor et al., 1968). As a next step, combinations of these drugs have been designed to enhance response, ending in rather disappointing results, with the exception of a combination of methotrexate and bleomycin (Conroy et al., 1976).

In contrast, the combination of BLM and MMC resulted in an excellent response to metastatic cervical cancer. The results are presented in this paper.

II. MATERIALS AND METHODS

A. Patients

From July 1974 to September 1977, 26 patients with metastatic cervical cancer have been treated with BLM and MMC in a sequential manner at the Hospital of the

Schedule of B-M Therapy

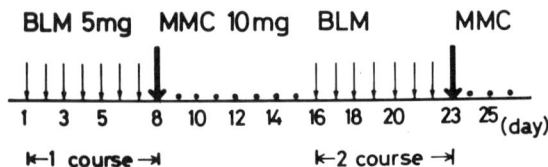

Fig. 1. An illustrated protocol of bleomycin and mitomycin-C (B-M) therapy.

National Institute of Radiological Sciences. Twenty-three patients among them, evaluated objectively, were entered in this study. All of the patients with histologically squamous carcinoma had distant metastases in lung, bone, liver, skin, lymph node, and other sites. They had received radical radiotherapy previously, but no chemotherapy.

B. Drug Regimen

The protocol for the combined use of BLM and MMC is illustrated in Fig. 1. BLM was administered by drip infusion at a daily dose of 5 mg for 7 consecutive days, followed by an intravenous injection of MMC at a dose of 10 mg on day 8. This is one course of BLM and MMC (B-M) therapy for remission induction. The course is repeated three or five times with 1 week rest periods between courses.

C. Evaluation of Response

Complete remission (CR) was defined as disappearance of all clinical evidence of tumor. Some tumors receiving B-M therapy tended to change into a scarlike appearance on the roentgenogram. Therefore, CR for the patients with these tumors was carefully identified by confirming no tumor regrowth over 3 months. Partial remission (PR) was defined as more than 50% decrease in tumor volume. Other responses were classified as no remission (NR).

III. RESULTS

A. Response to Treatment

As shown in Table I, overall response rate was 95.6%, which subdivided into 74% in CR and 21% in PR. Fifteen patients treated with B-M therapy alone were 73% in CR, 20% in PR, and 6% in NR. Another eight patients received simultanous or sequential combination radiotherapy of about 4,000 rads to some part of metastatic

TABLE I.   Response Rate (%) to B-M Therapy (Metastatic Cervical Cancer)[a]

	CR	PR	NR	CR+PR
Total	74 (17/23)	21 (5/23)	4 (1/23)	95.6
B-M alone	73 (11/15)	20 (3/15)	6 (1/15)	93.0
B-M + radiotherapy	75 (6/8)	25 (2/8)	0 (0/8)	100.00

[a] CR—complete response; PR—partial response; NR—no response.

lesion with B-M therapy. They had 100% total response rate, 75% CR rate, and 25% PR rate.

Table II shows the complete response rates of tumors in the various organs involved that were obtained by using only chemotherapy. Although there was a small number of patients, CR rate expressed in percentage was 100% (3/3) in skin, 75% (3/4) in liver, 71% (10/14) in lung, 66% (6/9) in bone, and 57% (4/7) in lymph node. These results show that it was difficult for patients whose tumors involved the lymph node to achieve CR. Such high and powerful response made it possible to eradicate all signs and symptoms within two B-M courses on the average (Miyamoto *et al.*, in press).

B.   Toxicity

Table III shows the toxic effects and their frequency in B-M therapy. The average doses of BLM and MMC used in this study for remission induction were 100 and 35 mg, respectively. The frequency of leukopenia and thrombocytopenia was 24 and 20%, respectively. The value seems not to be increased significantly compared with that in single-agent use of MMC. It must be carefully noted that lung fibrosis became more frequent with combination of both drugs than in single-agent use. These are dose-limiting toxicities to B-M therapy. Others were not dose-limiting except for allergic reactions and increases significantly compared with those in single-agent use of BLM (Blum *et al.*, 1973).

TABLE II.   Complete Response Rate to B-M Therapy

Metastatic site	Percentage response
Lung	71 (10/14)
Bone	66 (6/9)
Lymph node	57 (4/7)
Liver	75 (3/4)
Skin	100 (3/3)
Other sites	66 (2/3)

TABLE III.   Bleomycin-Mitomycin C (B-M) Toxicity

Toxicity	Frequency (%)
Leukopenia	24
(WBC < 2000/mm^3)	
Thrombocytopenia	20
(platelet < 7.5 x 10^4/mm^3)	
Lung fibrosis	8
Alopecia	12
Fever >38° C	8
Stomatitis	4
Proteinuria	4
Drug eruption and	16
hepatotoxicity	

C. Relapse and Retreatment

As shown in Table IV, all of the patients without maintenance therapy had re-currence 4.5 months after achievement of CR. However, oral administration of Carboquon at a daily dose of 0.5 mg for 1 to 6 months inhibited the recurrence efficiently. The patients with relapse due to insufficient B-M courses responded to the retreatment with B-M regimen as well as at first treatment, but finally had no CR because of the increased toxicities of both drugs.

D. Survivors and Cause of Death

There were 13 complete responders 1 year after B-M therapy was given. Each symbol depicted in Fig. 2 indicates one patient. Three patients among them (closed circle) died of lung fibrosis and perforation of a radiation ulcer in the esophagus and terminal ileum where irradiation had been delivered at an overdose within 4 months after the beginning of B-M therapy. Four patients (closed triangle) died of recurrence within 1 year. By introducing maintenance therapy, recurrence was suc-cessfully controlled, but complications due to radiotherapy and chemotherapy such as mycotic pneumonia and intestinal bleeding appeared. Three patients (closed square) with these complications died within 2 years. The other three patients (open circle) are still alive after 16, 28, and 40 months without the disease.

TABLE IV.   Recurrence Rate (%) of Complete Responders

Overall	35 (6/17)
Without maintenance	100 (6/6)
With maintenance	20 (2/10
Average remission duration of complete responders: 4.5 months	

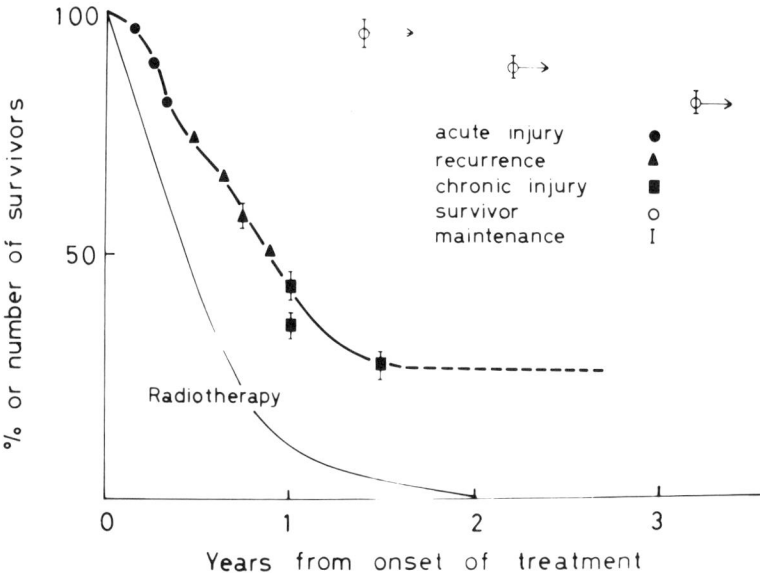

Fig. 2. Survival curve of 13 complete responders over 1 year after B-M therapy was given. Each symbol indicates one patient entered in the study. The deceased patients are shown in closed symbols of which each form implies the cause of death; circles represent acute injuries such as lung fibrosis and intestinal perforation, triangles represent recurrence, and squares represent chronic injuries such as mycotic pneumonia and intestinal bleeding. Open circles show the patients who are still alive. Vertical bars across the symbols indicate the addition of the maintenance therapy. The thin curve shows the survival rate of the patients with metastatic cervical cancer treated with radiotherapy alone.

Comparing these results with the survival rate of the patients with metastatic cervical cancer who had received radiotherapy alone (Morita *et al.,* 1975), the median survival time of the patients treated with B-M therapy was prolonged by 6 months, with three long-term survivors.

IV. DISCUSSION

Studies of B-M treatment of metastatic cervical cancer have revealed that there are two major problems on which our interest has to concentrate.

One is the question of the mechanism of the synergistic effect induced by the combination of the two drugs. On the basis of the cellular effects of the two drugs, the following possible explanations are proposed: (a) a consecutive BLM treatment may arrest most tumor cells in the G_2 period (Barranco *et al.,* 1973; Watanabe *et al.*, 1974), allowing some of them to move into the early stages of the next cycle and thus making the tumor cell population more susceptible to the action of MMC as a G_2-G_1 attacking agent (Ohara and Terasima, 1972); and (b) tumor cell killing effect may be potentiated by an unknown combined action of both agents. For the second assumption this author recently observed the notable experimental fact that the cell killing effect of BLM for HeLa cells was enhanced by administration of MMC both simultanously and consecutively (Miyamoto *et al.*, 1977).

The other problem is the several kinds of hazard to be guarded against, such as lung fibrosis, radiation ulcer, recurrence, and late complications during a series of this therapy. In addition to modifying the B-M regimen for better effect according to the basic studies mentioned above, we must make an effort (1) to protect against lung fibrosis in advance; (2) to rule out the patients who have a past history of over-irradiation to their intestinal canal; and (3) to determine the proper treatment dose and time of Carboquon which can be expected to prohibit recurrence and late complications.

As noted in the introduction of this paper, it is clear that nobody could expect patients with metastatic cervical cancer to be cured by conventional chemotherapy. However, the introduction of B-M therapy makes possible some hope for cure of the disease.

ACKNOWLEDGMENTS

The author thanks Drs. Takabe, Watanabe, Nakagima, Tanabe, and Terasima for their useful advice in clinical matters, and basic approach, the staff of the hospital for providing primary care to the patients involved in this study, and Miss Matzuda for typing the manuscript.

REFERENCES

Barranco, S. C., Luce, J. K., Romadahl, M. M., and Humphrey, R. M. (1973). *Cancer Res. 33,* 882.

Blum, R. H., Carter, S. K., and Agre, K. (1973). *Cancer 31,* 903.

Clasysse, A., Kenis, Y., and Mathe, G. (1976). *Cancer Chemotherapy.* Springer-Verlag, Berlin–Heidelberg–New York, p. 481.

Conroy, J. E., Lewis, G. C., Brady, L., Brodsky, I., Kuhn, S. B., Ross, J., and Nuss, R. (1976). *Cancer 37,* 660.

Miyamoto, T., Takabe, Y., Watanabe, M., and Terasima, T. *Cancer* (in press).

Miyamoto, T., Takabe, Y., Watanabe, M., Nakagima, Y., and Terasima, T. (1977). *Proc. Jpn. Cancer Assoc. 35,* 136.

Moor, G. E., Bross, I. J. D., and Ausman, R. (1968). *Cancer Chemother. Rep. 52,* 675.

Morita, S., Arai, T., and Kurisu, A. (1975). *Jpn. J. Cancer Clin. 21,* 621.

Ohara, H., and Terasima, T. (1972). *Gann 63,* 773.

Watanabe, M., Takabe, Y., Katzumata, T., and Terasima, T. (1974). *Cancer Res. 33,* 882.

Chapter 17

BLEOMYCIN IN TESTICULAR CANCER

Michael A. Friedman

I. INTRODUCTION

This brief review of bleomycin (BLM) in testicular cancer serves as an overture to the discussions which follow. Broad themes will be introduced here which will be elaborated upon in the succeeding presentations.

The unquestioned importance of BLM in current combination drug programs for patients with testicular cancer is demonstrated by the fact that this drug is included in almost all therapeutic programs. There are several reasons for BLM's popularity: (1) the theoretical advantages of BLM conbined with vincristine (VCR) or vinblastine (VLB) as described by Barranco and Humphrey (1971); (2) the absence of significant BLM marrow toxicity which allows for its combination with full doses of other effective but hematotoxic agents; (3) the variety of schedules and routes available for its administration; and (4) the empirical evidence that BLM is effective as both a single agent and in combination with other drugs.

II. HISTORY

It is only within the past several years that BLM has been successfully employed in treating these patients. To place this drug in its proper historical perspective, I have outlined the evolution of chemotherapy of testicular cancer in Fig. 1 and have

TABLE I. Chemotherapy Protocols for Carcinoma of the Testis [a]

Study	Therapy (mg/m^2)	D	Fr	N	CR (%)	PR (%)	Comments
SWOG 7303	VLB 7.5	D1+D2		48	50	24	MDR 49 wk
	BLM 15		q 21 d				
	VCR 2	D1+D8+D15		22	30	30	51 wk
	BLM 15 (6 hr later)	D1–4	q 21 d				
	ACT D .35						
Blom and Brodovsky (1976)	ACT D .4	D1–5		42	12	10	Overall survival not significantly different with short MDR
	ACT D .4	D1–5		42	19	50	
	VCR 1	D1–8					
	BLM 15	D1+D8+D15					
Burgess et al. (1975)	ADM 75	D1		25	28	51	
	VCR 1	D1+D8+D15	q 21 d				

Reference	Regimen	D	Fr	N	CR	PR	Comments
Daniels (1976)	CYT 7 mg/kg MITH 0.05 mg/kg VLB .075 mg/kg BLM .4 mg/kg	D1-3 D1+D3+D5 D1-4 D1-5	q 21-28 d	11	36		
	ACT D .01 mg/kg MTX .5 mg/kg CYT 10 mg/kg VCR .025 mg/kg	D1-5 D1 D1+D5	q 21-28 d	12	41		
Samuels et al. (1977)	COMF-BLM CYT 200 D VCR 2 MTX 15 5FU 400 BLM 300	D1+D8 D1-5 D1-8	q 28 d	35	43	20	Extragonal tumors
Samuels et al. (1976)	VB-1 VLB 0.2-0.3 mg/kg BLM 15-20	D1+D2	q 28 d	26	27		Survival better for VB-3
	VB-3 VLM 0.2-0.3 mg/kg BLM 30 mg/d infusion	D1+D2 D2-6	q 28 d	34	58		benefit demonstrated for embryonal tumors

a D = day number; Fr = frequency; N = number of patients; CR = complete response; PR = partial response; MDR = median duration response.

TABLE I – continued

Study	Therapy (mg/m²)	D	Fr	N	CR (%)	PR (%)	Comments
Samuels et al. (1977)	VB-3 VLB 0.2–0.3 mg/kg BLM 30 infusion	D1+D2 D2–6	q 28 d	89	65		Embryonal terato-carcinoma (survival not different). Minimal pulmonary metastases = 18/20 CR. Advanced pulmonary metastases = 15/31 CR. Abdominal metastases = 9/21 CR.
SWOG 7610	VLB 9–12 BLM 15 CDDP 10–15 + CHL 7–10 ACT 1–1.5 VLB 9–12	D1 D1–5 D1 D30	q 28 d x 4 x 2 wk				Stage III (in progress)
Einhorn et al. (1976)	CDDP 20 VLB 0.2 mg/kg BLM 30 mg/wk x 12 (6 hr post VLB) + Maintenance VLB 0.3 mg/kg + BCG	D1–5 D2+3	q 21 d	20	75	25	Median disease-free time 9 mo.

Reference	Regimen		Schedule				Chemotherapy preoperatively
Memo et al. (1977)	VLB 4 BLM 15 x 2 wk → CDDP 20 VCR 1.4 ACT D .35 → Surgical resection	D1+D2 D1–5 D1 D1–4	q 21 d x 7 wk	6	3	3	
Cvitkovic et al. (1977) –Silvay et al. (1973)	<u>VAB I</u> BLM 0.4 mg/kg VLB 0.025–0.05 mg/kg ACT D 0.0075– 0.015 mg/kg	D1–3 D1–3 D1–3	q 7–14 d	71	14	22	NED[b] = 12%

–Cvitkovic et al. (1975)	<u>VAB II</u>
	BLM 0.5 mg/kg infusion
	VLB 0.06 mg/kg
	ACT D 0.02 mg/kg
	CDDP 1 mg/kg
	  then
	VLB
	ACT D (or CDDP q 3 wk)
	BLM
	  and reinduction
		D1–7
		D1
		D1
		D8
			q wk
			q 3 mo
				51	58	17	NED = 23%

[b] NED = no evident disease.

TABLE I – continued

Study	Therapy (mg/m²)	D	Fr	N	CR (%)	PR (%)	Comments
Cvitkovic et al. (1977)	VAB III			80	63	25	NED = 63%; only 2/192 fatal toxicities overall
Cvitkovic, Hayes, and Golbey (1976)	BLM 20 d infusion	D1–7					
	VLB 4	D1					
	CYT 600	D1					
	ACT DL	D1					
	CDDP 120	D8					
	then						
	VLB 4		q 21 d				
	CHL 4	D1–15	q 21 d				
	alternating						
	ACT	D1					
	ADR 45						
	CDDP 50						
Merrin (1977)	Induction			28	68	32	16/28 NED at 3–18 mo.
	BLM 420						
	VLB 2 mg/kg						
	CDDP 4 mg/kg (4 wk)						
	PRED 20 mg/D →						
	Consolidation						
	ACT D 5 (6 wk)						
	VCR 6						
	CDDP 6 mg/kg		q 6 wk				
	ACT D 2.5						
	CDDP 1 mg/kg		q 3 wk				

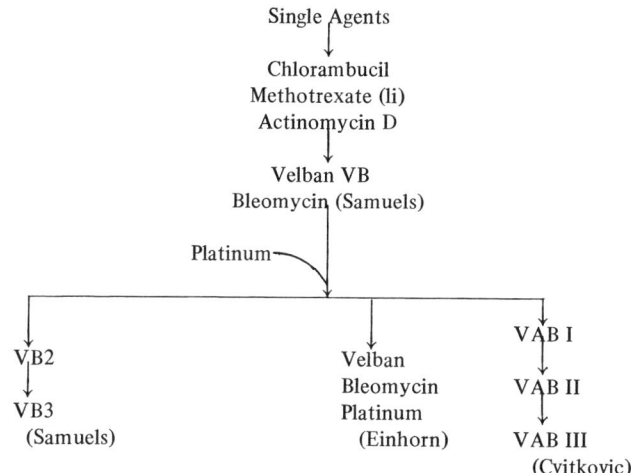

FIG. 1. The development of chemotherapy programs for testicular cancer.

begun with the initial phase II efforts which identified active single agents. These activities, in turn, led to combination drug trials. Programs such as "Li's triple therapy" (Li *et al.*, 1960) were initially promising because they resulted in increasing numbers of objective tumor regressions, but disease was controlled for long periods of time in only relatively few patients. However, the introduction of high dosage VLB plus BLM by Samuels *et al.* (1973) resulted in significantly increased rates of complete response (CR) and long-term control. The identification of *cis*-dichloro-diammine platinum (CDDP) as an active agent was the next important development in the chemotherapy of this disease and led to the major effective programs in current use. The three main protocols now actively being pursued are natural extensions of previous activities. Samuels *et al.* (1975) have logically explored modifications of schedule and dosage of VLB and BLM (VB2 and VB3). Cvitkovic and his co-workers at the Memorial Sloan-Kettering Cancer Center have employed successively more complicated and effective multidrug programs [VAB (Silvay *et al.*, 1973), VAB II (Cvitkovic *et al.*, 1976), and VAB III (Cvitkovic *et al.*, 1977)]. Einhorn and his colleagues (1976) have used the simplest combination scheme of BLM and VLB and CDDP. Although these combination drug programs produce significant toxicities, the majority of patients treated have CRs.

These regimens, as well as other selected studies, are outlined in Table I. Many of the studies appear to be similar in terms of drugs and schedules and many offer a greater than 50% possibility of CR with an acceptable duration of that response. Unfortunately, however, no concurrent ongoing comparisons have been made among the major programs; rather, data have been compared retrospectively. In order to make conclusive comparisons among the major programs in terms of toxicity or efficacy, each patient's type and extent of disease must be known; and these data, for the most part, have been lacking in published series.

It is currently known that the site and extent of malignant disease are of prognostic significance. Samuels and his associates (1977a,b) have demonstrated that

TABLE II. Chemotherapy Protocols for Carcinoma of the Testis [a]

Study	Therapy (mg/m^2)	D	Fr	N	CR (%)	PR (%)	Comments
SWOG 5256	XRT (1 mo. rest), then						Stage 1B and II (in progress)
	VLB 7.5	D1	q 21 d				Tolerable toxicity to date
	BLM 15	D2+D5					
	VLB 7.5	D1	q 21 d				
	BLM 15	D2–5					
		3 wk rest, XRT then chemotherapy					
SEG 76 GUO 103	XRT						Stage I and II (in progress)
	XRT +						
	CDDP 10	D1–5	q 28 d x 4				
	VLB 15	D1+D2					
	BLM 15 (infusion) → maintenance	D1+D5					
Merrin et al. (1976)	VLB 0.1–0.15 mg/kg	D1–7, 15–21	wk 1 + 3	16	77	13	With surgery
	BLM 30 mg/d infusion	D1+D8+D15					
	CDDP 10 →						
	CDDP 10						
	ADM 60						
	CYT 800 →						
	ACT D 2.5		q 6 wk				
	CYT 800		q 6 wk				

[a] D = day number; Fr = frequency; N = number of patients; CR = complete response; PR = partial response; MDR = median duration response.

VLB + BLM are more effective in patients with minimal pulmonary metastases than in those with more advanced lung metastases, and that these patients fare better than those with advanced abdominal metastases. Additionally, Samuels *et al.* (1976) have provided preliminary information correlating the histologic cell type of the tumor with response to VB1 and VB3 therapy. Unfortunately, this type of biologic data is not sufficiently available for all the therapy programs described.

Because these drug programs are so effective in patients with advanced disease, they have been applied as adjuvant treatment in conjunction with radiation therapy and surgery. For example, both the Southwest Oncology Group (SWOG Protocol 7525) and the Southeastern Oncology Group (SEG Protocol 76 GUO 103) have initiated multimodal trials of VLB + BLM ± radiotherapy (RT) for patients with stage IB and II disease. Merrin (1977) (Table II) has employed a more complicated multiple drug program in association with "cytoreductive surgery" and has reported promising initial results.

III. UNRESOLVED QUESTIONS

Encouraging results have generated enormous and appropriate enthusiasm; however, the following critical questions remain unresolved.

1. What are the long-term toxicities (currently unappreciated) inherent in these combination drug programs? This question is of less concern for patients with obvious gross disseminated disease than for those patients treated for suspected microscopic occult disease. Toxicities that are acceptable for patients with known metastatic disease (who predictably will not survive long) may not be acceptable for those who may be free of disease predictably after surgical treatment. We must begin even now to concentrate on devising therapies which are less toxic and less damaging to kidney, hearing, lung, and immunologic function.

2. Is it the number of active drugs or how intensely the drugs are used that most accurately correlates with long-term control of disease? Intensive programs using high-dosage VLB + BLM and VLB + BLM + CDDP are clearly very effective. When more drugs are employed, to administer them sequentially (as in Cvitkovic's or Merrin's approach) appears to be more efficacious than to use them concurrently. When several active agents are given simultaneously, the necessary proportional dosage reductions may impair the overall impact of the drugs on the disease.

3. How do we modify the CR rate to make it equal the "cure" rate? To move toward "cure" we must first analyze both the nature of failure in the treated patients (i.e., site, lesion cell type, previous therapy) and the time of failure (i.e., during or after therapy) in order to employ the many therapeutic options that are available to prevent such failures. Our knowledge must become sophisticated enough to allow the stratification of patients into higher- and lower-risk groups, and we must design studies to provide these data.

4. With such effective therapies available, can we now learn something more fundamental about the general aspects of tumor biology? With testicular cancer as a specific model, employing serologic markers (e.g., B-hcG, AFP, or polyamines) we

perhaps can develop a better intellectual model of neoplastic disease. Additionally, with such effective modalities available, we may find answers to specific immunologic questions.

We are no longer searching for effective primary modalities to treat testicular cancer. Instead, we are turning our attention to finding effective means of decreasing toxicity and integrating the modalities of surgery, radiation (XRT), and drugs. The unresolved questions will not be easy to answer, and unless large-scale cooperative trials can be initiated these questions will remain only partially resolved for many years to come.

REFERENCES

Barranco, S. E., and Humphrey, R. M. (1971). *Cancer Res. 31*, 1218.

Blom, J., and Brodovsky, H. S. (1976). *Proc. Am. Assoc. Cancer Res. 17*, 290, C-213.

Burgess, M. A., Einhorn, L. H., and Gottleib, J. A. (1975). *Proc. Am. Assoc. Cancer Res. 16*, 244, No. 1094.

Cvitkovic, E., Hayes, D., and Golbey, R. (1976). *Proc. Am. Assoc. Cancer Res. 17*, 296, C-237.

Cvitkovic, E., Cheng, E., Whitmore, W. F., and Golbey R. B. (1977). *Proc. Am. Assoc. Cancer Res. 18*, 324, C-232.

Daniels, J. R. (1976). *Proc. Am. Assoc. Cancer Res. 17*, 282, C-181.

Einhorn, L. H., Furnas, B. E., and Powell, N. (1976). *Proc. Am. Assoc. Cancer Res. 17*, 240, C-13.

Li, M. C., Whitmore, W. F., Golbey, R., and Grabstald, H. (1960). *J. Am. Med. Assoc. 1974*, 1291.

Memo, R., Wise, H., Metz, E., and Neidhart, J. (1977). *Proc. Am. Assoc. Cancer Res. 18*, 92, No. 368.

Merrin, C. (1977). *Proc. Am. Assoc. Cancer Res. 18*, 298, C-128.

Merrin, C., Takita, H., Weber, R., Wajsman, Z., Baumgartner, G., and Murphy, G. P. (1976). *Cancer 37*, 20.

Samuels, M. L., Johnson, D. E., and Holoye, P.Y. (1973). *Proc. Am. Assoc. Cancer Res. 14*, 23, No. 89.

Samuels, M. L., Holoye, P. Y., and Johnson, D. E. (1975). *Cancer 36*, 318.

Samuels, M. L., Boyle, L. E., Holoye, P. Y., and Johnson. D. E. (1976). *Proc. Am. Assoc. Cancer Res. 17*, 98, No. 392.

Samuels, M. L., Boyle, L. E., Nicholson, G. L., Smith, T., and Johnson, D. E. (1977a). *Proc. Am. Assoc. Cancer Res. 18*, 147, No. 585.

Samuels, M. L., Lanzotti, V. J., Holoye, P. Y., and Howe, C. D. (1977b). *Proc. Am. Assoc. Cancer Res. 18*, 146, No. 584.

Silvay, O., Yagoda, A., Wittes, R., Whitmore, W., and Golbey, R. (1973). *Proc. Am. Assoc. Cancer Res. 14*, 68, No. 271.

Chapter 18

COMBINATION CHEMOTHERAPY WITH Cis-DIAMMINEDICHLOROPLATINUM, VINBLASTINE, AND BLEOMYCIN IN DISSEMINATED TESTICULAR CANCER: AN UPDATE

Lawrence H. Einhorn

I. INTRODUCTION

Although testicular cancer accounts for only 1% of all malignant tumors in males, it ranks first in incidence of cancer deaths in the 25–34 age group (MacKay and Sellers, 1966). Thus cancer of the testis has a significant impact on the social, economic, and emotional status of this young population.

Radiotherapy is the treatment of choice for pure seminoma, as this tumor is very radiosensitive, producing a 90–95% cure rate, and retroperitoneal node dissection is rarely indicated (Maier *et al.*, 1968). Indeed, radiotherapy for metastatic lesions produces an excellent 55% 5-year survival (Freedman and Purkayastha, 1960). However, the treatment for nonseminomatous germinal neoplasms has produced much less satisfactory results with considerably more controversy as to the preferred treatment for all stages of disease.

In 1960, Li and associates introduced the first major thrust of chemotherapy in advanced testicular cancer with the combination of actinomycin-D, chlorambucil, and methotrexate (Li *et al.*, 1960). Subsequent studies confirmed a 50–70% response rate, which included a 10–20% complete remissions (Ansfield *et al.*, 1969; MacKenzie, 1966). The past 15 years have also seen the development of many new agents with substantial activity, notably vinblastine (Samuels and Howe, 1970), bleomycin (Blum *et al.*, 1973), and mithramycin (Kennedy, 1970). One of the major significant achievements of these single-agent studies was not only the demonstration that a complete remission could be obtained in disseminated testicular cancer, but that approximately half of those complete remissions were permanent cures (Ansfield *et al.*, 1969; MacKenzie, 1966; Samuels and Howe, 1970; Kennedy, 1970). Most relapses occurred within 2 years of initiation of chemotherapy.

Combination chemotherapy has produced excellent long-term complete remissions in other chemosensitive tumors such as Hodgkin's disease (DeVita *et al.*, 1970). Likewise, most recent attempts at improved chemotherapy in testicular cancer have been with combination chemotherapy. One of the most widely used combinations has been vinblastine plus bleomycin (Samuels *et al.*, 1975).

Cis-diamminedichloroplatinum is one of a group of coordination compounds of platinum identified by Rosenberg *et al.* (1965) which strongly inhibits bacterial replication. This agent has significant activity in refractory advanced testicular cancer, and furthermore, it is ideal for combination chemotherapy because of its relative lack of myelosuppression (Higby *et al.*, 1974).

In 1974, we began a study utilizing vinblastine, bleomycin, and (*cis*-diamminedichloroplatinum in disseminated testicular cancer. The primary goal was to increase the complete remission rate and potential cure rate. The results of treatment of the first 50 patients are the subject of this report.

II. MATERIALS AND METHODS

Fifty patients with germ cell tumors of the testis were the subjects of these studies. The median age was 26 with a range of 15 to 63. All had metastatic measurable disease and were no longer amenable to attempts at surgical cure. Three patients died within 2 weeks of initiation of chemotherapy and were considered inevaluable. The drug regimen was administered according to the schedule shown in Table I.

TABLE I.   Platinum + Vinblastine + Bleomycin

---

1. Platinum 20 mg/m^2 IV (over 15 minutes) daily x 5 once every 3 weeks for three courses
2. Bleomycin 30 U IV push weekly x 12
3. Vinblastine 0.2 mg/kg IV push daily x 2 every 3 weeks
   a. Vinblastine given 6 hours prior to bleomycin
   b. After five courses (12 weeks) of vinblastine, maintenance therapy consisted of vinblastine 0.3 mg/kg IV push every 4 weeks and BCG by scarification 1, 2, and 3 weeks after each dosage of vinblastine
   c. Therapy to be continued for a total of 2 years

Platinum was given as a 15 minute IV infusion for 5 consecutive days (days 1–5) every three weeks for three courses. Eight patients were given additional courses of platinum because they had no significant nephrotoxicity and had persistent evidence of residual disease after the first three courses. Vinblastine was given on days 1 and 2 in a total dosage of 0.4 mg/kg for a total of five courses, and then given as a single injection in a dosage of 0.3 mg/kg every 4 weeks for a total of 2 years of therapy. Bleomycin was given on days 2, 9, and 16 of each platinum course, and was given with the platinum 6 hours after vinblastine and then given weekly for a total of 12 weeks. Vinblastine and bleomycin were used in a sequential combination in an attempt to synchronize neoplasm with vinblastine for subsequent destruction by bleomycin, with the bleomycin being given 6 hours after vinblastine (Livingston et al., 1973). Bleomycin was shown to be most effective in killing Chinese hamster ovary cells in mitosis (Barranco and Humphrey, 1971), and since vinblastine, like vincristine, also produces an arrest in the mitotic phase of the cell cycle, vinblastine and bleomycin were used in sequential combination for potential maximal tumor destruction by bleomycin. The bleomycin was stopped at a total dosage of 360 u because this drug can cause cumulative pulmonary fibrosis.

Bacillus Calmette–Guerin (BCG) immunotherapy was started after completion of the 12 weeks of bleomycin in those patients who achieved complete remission, and was given by scarification 1, 2, and 3 weeks after each vinblastine injection for a total of 4 months and thereafter was given 1 and 3 weeks after each vinblastine injection. This immunotherapy was used in an attempt to augment host cell-mediated immunity and prolong the duration of remission and improve the prospects for total cell kill and eventual cure, as has been demonstrated in other diseases (Gutterman et al., 1974a, b). However, because of the serious question as to whether immunotherapy is of any value, BCG was deleted 15 months ago; thus far, we have had no relapses of complete remissions utilizing vinblastine alone for maintenance therapy, and thus it appears unlikely that BCG contributed any significant therapeutic advantage.

The criterion for a partial response was a decrease of 50% or more in the sum of the products of diameters of all measurable lesions. A complete response was defined as a complete disappearance of all clinical, radiographic, and biochemical evidence of disease, including normal whole lung tomograms and serum HCG and alpha-fetoprotein by radioimmunoassay, and normal abdominal CAT scan and ultrasound.

Blood cell counts, platelet counts, and differentials were determined weekly for all patients, and liver and renal function tests were performed every 3 weeks. Arterial blood gases and pulmonary functions were performed every 3 weeks while patients were on bleomycin. Tumor measurements were recorded at least every 3 weeks, and appropriate radiologic and biochemical studies, including radioimmunoassay alpha-fetoprotein and beta subunit of HCG were repeated every 6–8 weeks.

III. RESULTS

Fifty patients with disseminated testicular cancer were the subject of this study. Two patients died within 1 week of institution of chemotherapy, and a third patient died at home 2 weeks after initiation of chemotherapy, all presumably due to massive tumor, leaving 47 evaluable patients.

Thirty-three of 47 patients (71%) achieved complete remission. Four patients died in complete remission. Two of these deaths were due to gram-negative sepsis, one from bleomycin-induced pulmonary fibrosis, and one from multiple small-bowel fistulae and obstruction secondary to previous surgery. One of the above two deaths from gram-negative sepsis was from Klebsiella pneumonia in a chronic alcoholic who had no evidence of leukopenia during this episode.

Only five of these 33 complete remissions have relapsed. One patient relapsed on maintenance therapy with recurrent pulmonary disease and died shortly thereafter; a second patient refused any form of maintenance therapy and developed rapidly progressing pulmonary metastases and died within 24 hours of readmission; three other relapses occurred on vinblastine + BCG maintenance therapy, and two of these three patients are back in complete remission with reinduction with platinum + adriamycin (60 mg/m^2) + vincristine + bleomycin. Four of these five relapses occurred within 9 months of initiation of chemotherapy, and the other relapse occurred at 17 months.

In addition, five of the 12 partial remissions were rendered disease-free following surgical removal of residual disease after significant reduction of tumor volume with chemotherapy. Three of these five patients had complete removal of a teratoma, one via thoracotomy and two via laparotomy, and all three of these patients remain alive and disease-free on maintenance therapy for 18$^+$ to 33$^+$ months following their surgery. The other two patients had residual embryonal and choriocarcinoma removed completely at laparotomy, but both eventually died with progressive tumor. These two patients received maintenance vinblastine, and we now feel that such patients with residual embryonal, teratocarcinoma, or choriocarcinoma, even after complete surgical removal, should be "reinduced" with platinum + vinblastine + bleomycin rather than just going on vinblastine alone. Thus, the chemotherapy regimen of cis-diamminedichloroplatinum, vinblastine, and bleomycin produced 70% complete and 30% partial remissions in 47 evaluable patients. With the addition of surgical removal of residual disease in five of the partial remissions, an 81% overall disease-free status was obtained. Thirty-four of these 47 patients remain alive and 28 remain alive and continuously disease-free from 13$^+$ to 39$^+$ months.

TABLE II. Classification of Primary Tumor

Dixon-Moore	Histology	No. of Patients	CR%
I	Pure Seminoma	4	50
II	Embryonal, with or without seminoma	25	84
III	Teratoma	2	50
IV	Teratocarcinoma with embryonal or choriocarcinoma	9	44
V	Choriocarcinoma with embryonal carcinoma	5	60
	yolk sac	2	100

TABLE III. Extent of Disease

A. Minimal pulmonary disease—no more than five metastases in each lung field with maximum diameter less than 2.0 cm
B. Advanced pulmonary disease—any mediastinal or hilar mass, pleural effusion, or intrapulmonary mass greater than 2.0 cm
C. Minimal abdominal disease—minimal pulmonary disease plus positive lymphangiogram with no ureteral displacement
D. Advanced abdominal disease—palpable mass, liver metastases, ureteral displacement with or without obstructive uropathy, and inferior vena cava distortion by metastatic nodes
E. Elevated beta-HCG with no other evidence of disease

The relationship of histology to response to chemotherapy is shown in Table II. Excellent complete remission rates were seen in all cell types, although there was a suggestion of a lower complete remission rate in teratocarcinoma and choriocarcinoma. Obviously these numbers are too small to allow any valid conclusions concerning histology and complete remission; however, it was our impression that the lower complete remission rates in these histologies were primarily due to more extensive disease. Samuels *et al.* (1975) have devised a classification for extent of disease (defined in Table III), and the relationship of extent of disease to complete remission is shown in Table IV. Twenty of 22 patients with minimal disease (groups A, C, and E) achieved complete remission with this chemotherapy, and 18 of these patients are presently alive and disease-free.

The relationship of prior therapy to complete remission is shown in Table V. There was a lower complete remission rate in patients with prior radiotherapy, and these patients had considerably more prolonged and severe hematological and gastrointestinal toxicity.

Radioimmunoassay alpha-fetoprotein was elevated in 40% of the patients and beta-HCG was elevated in 75% of these patients. Only three patients failed to have one of those two markers elevated. Generally speaking, we tended to see a one log reduction in these tumor markers with each course of *cis*-platinum therapy. Eight patients received more than three courses of platinum. Each of these patients had extensive pulmonary (± abdominal) disease and achieved significant cytoreduction clinically, radiographically, and biochemically with each preceding course, but still

TABLE IV. Extent of Disease

	No. of Patients	CR%
A. Minimal pulm. disease	10	80
B. Advanced pulm. disease	9	67
C. Minimal abd. and pulm. disease	9	88
D. Advanced abd. disease	16	50
E. Elevated HCG alone	3	100

TABLE V. Prior Therapy

	No. of patients	Complete remissions (%)
Surgery alone	21	76
Surgery + chemoprophylaxis	9	88
Surgery + chemotherapy (for metastatic disease)	10	70
Surgery + radiotherapy	3	33
Surgery + chemotherapy + radiotherapy	4	25

had not yet achieved a complete remission. Five of these patients received a fourth course of platinum; three of these five patients achieved a complete remission with this course and have all remained in complete remission for over 12 months. The other two patients did not achieve complete remission, but the fourth course did normalize their tumor markers and they both have remained in partial remission for over a year. The three patients who had more than four courses of cis-platinum achieved further cytoreduction, but never achieved complete remission.

Toxicity could be best described by separating this three-drug combination into its individual components:

Cis-platinum caused moderate to severe nausea and vomiting in all patients during each 5 day course. During the first year of this study intravenous hydration was only employed for very severe nausea and vomiting. Although only three of these earlier patients had significant azotemia (blood urea nitrogen greater than 50 mg% and/or serum creatinine greater than 3.0 mg%), many of these earlier patients now have a 25 to 50% reduction from their baseline creatinine clearance and have serum creatinines of 1.5 to 2.0 mg%. None of these patients shows progressive nephrotoxicity or azotemic symptomatology, and the long-term effects of cis-platinum on renal function are still being studied. One patient required hemodialysis for acute renal failure and is the subject of a separate case report (Crooke *et al.*, 1977). In the past 18 months we have been employing vigorous intravenous hydration on all patients during each course of cis-platinum utilizing 100 cc/hour of normal saline for 12 hours prior to administration of chemotherapy (prehydration) and then continuous saline hydration during all 5 days of cis-platinum administration. Since we have been utilizing this form of intravenous hydration, we have only rarely encountered any of the above biochemical manifestations of platinum nephrotoxicity. We have not employed mannitol diuresis in any of our patients. Although occasional patients had a decrease in high-frequency hearing, there were no observed clinical audiological abnormalities. Mild hyperuricemia and hypokalemia were occasionally seen, but were not a clinical problem.

Bleomycin produced fever, chills, and cutaneous striae in all patients, but these were not a clinical problem and did not require alteration of the bleomycin dosages. All patients had significant alopecia and most had weight loss (from cis-platinum and bleomycin) during the 12 weeks of bleomycin. The average weight loss was 20 lb. No patient required intravenous hyperalimentation, and all patients completely regained their weight after the completion of bleomycin. There was one death from bleomycin pulmonary fibrosis; there were no other cases of clinically significant pulmonary fibrosis.

Vinblastine produced myalgia in half of the patients. Although this was occasionally severe enough to require narcotic analgesics during the first 12 weeks of therapy, it was not a clinical problem during maintenance therapy with the lower dosage (0.3 mg/kg) of vinblastine. Anemia and thrombocytopenia were observed in several patients but no patient had thrombocytopenic bleeding or required platelet transfusions. Only four patients experienced thrombocytopenia below 100,000 and these were all patients who had had prior radiotherapy. Anemia was more of a problem, especially in patients who had had prior radiotherapy. Packed red blood cell transfusions were required periodically on four patients during the first several months of therapy, and four of these patients had received prior radiotherapy. Leukopenia also was more severe and prolonged in patients with prior irradiation and they were started on a lowered dosage of vinblastine (0.15 mg/kg for 2 consecutive days). The most serious side effect, which was seen in all patients, was sever leukopenia. The nadir of the white blood count usually was 1000 between days 7 and 14. Eighteen patients required hospitalization for presumed sepsis with granulocytopenic fever and were cultured and started on antibiotic coverage with broadspectrum antibiotics. Seven of these patients had documented Gramnegative sepsis and one of these patients died of sepsis.

BCG immunotherapy caused local erythema, pruritus, fever, and myalgia but was generally well-tolerated by all patients except one who had severe local reactivity and an ulcerated regional lymph node requiring cessation of the BCG.

Despite the aforementioned significant toxicity, this occurred primarily during the 12 weeks of remission induction therapy. Maintenance therapy with vinblastine and BCG was well-tolerated and all patients regained their hair growth and weight during this period. No patient required hospitalization for complications of therapy during vinblastine and BCG maintenance and all were able to continue school or work full time.

IV. DISCUSSION

Since the original report by Li *et al.* in 1960 demonstrating activity of chemotherapy in disseminated testicular cancer, there have been numerous clinical trials evaluating a variety of drugs in these diseases (Table VI). Although it is not possible to extract present survival data on all patients reported in Table VI, there does appear to be a general trend revealing that over 50% of all complete remissions in disseminated testicular cancer have prolonged survival and potential cure. Indeed, in testicular cancer in general, most relapses occur within 2 years of initiation of chemotherapy or surgery (Nefzger and Mostofi, 1972; Lefevre *et al.*, 1975). It seems quite reasonable to expect that many of the patients in this study who are currently alive and disease-free will be cured of their malignancy.

TABLE VI. Results with Chemotherapy in Disseminated Testicular Cancer

Author	Treatment	Total Patients	Complete Remissions	Prolonged survivors[a]
Wyatt and McAninch (1967)	Methotrexate	10	4 (40%)	4
MacKenzie (1966)	Actinomycin-D (alone or in double or triple therapy	154	24 (16%)	13
Mendelson and Serpick (1970)	Cyclophosphamide + vincristine + methotrexate + fluorouracil (COMF)	17	5 (29%)	1
Jacobs (1970)	Vincristine + actinomycin-D + cyclophosphamide (VAC)	58	7 (12%)	4
Kennedy (1970)	Mithramycin	23	5 (22%)	5
Samuels and Howe (1970)	Vinblastine	21	4 (19%)	2
Samuels et al. (1975)	Vinblastine + bleomycin	23	9 (39%)	–
Golby et al. (1977)	VAB III	80	50 (63%)	23 (46%)

[a] Refers to those patients remaining alive and disease-free at the time of publication.

Generally speaking, the only meaningful response for the patient has been complete remission, as partial remissions were usually of brief duration. However, it is noteworthy that of our 14 patients who achieved partial remission, five had significant enough reduction of tumor volume to make an attempt at surgical removal of residual disease feasible, and three of these five patients remain alive and disease-free 18^+ to 33^+ months following their surgery. Three of the other nine partial remissions have remained in their original partial remission for 16^+, 22^+, and 30^+ months. The median duration of partial remission was 11 months. Aggressive chemotherapy appears capable of changing the histology to a more mature and benign form, as has been previously reported (Willis and Hejdu, 1973; Merrin et al., 1976), and this may be partly responsible for the prolonged duration of partial remissions seen in some of the patients.

The rationale behind combination chemotherapy is to combine antineoplastic drugs which are all individually active against the specific tumor, exhibit different toxicities, have different mechanisms of action, and have demonstrated clinical synergism. Vinblastine, bleomycin, and cis-platinum all have activity against testicular cancer as single agents (Samuels and Howe, 1970; Blum et al., 1973; Higby et al., 1974). These three agents have individual and separate side effects, with the dose-limiting toxicity of vinblastine, bleomycin and cis-platinum being leukopenia, pulmonary fibrosis, and nephrotoxicity, respectively. Vinblastine, a vinca alkaloid, produces a mitotic arrest (Creasey, 1968). Bleomycin combines with DNA in the presence of a sulfhydryl compound of hydrogen peroxide, resulting in a decrease of the DNA melting point and scission of the DNA strands (Hagai et al., 1969). Cis-platinum produces inhibition of DNA synthesis, possibly through template inactivation (Harder et al., 1976). The combination of vinblastine and bleomycin appears to represent a truly synergistic combination as the complete remission rate for this two-drug combination is higher than would be predicted from the single-agent data of the two drugs (Samuels and Howe, 1970; Blum et al., 1973).

Patients with testicular cancer are clinically staged as follows (Boden and Gebbs, 1951):

Stage A – tumor confined to the testis, with or without adnexal invasion

Stage B – tumor metastatic to retroperitoneal lymph nodes but not beyond

Stage C – tumor metastatic to a site other than retroperitoneal lymph nodes

The surgical cure rate for stage A testicular cancer with orchiectomy plus bilateral retroperitoneal node dissection has been 90-100% (Donohue and Einhorn, in press; Staubitz et al., 1974), and there clearly is no need for consideration of postoperative adjuvant therapy on such patients. However, patients with stage B disease have variably been reported to have only 30 to 60% cure rates with surgery alone, and such patients have been considered for postoperative irradiation (Maler and Sulak, 1973). However, the recent series by Staubitz et al. (1974) which represented a study of orchiectomy plus transabdominal bilateral retroperitoneal dissection with no postoperative therapy, achieved a 75% 3-year survival for patients with stage B disease and a 93% 3-year survival rate for stage A disease, with an overall 88% 3-year and 81% 5-year survival. Although seminoma is a highly radiosensitive tumor, the nonseminomatous testicular cancers are considerably less radiosensitive and there is no evidence that radiotherapy improves survival in these patients when used postoperatively. (Skinner and Leadbetter, 1971). Although recent radiotherapy studies utilizing the "sandwich" technique (lymphadenectomy combined with preoperative and postoperative radiotherapy) have produced better results than previous radiotherapy studies (Nicholson *et al.*, 1974), they are still no better than the results of an adequate surgical procedure alone (Staubitz *et al.*, 1974). Although one could argue that a randomized prospective clinical study would be required comparing bilateral retroperitoneal node dissection to the sandwich technique to fully answer the question as to the role of radiotherapy in nonseminomatous testicular cancer, we feel that there is no indication for such a study. A certain percentage of such patients (probably 20–40%) are going to relapse and require aggressive chemotherapy regimens such as *cis*-platinum, vinblastine, and bleomycin for metastatic disease. Bone-marrow depression has prevented the full use of myelosuppressive chemotherapeutic agents in patients who have recurrent disease after radiotherapy (Nicholson *et al.*, 1974), and indeed we have found it impossible to administer full dosage vinblastine in our patients who had prior radiotherapy, and subsequently we start such patients on a 25–50% dosage reduction of vinblastine. Even using such precautions, these patients have had severe and prolonged myelosuppression. Furthermore, there is a significantly higher incidence of small bowel obstruction and gastrointestinal bleeding in such patients, and Samuels has recently reported radiation strictures requiring surgical intervention in four patients treated with surgery and radiotherapy who subsequently relapsed and were treated with vinblastine and bleomycin (Samuels *et al.*, 1976). Furthermore, the radiotherapy field frequently encompasses the mediastinum, which increases the incidence of bleomycin-induced pulmonary fibrosis (Einhorn *et al.*, 1976). It is not known at the present time whether or not patients who have had abdominal radiotherapy have an increased incidence of platinum nephrotoxicity. Thus, we feel that there is no evidence for improved survival with radiotherapy in nonseminomatous testicular cancer, and that such therapy can significantly increase the morbidity and mortality of subsequent aggressive chemotherapy, should it eventually be needed.

Although the treatment of choice for seminoma is orchiectomy plus radiotherapy, a word of caution is necessary. Patients who have a "pure seminoma" diagnosed by orchiectomy should not have an elevated beta-HCG or alpha-fetoprotein level, as such patients have nonseminomatous elements present elsewhere and their cases should be managed as nonseminomatous testicular cancers (Lange *et al.*, 1976).

It is attractive to consider adjuvant aggressive chemotherapy with regimens such as *cis*-platinum, vinblastine, and bleomycin in stage B nonseminomatous testicular cancer. Clearly this three-drug regimen has significant activity in stage C disease, and many patients with stage B disease will relapse following surgery. The use of adjuvant aggressive combination chemotherapy will certainly lower the recurrence rate, but only a randomized prospective study could determine if it would improve the survival in stage B nonseminomatous testicular cancer. There is a certain morbidity and mortality associated with such chemotherapy, and it is our feeling that we can avoid such aggressive chemotherapy in most patients with stage B disease without lowering the survival probability by following the patients postoperatively once a month for the first year with chest x-ray and beta-HCG and alpha-fetoprotein determinations. This allows us to find relapses at a relatively early time when the patients have minimal stage C disease, and institute chemotherapy with *cis*-platinum, vinblastine, and bleomycin at that time with a very high probability of complete remission. Twenty of 22 patients with "minimal" disease (Table III) achieved complete remission and the only two patients failing to achieve complete remission were patients heavily treated with previous chemotherapy. It is noteworthy in this series that all eight patients treated with actinomycin-D chemoprophylaxis who eventually relapsed (all within 1 year of initiation of actinomycin-D) achieved complete remission and are presently alive and disease-free following institution of *cis*-platinum, vinblastine, and bleomycin chemotherapy. One patient had the rare clinical situation of developing recurrent advanced pulmonary metastases 7 years after completion of a course of adjuvant actinomycin-D, and this patient failed to achieve complete remission.

Our experience with this regimen of combination chemotherapy in 50 patients with advance testicular cancer allows us to suggest the following guidelines:

1. The goal of therapy in all patients should be complete remission, and if a clinical complete remission is not achieved after three courses of *cis*-platinum in a responding patient with no significant nephrotoxicity, a fourth course should be given. We have found no value in exceeding four courses. Most patients achieved a clinical complete remission by the end of two courses of *cis*-platinum.

2. If a clinical complete remission has not been achieved with chemotherapy, surgical excision of residual disease should be considered if feasible. The two clinical situations in which this occurs are: (a) Complete disappearance of pulmonary metastases except for a solitary residual nodule or nodules confined to a single lobe of the lung; wedge resection is the preferred surgical approach. (b) Complete disappearance of all supradiaphragmatic disease in a patient who initally presented with a large palpable abdominal mass. It has been our policy to do an exploratory laparotomy with removal of any residual tumor in all such patients who initially presented with stage C disease and a large palpable abdominal mass following the 12 weeks of bleomycin therapy. We have done seven such surgical explorations; four patients had complete excision of residual tumor and three others had no evidence of remaining abdominal tumor. Interestingly, one of these patients had a persistent palpable abdominal mass which was removed at surgery and proven to be fibrous tissue only. Thus, as has been previously reported (Comisarow and Grabstald, 1976), the presence of a persistent retroperitoneal mass in this circumstance does not invariably mean the presence of persistent malignant tissue. We have not felt it necessay to do laparotomies or retroperitoneal node dissection in any of the other patients in this series, despite the fact that many of them had evidence of abdominal disease initially.

3. The major toxicity with this therapeutic regimen has been the significant

leukopenia and potential granulocytopenic sepsis secondary to vinblastine. It is quite possible that we could achieve the same therapeutic results without such significant leukopenia and potential sepsis by starting with a 25% reduction in the vinblastine dosage. This question is currently being evaluated at this institution in a randomized prospective study, and although the numbers are small thus far, we have achieved the same disease-free rate with the lowered dosage of vinblastine (11/13 with 0.3 mg/kg of vinblastine versus 12/13 with 0.4 mg/kg of vinblastine). Any patient who has had prior irradiation should have a 25-50% dosage reduction of vinblastine.

4. It has been our practice to hospitalize any patient with a temperature above 38.3 °C and less than 1000 granulocytes/mm^3, obtain appropriate cultures, and institute broad-spectrum antibiotic coverage with cephalothin and carbenicillin. We try to avoid gentamicin in this situation because of the possible synergistic renal tubular damage between *cis*-platinum and aminoglycoside antibiotics. Some of the more significant transient nephrotoxicity in our earlier patients was seen in this clinical situation where gentamicin was used.

5. Vigorous attention is paid to saline hydration, regardless of the patient's oral intake. All patients receive 100 cc/hour normal saline intravenous hydration for 12 hours prior to institution of the chemotherapy and for the entire 5 day course of *cis*-platinum.

This regimen has produced the highest complete remission rate in testicular cancer reported thus far. Furthermore, chemotherapy can significantly alter the course of this disease, even when a complete remission is not seen. Present aggressive chemotherapy regimens appear to be capable of changing the histology to a more benign form and transferring previously inoperable patients (who fail to achieve a chemotherapy complete remission) to potentially operable and hopefully curable patients.

The results of recent regimens and this regimen clearly indicate that disseminated testicular cancer is a disease very responsive to chemotherapy, and many patients are probably curative, even with far-advanced disease. The complete remission rate of 70% and overall disease-free status of 81% is as high as has been seen in any adult malignancy treated with chemotherapy.

REFERENCES

Ansfield, F. J., Korbitz, B. D., Davis, H. L., Jr., and Ramirez, G. (1969). *Cancer 24*, 442–446.
Barranco, S. C., and Humphrey, R. M. (1971). *Cancer Res. 31*, 1218–1223.
Blum, R. H., Carter, S., and Agre, K. (1973). *Cancer 31*, 903–914.
Boden, G., and Gebbs, R. (1951). *Lancet 2*, 1195–1197.
Comisarow, R. H., and Grabstald, H. (1976). *J. Urol. 115*, 569–571.
Creasy, W. (1968). *Fed. Proc. 27*, 760.
Crooke, S. T., Luft, F., Broughton, A., *et al.* (1977). *Cancer* (in press).
DeVita, V. T., Serpick, A. A., and Carbone, P. P. (1970). *Ann. Intern. Med. 73*, 881–895.
Donohue, J., and Einhorn, L. (1978). *J. Urol.* (in press).
Einhorn, L. H., Krause, M., Hornback, N., *et al.* (1976). *Cancer 37*, 2414–2416.
Freedman, M., and Purkayastha, M. C. (1960). *Am. J. Roentgenol., Radium Ther. Nucl. Med. 83*, 25–42.

Golby, R. B., *et al.* (1977). Bleomycin Symposium, San Francisco, October 21.

Gutterman, J. U., Mavligit, G., Gottlieb, J. A., *et al.* (1974a). *N. Engl. J. Med. 291*, 592–597.

Gutterman, J. U., Rodriguez, V., Mavligit, G., *et al.* (1974b). *Lancet 2*, 1405–1409.

Harder, H. C., Smith, R. G., and LeRoy, A. (1976). *Proc. Am. Assoc. Cancer Res. 17*, 80.

Higby, D. J., Wallace, H. J., Albert, D. J., and Holland, J. F. (1974). *Cancer 33*, 1219–1225.

Jacobs, E. (1970). *Cancer 25*, 324–332.

Kennedy, B. J. (1970). *Cancer 26*, 755–766.

Lange, P. H., McIntire, R., Waldmann, T. A., *et al.* (1976). *New Engl. J. Med. 295*, 1237–1240.

Lefevre, R. E., Levin, H. E., Banowsky, L. H., *et al.* (1975). *Urology 6*, 588–593.

Li, M. C., Whitmore, W. F., Golbey, R., and Grabstald, H. (1960). *J. Am. Med. Assoc. 174*, 145–153.

Livingston, R. B., Bodey, G. P., Gottlieb, J. A., *et al.* (1973). *Cancer Chemother. Rep. 57*, 219–224.

MacKay, F. N., and Sellers, A. H. (1966). *Can. Med. Assoc. J. 94*, 889–899.

MacKenzie, A. R. (1966). *Cancer 19*, 1369–1376.

Maier, J. G., Mittemeyer, B. T., and Sulak, M. H. (1968). *J. Urol. 99*, 72–78.

Maier, J. G., and Sulak, M. H. (1973). *Cancer 32*, 1212–1226.

Mendelson, D., and Serpick, A. A. (1970). *J. Urol. 103*, 619–623.

Merrin, C., Takita, H., Weber, R., *et al.* (1976). *Cancer 37*, 20–29.

Nagai, K., Suzuk, H., Tanaka, N., *et al.* (1969). *J. Antibiot. 22*, 624–628.

Nefzger, M. D., and Mostofi, F. K. (1972). *Cancer 30*, 1225–1232.

Nicholson, T. C., Walsh, P. C., and Rotner, M. B. (1974). *J. Urol. 112*, 109–110.

Rosenberg, B., VanCamp, L., and Krigas, T. (1965). *Nature 205*, 678–699.

Samuels, M. L., and Howe, C. D. (1970). *Cancer 25*, 1009–1017.

Samuels, M. L., Johnson, E. E., and Holoye, P. Y. (1975). *Cancer Chemother. Rep. 59*, 563-570.

Samuels, M. L., Lanzotti, V. J., and Holoye, P. Y. (1976). *Proc. Am. Soc. Clin. Oncol. 17*, 266.

Skinner, D. G., and Leadbetter, W. F. (1971). *J. Urol. 106*, 84–93.

Staubitz, W. J., Early, K. S., Magoss, I. V., *et al.* (1974). *Urology III*, 205–209.

Willis, G. W., and Hajdu, S. I. (1973). *Am. J. Clin. Pathol. 59*, 338–343.

Wyatt, J. K., and McAninch, L. H. (1967). *Can. J. Surg. 10*, 421–426.

Chapter 19

DEVELOPMENT OF CHEMOTHERAPY PROGRAMS CONTAINING VINBLASTINE, BLEOMYCIN, ADRIAMYCIN AND *Cis*-DICHLORODIAMMINEPLATINUM(II)

Siegfried Seeber
Max E. Scheulen
Rainhardt Osieka
Klaus Höffken
Carl G. Schmidt

This report summarizes our experience with continuously developed chemotherapy programs for metastatic testicular teratomas from 1968 to 1977. It will be demonstrated that new therapeutic regimens based on the vinblastine-bleomycin combination as initiated by Samuels *et al.* (1975, 1976b) and on the combination of adriamycin and *cis*-dichlorodiammineplatinum(II) are therapeutically superior to earlier programs mainly based on actinomycin-D.

I. PATIENT POPULATION

Between 1968 and mid-1977 about 280 patients with metastasizing testicular teratomas were seen at the West German Tumor Center in Essen. Early in this period (1968 to 1973), almost 80% of the patients had advanced metastatic disease (clinical stages III and IV). More recently, however, patients were referred earlier, and in 1976–77 about 50% of the patients presented as stage II. The clinical stages were assigned as follows (modified after Castro, 1972).

TABLE I. Testicular Teratomas: Incidence of Histological Categories (Dixon and Moore) in Total Study Populations [a]

I.	Embryonal pure or with seminoma	32 (17%)
II.	Teratocarcinoma pure or with seminoma	63 (34%)
III.	Teratocarcinoma pure or with embryonal or choriocarcinoma	58 (32%)
IV.	Choriocarcinoma pure or with embryonal	31 (17%)
	total	184

[a] West German Tumor Center, Essen.

Stage I: Disease limited to testis; no evidence of invasion of spermatic cord or capsule.

Stage II: Regional lymphatic spread including tumor in the spermatic cord, iliac, inguinal or periaortic nodes.

Stage IIA: Retroperitoneal spread totally resectable by lymphadenectomy (as judged by surgeon or urologist).

Stage IIB: Retroperitoneal lymph nodes not completely resectable at laparotomy. Advanced abdominal disease with palpable masses or ureteral displacement or obstructive uropathy.

Stage III: Extension of disease beyond diaphragm but still confined to lymphatic system.

Stage IV: Visceral metastases (lungs, liver, gastrointestinal tract, brain).

The overall incidence of the histological categories of Dixon and Moore (1952) within the study groups of this report is presented in Table I. Pure seminomas were excluded, as their incidence within the total patient population was below 10%. This histological distribution differs from other large series mainly by its higher incidence of the Dixon and Moore group No. 3 (teratocarcinoma) and a lower percentage of embryonal carcinomas (Samuels *et al.*, 1976b).

II. TREATMENT PROGRAMS AND RESULTS

A. Early Actinomycin-D Programs

1. Actinomycin-D Monotherapy (Höffken et al., 1976)

Twenty-one stage IV patients (1968-69) were treated with 1 mg actinomycin-D for 4-5 days every 2-4 weeks, depending on myelosuppression. Most patients

TABLE II. Actinomycin-D–Monotherapy in Stage IV [a]

Response	N	%	Duration of response (months)
Complete responders	1/21	5	> 70
Partial responders	3/21	14	(2, 2, 22)

[a] Testicular Teratomas at the West German Tumor Center, Essen (1968 - 1971) (Höffken *et al.*, 1974).

TABLE III.

Actinomycin-D	0.5–1.0 mg IV daily x 5
Vinblastine	10 mg IV day 1
Methotrexate	10 mg IV days 1 and 2
Cyclophosphamide	100–200 mg daily p. o.

q. 4–6 weeks

belonged to the prognostically unfavorable Dixon and Moore categories 3–5; 6/21 patients had prior irradiation to abdominal masses. Only one patient (5%) achieved complete remission and is still alive 6 years after onset of treatment. The overall response rate was 19% and lower than in other monotherapeutic studies with actinomycin-D, indicating the unfavorable patient selection of our early series (Table II).

2. Combination of Actinomycin-D, Vinblastine, Methotrexate, and Cyclophosphamide (Höffken et al., 1974)

Fifty-one consecutive patients with disseminated nonseminomatous testicular cancer were treated with a four-drug regimen as detailed in Table III. The results of this chemotherapy program are shown in Table IV. In summary, with actinomycin-D programs the complete remission rate was below 10% and an objective response rate of maximally 40% was achieved, with a very short median duration of remissions for complete and partial responders (4–5 months).

B. Bleomycin-Containing Combinations

1. The "ABO" Program (Burgess et al., 1975; Seeber et al., 1975)

A combination consisting of adriamycin, bleomycin, and vincristine for the treatment of metastatic germ cell tumors was first reported by Burgess et al. (1975). Objective responses (50%)|were observed in 20/25 patients (80%), with 7/25 (28%)

TABLE IV. Combination Chemotherapy with Actinomycin-D, Vinblastine, Methotrexate, and Cyclophosphamide for Stage IV Testicular Teratomas [a]

		N	%	Median durations (months)
A.	Without previous chemotherapy			
	Complete responders	1/36	3	5
	Partial responders	14/36	39	4.5
B.	With previous chemotherapy			
	Complete responders	1/15	7	1
	Partial responders	6/15	40	3.9
Overall response:	2/51 CR (4%)			
	20/51 PR (38%)			

[a] West German Tumor Center Essen, 1968–1973 (Höffken et al., 1974).

TABLE V. "ABO" for Testicular Teratomas [a]

Adriamycin	75 mg/m^2	
Vincristine	1 mg	IV on day 1 q. 3 weeks
Bleomycin	15 mg	

[a] West German Tumor Center

complete responses; 3/7 complete responders and 8/13 partial responders had previously received radiotherapy and chemotherapy with actinomycin-D and/or other agents. The median duration of partial remissions had been 4 months; within the group of complete responders three long-term remissions (>12 months) were reported.

Between 10/74 and 9/75, 22 patients with stage III or stage IV testicular teratomas were treated at our clinic with a similar regimen, which is presented in Table V. The results of this protocol, which allowed chemotherapy on an outpatient basis, have been reported previously (Seeber et al., 1975) and are updated in Table VI.

Although the dose schedule for bleomycin was probably not optimal, this series showed a considerable improvement in therapeutic results in a patient population which was comparable to our previous actinomycin-D series. Of special interest were the long-term results in this group of patients, with three complete responders disease-free after 24 months and five other patients alive 10, 11, 18, 21, and 26 months after onset of treatment, when analyzed in 1976 (Gallmeier et al., 1976). Histologically, 4/7 complete responders belonged to the Dixon and Moore No. 3 category (teratocarcinoma, pure or with seminoma), 2/7 had embryonal carcinomas, and one patient had a No. 4 Dixon and Moore category tumor (teratocarcinoma with choriocarcinoma). It should be pointed out that none of the complete responders had presented with palpable abdominal masses. Toxicity in this outpatient series was minimal and mainly related to adriamycin side effects (nausea, alopecia). Severe myelosuppression occurred in one out of 22 patients who had previous paraortal irradiation of 4000 rads (Seeber et al., 1975).

2. The "VeBa" Program

Encouraged by the results of the velban-bleomycin continuous infusion program of Samuels et al. (1975) and because of our own impression of a significant therapeutic

TABLE VI. Adriamycin, Bleomycin, and Vincristine
in Stage IV Metastasizing Teratomas [a]

	N	%	Duration of response (months)
Complete responders	7/22	32	2, 4, 6, 10, 22, 25, 40+
Partial responders	6/22	27	5
Total	13/22	59	

[a] West German Tumor Center, Essen.

TABLE VII. Velban, Bleomycin, and Adriamycin ("VeBa")
for Metastasizing Testicular Teratomas

Adriamycin	40 mg/m²	IV push on day 1
Vinblastine	10 mg/m²	IV push on day 1
Bleomycin	30 mg/m²	Continuous infusion, days 1 and 2

contribution of adriamycin alone (Monfardini *et al.*, 1972) and in combination (Seeber *et al.*, 1975) in metastatic testicular cancers, we began a study at our clinic in 1975 combining velban, bleomycin, and adriamycin (Table VII). Because of the overlapping bone-marrow toxicity of adriamycin and vinblastine, the doses of both drugs were reduced, when compared to the VB protocol (bleomycin [Samuels *et al.*, 1975]) and the ABO regimen (adriamycin [Seeber *et al.*, 1975]). The early results of this phase II study, which had encompassed 17 patients, indicated that this probably was not a good compromise. Although the overall response rate of this interim program was again improved in comparison to our previous series (70% CR and PR), the medium duration of all responses was only about 4 months, and the rate of complete remissions was low. This study was therefore terminated and replaced by a velbane–bleomycin–DDP program in early 1976 (see Section II, B, 4). It is concluded —and this was also reported by Kardinal *et al.* (1976)—that the combination of bleomycin, adriamycin, and vinblastine at the dose levels investigated cannot be recommended as primary therapy for advanced testicular tumors.

3. DDP-Monotherapy in Metastasizing Testicular Teratomas Refractory to Actinomycin-D, "ABO" and "VeBa" Programs (Osieka et al., 1976a,b)

Cis-dichlorodiammineplatinum(II) (NSC-119875; supplied by the NCI) was investigated as a second-line drug, designated for failures of our previous actinomycin-D

TABLE VIII. Treatment of Metastasizing Testicular Teratomas
with *Cis*-Diamminedichloride Platinum (NSC - 119875)[a]

Response to previous therapy	Response to DDP
Progressive disease: 5	Partial remissions: 3 Progressive disease: 2
No change: 2	No change: 1 Progressive disease: 1
Partial response: 8	Complete remissions: 1 Partial remissions: 4 No change: 2 Progressive disease: 1
total: 15 patients: 1 CR, 7 PR, 3 NC, and 4 PD	

[a] West German Tumor Center, Essen (Osieka *et al.*, 1976).

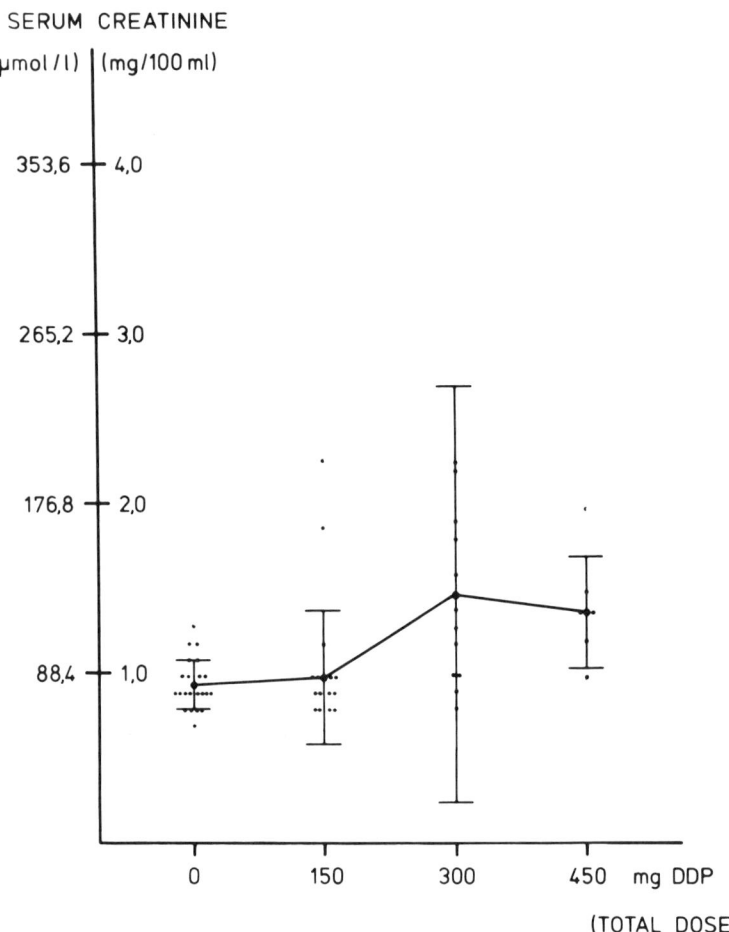

Fig. 1. Changes of serum creatinine in patients with metastasizing testicular teratomas after chemotherapy with *cis*-dichlorodiammineplatinum(II).

programs, the "ABO" and the "VeBa" series. The results have been previously presented by Osieka *et al.* (1976a, b). The treatment schedule called for intravenous push injections of the platinum compound at a single daily dose of 20 mg/m² on 5 consecutive days, which was to be repeated every 4 weeks. Drug toxicity was to be monitored by biweekly controls of serum creatinine, transaminases and electrolyte levels, WBC and thrombocyte counts. Audiograms were to be performed every other month. The results of this study are summarized in Table VIII.

Altogether, 22 patients were finally evaluable in this monotherapeutic trial, with one complete responder, 14 partial remissions, two "no change" courses, and five progressions, resulting in an overall response rate of 68% in a highly unfavorable patient

TABLE IX. Velban, Belomycin, and *cis*-DDP
for Metastasizing Testicular Teratomas

Vinblastine	0.4 mg/kg (divided into two IV doses, days 1 and 2)
Bleomycin	30 mg/day x 5 (continuous infusion)
Cis-DDP	18 mg/m²/day x 5 (max. 3 x 10 mg/day) daily IV injections

population with acquired resistance to combination chemotherapy (Osieka *et al.*, 1976b). Most of the patients (18/22) had massive pulmonary disease. Nephrotoxicity, as determined by a reduced serum creatinine clearance, occurred in 7/22 patients and was only partly reversible. The average increase of serum creatinine as a function of the total dose of *cis*-platinum is shown in Fig. 1. In the meantime, the schedule for DDP has been changed in that the drug is given at 18 mg/m²/day (x5) in three divided IV doses (at maximum 3 x 10 mg/day). By this measure and by a daily oral uptake of 3-4 liters of fluid, nephrotoxicity has been largely avoided without demonstrable loss of cytostatic activity. Such a decrease of efficacy had been noted when the platinum dose was temporarily reduced to 12 mg/m²/day (x5).

4. The Velban-Bleomycin-DDP Combination

This combination has been a consequence of the striking data reported for the velban-bleomycin combination (Samuels *et al.*, 1975, 1976b) and the impressive monotherapeutic results with *cis*-DDP (Osieka *et al.*, 1976b). A phase I clinical trial with a combination of these drugs was first published by Samson *et al.* (1976). At our clinic, a phase II study was initiated in early 1976, based on a regimen as presented in Table IX.

The tolerance of the continuous bleomycin infusion was significantly improved by the addition of IV prednisone (50 mg Solu-Decortin H, Merck, Darmstadt, added

TABLE X. Vinblastine, Bleomycin, and *Cis*-DDP
in Stage IV Testicular Teratomas [a]

A. Without prior chemotherapy (N = 24)			
Complete remissions	9	(38%)	} 92%
Partial remissions	13	(54%)	
No change	1		
Progression	1		
B. With prior chemotherapy (N = 19)			
Complete remissions	5	(26%)	} 73%
Partial remissions	9	(47%)	
No change	1		
Progression	4		

[a] West German Tumor Center, Essen

TABLE XI. Vinblastine–Bleomycin (VB 3) versus Adriamycin–DDP in Stage IV Testicular Teratomas. A Randomized Monoinstitutional Phase III Study

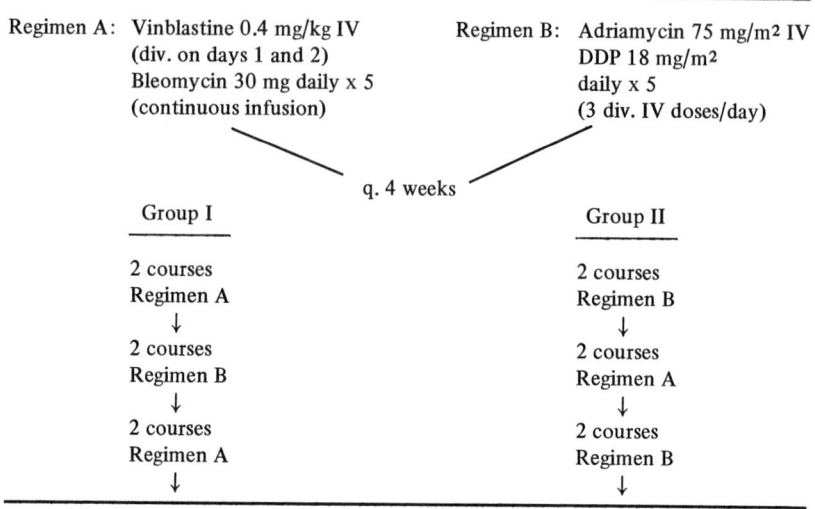

Regimen A: Vinblastine 0.4 mg/kg IV
(div. on days 1 and 2)
Bleomycin 30 mg daily x 5
(continuous infusion)

Regimen B: Adriamycin 75 mg/m² IV
DDP 18 mg/m²
daily x 5
(3 div. IV doses/day)

q. 4 weeks

Group I

2 courses
Regimen A
↓
2 courses
Regimen B
↓
2 courses
Regimen A
↓

Group II

2 courses
Regimen B
↓
2 courses
Regimen A
↓
2 courses
Regimen B
↓

to each 500 ml of the bleomycin infusion = 100 mg Solu-Decortin H/24 hours).

Until April 1977, 43 patients were initially treated with this regimen. The results are listed in Table X. When the complete responders were analyzed for histology, the following distribution, which did not differ significantly from our total patient population, was noted: pure embryonal carcinoma or with seminoma: 2, pure teratocarcinoma or with seminoma: 5, teratocarcinoma with embryonal carcinoma or

TABLE XII. Velban-Bleomycin and Adriamycin-DDP in Stage IV Testicular Teratomas. Preliminary Data with Alternating Schedules

	N	Response	
Group I			
(start with VB3)	12	10/11	CR: 2
		too early: 1	PR: 8 (6 still improving)
Group II			
(start with Adm/DDP	6	3/4	CR: 1
		too early: 2	PR: 2

	N	Response (total)[a]	Response after failure of alternative program
VB3 courses (total)	28	23/28 = 82%	1/1
Adm/DDP courses	16	12/16 = 75%	1/1

[a] Responders remaining NED are included.

with carcinoma: 4, pure choriocarcinoma: 1, not classified: 2. Among the 14 complete remissions three were very short in duration (6-8 weeks) and all of them belonged to the Dixon and Moore No. 4 or No. 5 categories.

No data are available for the medium duration of response related to this velban-bleomycin-*cis*-DDP combination since our protocol (approved by the NCI) did only call for three courses of this combination as an inductive treatment, followed by three courses of adriamycin (80 mg/m², day 1) and DTIC (250 mg/m², days 1-5) at monthly invervals. For responders, the protocol provided for a third phase of chemotherapy based on high-dose cyclosphamide (2 Gm/m² IV every 4 weeks [Buckner *et al.*, 1974]). However, when 8/13 patients had relapsed under adriamycin-DTIC, the protocol had to be changed in that the velban-bleomycin combination of the induction phase (with or without DDP depending on renal function) was continued and only changed at relapse or progression.

5. Vinblastine–Bleomycin and Adriamycin-DDP in Testicular Teratomas: A Randomized Phase III Study

Since most of the patients with clinical stage IV disease require chemotherapy for periods between 18 and 24 months, cumulative tissue toxicity becomes one of the major obstacles and limits the use of combinations such as the velbane–bleomycin program. This has led us to the use of alternating schedules of two similarly effective combinations, with two main goals: (a) delay of cumulative tissue toxicity, and (b) delay of acquired resistance to the four individual drugs. (Table XI)

The following questions were to be answered by this study:

a.   What is the therapeutic value of adriamycin-DDP in various histologies of testicular teratomas as compared to the established velban–bleomycin combination?

b.   How are the patterns of cross-resistance between both regimens in relation to the histological subclassification?

c.   Is it possible to delay acquired resistance and to increase complete remissions by alternating schedules?

d.   To what extent can cumulative side effects be avoided or delayed by these programs?

Since this study was initiated only in February 1977, the limited number of patients can provide only preliminary data, which are summarized in Table XII. Apparently, adriamycin-DDP has comparable cytostatic activity in these tumors. Thus far, one primary treatment failure was noted in each of the two groups which responded to the alternative regimen. The patient who failed on adriamycin-DDP had choriocarcinoma; the patient who initially failed on velban–bleomycin had teratocarcinoma.

Although these early figures do not allow final conclusions, the preliminary data suggest that the two programs which have similar efficacy probably are not, or are only partially, cross-resistant in metastasizing testicular tumors. Since already one single course of velban–bleomycin or adriamycin-DDP could achieve a tumor reduction as shown in Fig. 2, higher numbers of complete responders and cure should be achieved in the near future.

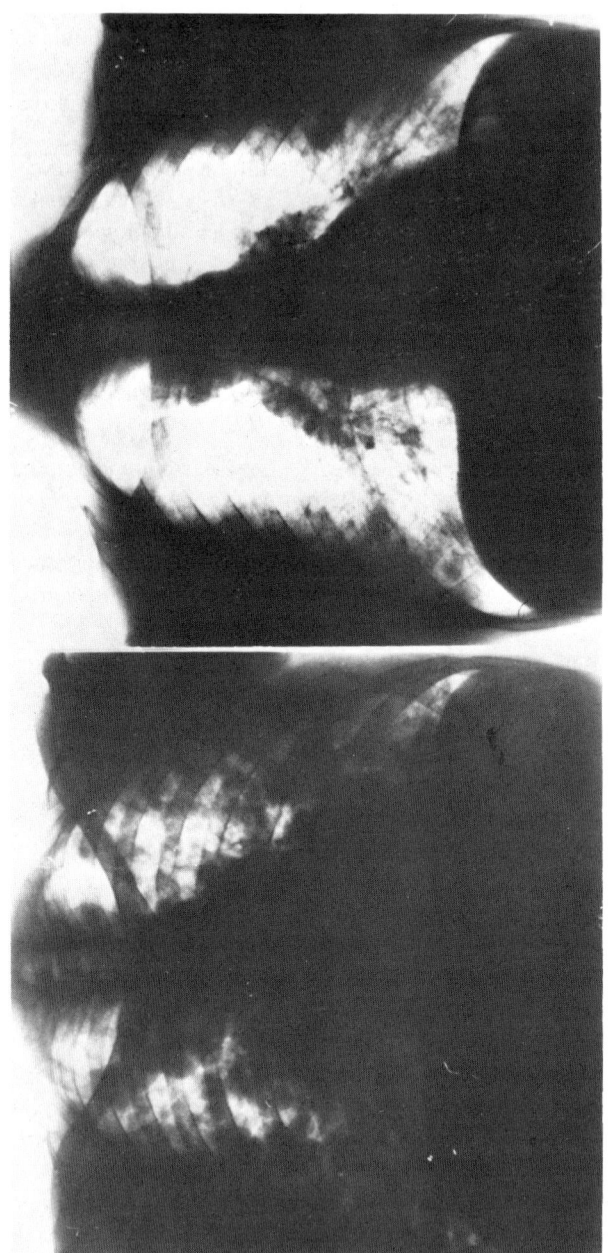

Fig. 2. Partial remission of metastasizing teratocarcinoma (patient H. H.) after one course of velban-bleomycin.

6. Chemotherapy of Stage IIB Testicular Teratomas

Patients with retroperitoneal disease offer special problems regarding therapy. As already defined above, the clinical stage IIB included all patients with histologically proven, positive retroperitoneal lymph nodes which were not totally or not at all resectable at laparotomy (stage IIA: positive nodes, but completely resectable). This clinical category is largely heterogenous, and a further distinction should be made between patients with palpable masses and those who are without palpable evidence of disease. This seems to be important, since additional radiotherapy may play a different role in these two types of patients and because chemotherapeutic cure appears to be directly related to the net tumor burden (Samuels *et al.*, 1976). Therefore, patients with palpable abdominal masses were classified as stage IIIB-4 by these authors, suggesting that the prognosis of these cases was worse when compared to patients with minimal pulmonary disease (IIIB-2) or even advanced pulmonary disease (IIIB-3 ⟨Samuels *et al.*, 1976b⟩).

Since October 1976, 23 patients with stage IIB disease were treated with alternate schedules of vinblastine–bleomycin and adriamycin-DDP. This chemotherapy is planned monthly for 1 year, and the regimens are changed every other month. Out of 23 patients, 12 patients have already been under study for at least 6 months, with only 2/12 showing progressive disease. These two patients belong to the group with palpable masses. No progression was seen in 8/8 patients without palpable disease (Table XIII).

III. SUMMARY AND CONCLUSIONS

Considerable progress has been made in the chemotherapy of metastasizing testicular cancers after velban, bleomycin, adriamycin, and DDP were introduced. At our clinic the overall response rate has been improved from 30–40% in 1973 up to 90% in 1977 in a comparable patient population. Complete remissions were increased

TABLE XIII. Chemotherapy of Testicular Teratomas (Stage IIB: Retroperitoneal Tumor after Lymphadenectomy) with Alternating Schedules of Vinblastine–Bleomycin and Adriamycin–DDP [a]

Number of patients		Progression at 6 months	Time NED (months) or without progression
All	23		
Evaluable [b]	12		
Without palpable masses	8	0	9+, 9+, 7+, 6+, 6+, 7+, 6+, 7+
With palpable masses ("stage IIC")	4	2	6, 4, 6+, 6+

[a] West German Tumor Center, Essen.
[b] Only patients receiving chemotherapy for at least 6 months were evaluable.

from 5% to 30–40% within the same period, and the number of patients who might have a chance of being finally cured at last seems to be slowly growing. Our results also indicate that the adriamycin-DDP combination may be of similar usefulness as has been already documented for the velban-bleomycin program. So far, there is no hint of a cross resistance between the two programs. A phase III study, to which some 30–40 new patients with stage IV teratoma are accruing per year, has been initiated in order to define (a) the comparative objective response rates of velban-bleomycin versus adriamycin-DDP within the different histological types of testicular teratomas, and (b) the value of alternating schedules in delaying cumulative tissue toxicity and acquired chemotherapy resistance. With regard to the clinical stage II, it seems to be advisable that this category should be further subdivided to the size of the residual tumor after lymphadenectomy. After 6 months, preliminary data indicate that chemotherapy with vinblastine–bleomycin and adriamycin-DDP may improve the prognosis of patients in the clinical stages IIB and IIC, especially when other measures (second surgery, irradiation) are included into the individual treatment concepts.

REFERENCES

Buckner, C. D., Clift, R. A., Fefer, A., Funk, D. D., Glucksberg, H., Neiman, P. E., Paulsen, A., Storb, R., and Thomas, E. D. (1974). *Cancer Chemother. Rep.* Part 1 *58*, 709–714.

Burgess, M. A., Einhorn, L. H., and Gottlieb, J. A. (1975). *Proc. Am. Assoc. Cancer Res., Am. Soc. Clin. Oncol. 16*, 244, ASCO abstr.

Castro, J. R. (1972). In Johnson, D. E. (Ed.), *Testicular Tumors.* Huber, Bern, Stuttgart, Vienna, pp. 181–201.

Dixon, F. J., and Moore, R. A. (1952). *Atlas of Tumor Pathology,* Section 8, Fascicle 31b and 32. Armed Forces Institute of Pathology, Washington, D.C.

Gallmeier, W. M., Osieka, R., Seeber, S., Bruntsch, U., Hossfeld, D. K., Böhlandt, D., and Schmidt, C. G. (1976). *Verh. Dtsch. Ges. Inn. Med. 82*, 1760–1763.

Höffken, K., Tingelhoff, J., Hornung, G., and Schmidt, C. G. (1974). *Z. Krebsforsch. 82*, 307–328.

Höffken, K., Tingelhoff, J., Seeber, S., and Schmidt, C. G. (1976). *Urol. Ausg. A 15*, 61–66.

Kardinal, C. G., Jacobs, E. M., Bull, F., Bateman, J. R., and Pajak, T. (1976). *Cancer Treatment Rep. 60*, 953–954.

Monfardini, S., Bajetta, E., Musumeci, R., and Bonadonna, G. (1972). *J. Urol. 108*, 293–296.

Osieka, R., Bruntsch, U., Gallmeier, W. M., Seeber, S., and Schmidt, C. G. (1976a). In *Chemotherapy. Proceedings of the 9th International Congress of Chemotherapy, London, 1975,* Vol. 8, *Cancer Chemotherapy,* Part 2. Hellman, K., and Connors, T. A. (Eds.). Plenum, New York and London.

Osieka, R., Bruntsch, U., Gallmeier, W. M., Seeber, S., and Schmidt, C. G. (1976b). *Dtsch. Med. Wochenschr. 101*, 191–195.

Samson, M. K., Baker, L. H., Devos, J. M., Duroker, T. R., Izbicki, R. M., and Vaitkevicius, V. K. (1976a). *Cancer Treatment Rep. 60*, 91–97.

Samuels, M. L., Johnson, D. E., and Holoye, P. Y. (1975). *Cancer Chemother. Rep.,* Part 1 *59*, 563–570.

Samuels, M. L., Lanzotti, V. J., Holoye, P. Y., Boyle, L. E., Smith, T. L., and Johnson, D. E. (1976b). *Cancer Treatment Rev. 3*, 185–204.

Seeber, S., Gallmeier, W. M., Höffken, K., Osieka, R., Bruntsch, U., and Schmidt, C. G. (1975). *Dtsch. Med. Wochenschr. 100*, 1319–1324.

Chapter 20

BLEOMYCIN IN COMBINATION WITH MOPP FOR THE MANAGEMENT OF HODGKIN'S DISEASE: SOUTHWEST ONCOLOGY GROUP EXPERIENCE

Charles A. Coltman, Jr.
Stephen E. Jones
Petre N. Grozea
Edward DePersio
Thomas E. Moon

I. INTRODUCTION

A. MOPP Alone

The management of advanced Hodgkin's disease is principally that of high-dose intermittent combination chemotherapy. Since the benchmark studies of DeVita and associates (1970) with MOPP chemotherapy, the Southwest Oncology Group (SWOG) has participated in a number of studies which have used MOPP chemotherapy for remission induction in patients with Stage III and IV Hodgkin's disease (Frei et al., 1973; Coltman et al., 1973) (Table 1). In the initial study, 178 patients were treated with six cycles of MOPP for remission induction, following which a random half of those who achieved complete response continued on MOPP every other month for a total of nine cycles (Frei et al., 1973). The complete response rate was 66% for all patients and 81% for those who had had no prior treatment. This result compared favorably with the NCI experience (DeVita et al., 1970). At the time of publication of the initial Southwest Oncology Group study (Frei et al., 1973) these data supported the hypothesis that maintenance therapy, for patients in complete

227

TABLE I. Oncology Group Studies in Advanced Hodgkin's Disease

Year	Study	Induction regimen	No. of patients	% CR	Survival at 3 Years (%)
1968–1969	SWOG 758	MOPP alone	178	66	50
1969–1971	SWOG 772	MOPP alone	206	62	59
1971–1974	SWOG 774	MOPP alone	44	70	62
		MOPP (CPF) [a]	28	64	60
		MOPP + high bleo	38	76	65
		MOPP + low bleo	118	84	81

[a] CPF—compromised pulmonary function.

response, was beneficial in terms of disease-free survival. Recent followup review of this study (Coltman et al., 1976) failed to show a survival advantage in patients maintained on chemotherapy with MOPP.

The second SWOG study (Coltman et al., 1973) involved MOPP alone for six cycles for remission induction followed by maintenance therapy with actinomycin D, methotrexate, or vinblastine for 18 months following complete remission. The complete response rate for 206 patients entered into the remission induction limb of the study was 62%, a figure which compared favorably with our initial study (Frei et al., 1973) with a complete response rate of 66%. The remission maintenance phase of this study showed no significant advantage over unmaintained remission for either of the three limbs. Thus, in 384 patients with advanced Hodgkin's disease treated on two major Southwest Oncology Group studies the overall complete response rate was 64%.

B. Bleomycin Alone

Bleomycin, a glycopeptide antibiotic produced by *streptomyces verticillis,* has been demonstrated to have activity as a single agent in the management of advanced Hodgkin's disease in 1971 by the Southwest Oncology Group (Haas et al., 1976). A response rate of 37% (11/27) in heavily pretreated patients was very encouraging for this single agent. Similar results were achieved by investigators in Japan (Kimura et al., 1972), Europe (Bonadonna et al., 1972), and England (Halnan et al., 1972). The latter investigators demonstrated activity of bleomycin in relatively low dose. All studies showed minimal myelosuppression, but rather the dose-limiting toxicity was a peculiar, occasionally fatal, pulmonary fibrosis which was associated with older patients and doses above 200 u/m^2. These characteristics made bleomycin the logical choice to add to prototype combination chemotherapy for advanced Hodgkin's disease.

II. MOPP PLUS BLEOMYCIN COMBINATIONS

A. Induction Regimen

The rationale for the initial MOPP plus bleomycin study (SWOG 774-MOPP 4) was based on the concept that this relatively nonmyelosuppressive antibiotic could be added to the intensively myelosuppressive MOPP regimen without significant additive toxicity, but with improvement in the overall complete response rate as well as survival. We chose to test two different test levels of bleomycin, in an attempt to establish a dose-response relationship, and, further, to determine whether or not bleomycin was active in low dose, as has been reported (Halnan *et al.*, 1972). Figure 1 shows the schema of this study, in which patients with advanced Hodgkin's disease, who did not have significant compromise of pulmonary function, were randomly assigned to MOPP alone or MOPP plus bleomycin in two different dose levels. A low dose of 2 u/m^2 on days 1 and 8 of the first six cycles of MOPP represented the MOPP plus low-dose bleomycin limb. A dose of 10 μ/M^2 on days 1 and 8 of the second through sixth cycles was administered following the administration of 5 u on days 1 and 8 of the first cycle of MOPP on the MOPP plus high-dose bleomycin limb. Because of bleomycin pulmonary toxicity, patients who were considered to have had significant compromise of pulmonary function were treated on a separate limb, for comparisons sake, with MOPP alone. This determination of significant compromise of pulmonary function on each patient was made jointly in telephone consultation between the principal investigator and the study coordinator.

TABLE II.   Distribution of Eligible Patients in MOPP 4 (SWOG 774)

	Total	MOPP alone	MOPP + LDB	MOPP + HDB	MOPP + CPF
Eligible	253	48	129	47	29
Evaluable	207	40	106	35	26
Partially evaluable	21	4	12	3	2
Not evaluable	25	4	11	9	1

Table II demonstrates the distribution of eligible patients into the four limbs of the study. A total of 253 eligible patients were entered into the study, of whom 228 were fully evaluable or partially evaluable, with 25 patients considered to be not evaluable. Partially evaluable patients included those who had inadequate trial because of toxicity, being lost to followup, or refused further therapy. Patients who were considered not evaluable are those who had major protocol violations for reasons other than toxicity or in whom data were inadequate to determine response and toxicity. It should be noted that randomization among the three limbs is significantly unbalanced (Table II). This imbalance occurred because when approximately 48 patients were randomized into each limb of the study, three patients on the MOPP plus high-dose bleomycin limb of the study died of irreversible myelosuppression. That limb of the study was immediately discontinued. At approximately the same time, because the complete response rate of the MOPP alone limb was comparable to our previous experience in 384 patients treated with MOPP alone (complete response rate 64%) (Frei *et al.*, 1973; Coltman *et al.*, 1973) and because it was unlikely that the complete response rate would ever achieve the level of MOPP plus low-dose bleomycin, the MOPP-alone limb of the study was also dis-

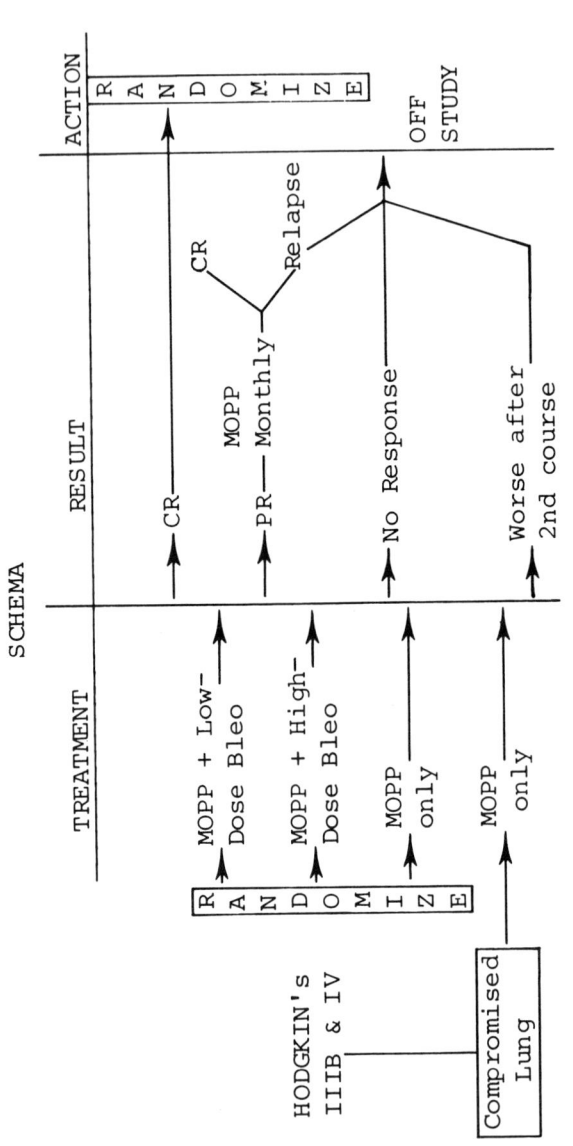

Fig. 1. MOPP 4 (SWOG 774) schema.

TABLE III. Response by Induction Regimen in MOPP 4 (SWOG 774)

Regimen	Total (%)	CR (%)	PR (%)
MOPP	44 (19)	31 (70)	6 (14)
MOPP + LDB [a]	118 (52)	99 (84)	14 (12)
MOPP + HDB	38 (17)	29 (76)	6 (16)
CPF	28 (12)	18 (64)	6 (21)

[a] $p = 0.076$.

continued. MOPP plus low-dose bleomycin was continued as a single arm, except that patients who had significant compromise of pulmonary function continued receiving the MOPP-alone option. This limb was continued in an attempt to firmly establish complete response rate with significant confidence. Twenty-eight (11.1%) of the 253 eligible patients were considered to have had significant compromise of pulmonary function and were analyzed independently.

B. Results

Table III shows the complete and partial response rate by induction regimen. The complete response rate for MOPP alone of $70 \pm 14\%$ (95% confidence interval for the true complete response rate) was comparable to our previous experience of 64% in a large number of patients (Frei *et al.*, 1973; Coltman *et al.*, 1973). MOPP plus low-dose bleomycin had a complete response rate of $84 \pm 7\%$ compared to $76\% \pm 14\%$ for MOPP plus high-dose bleomycin, $70 \pm 14\%$ for MOPP alone, and $64\% \pm 18\%$ for the compromised pulmonary function MOPP-alone limb. The difference in complete response rate between MOPP and MOPP plus low-dose bleomycin did not quite achieve the level of statistical significance ($p=0.076$). The complete plus partial response rate with MOPP plus low-dose bleomycin of 96% was statistically significantly greater than the complete plus partial response rate for MOPP alone of 84% ($p=0.03$). It is of considerable interest that the 28 patients treated on the compromised pulmonary function limb of the study had a complete response of 64%, exactly

TABLE IV. Pretreatment Characteristics versus Complete Response Rate in MOPP 4 (SWOG 774)

Characteristic	CR (%)	p Value
Marrow biopsy		0.009
Not biopsied	14 (61)	
Biopsied, neg.	127 (82)	
Biopsied, pos.	23 (64)	
Performance status		0.037
Asymptomatic, active	25 (76)	
Ambulatory, symptomatic	119 (82)	
Partially bedridden	15 (63)	
Completely bedridden	2 (40)	
Weight loss (>10% body wt.)		0.055
No	93 (83)	
Yes	74 (71)	

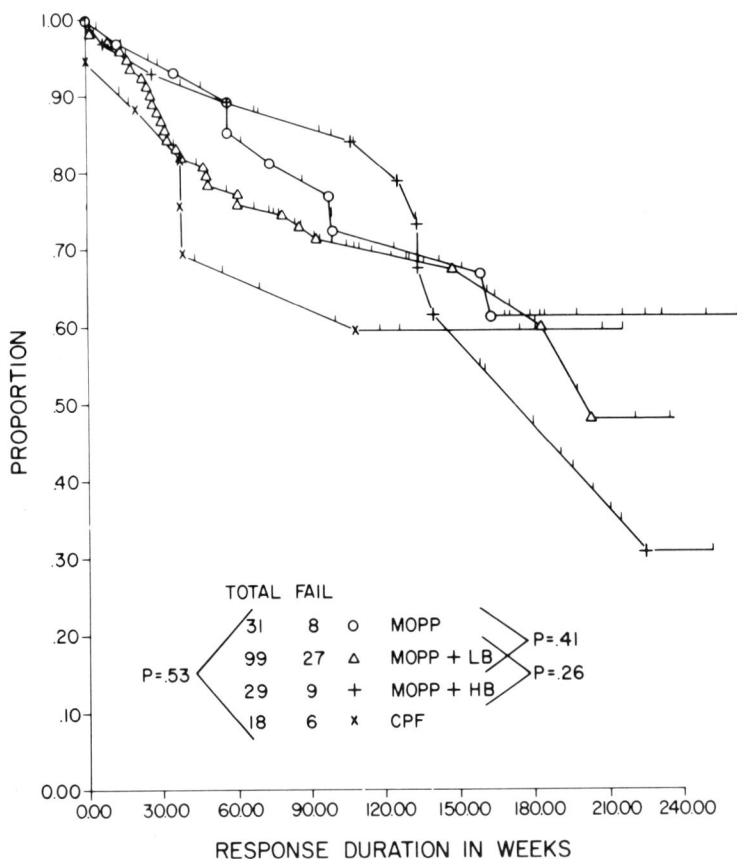

Fig. 2. MOPP 4 (SWOG 774) Complete response duration by induction treatment.

comparable to our previous MOPP alone experience (Table I), with a 3 year survival
similar to SWOG 772 (MOPP 1 and 2).

The median time to complete response is approximately 15 weeks with no significant difference in the three limbs ($p = 0.50$). Complete response rate was influenced
by three pretreatment characteristics (Table IV). A positive bone-marrow biopsy
adversely affected complete response rate ($p = 0.009$). Performance status, in which
patients were partially or completely bedridden, had a significantly adverse affect
on complete response rate ($p = 0.037$). Weight loss of >10% of the body weight over
the previous 6 months also lowered complete response rate ($p = 0.055$).

The duration of complete response data are available out beyond 5 years. Figure
2 shows the response duration curves and there are no statistically significant differences in these curves. The MOPP plus low-dose bleomycin limb just reached the
median duration of complete response at 200 weeks, the MOPP plus high-dose bleomycin at 165 weeks. The other two limbs have yet to reach their median and have

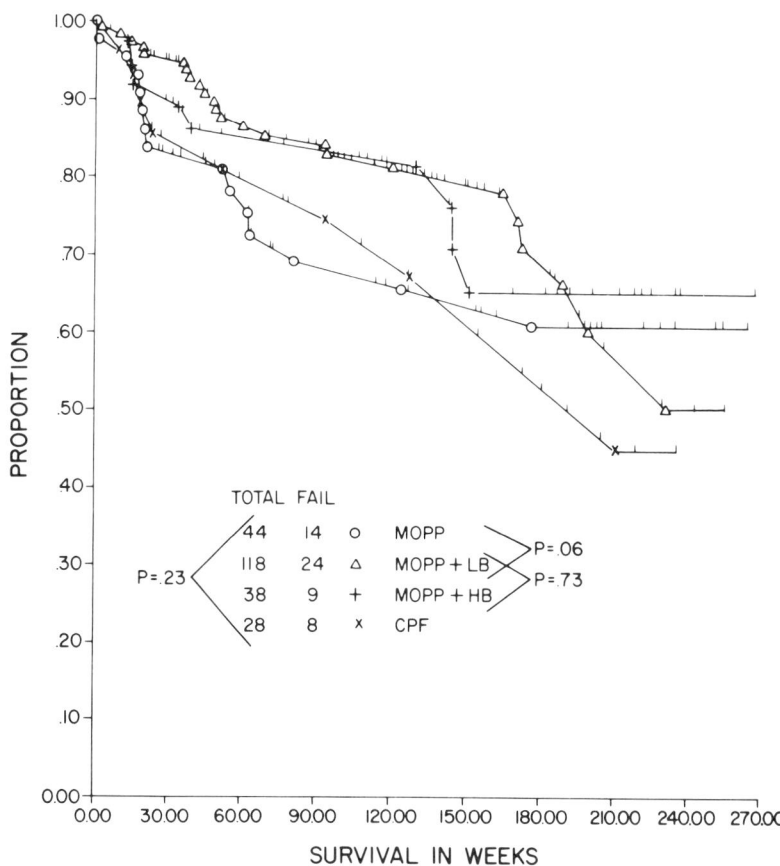

Fig. 3   MOPP (SWOG 774) survival by induction treatment.

plateaued above 60%. The survival curves are seen in Fig. 3 and there is suggestive evidence that the survival is better on the MOPP plus low-dose bleomycin limb than on the MOPP-alone limb (p = 0.06). There is no significant difference between MOPP plus low-dose bleomycin and MOPP plus high-dose bleomycin survival (p = 0.73).

If one examines the estimated survival, at 3 years, with MOPP alone, as administered in MOPP 1 and 2 (Table I), 50% of the patients were alive. This compares to 59% on the MOPP 3 study, 62% on MOPP alone, and 60% on MOPP (CPF) of the current study (MOPP 4-SWOG 774). On the other hand, the survival estimate at 3 years on the MOPP plus low-dose bleomycin limb of MOPP 4 (SWOG 774) is 81%. Thus, we have established a complete response rate for MOPP alone (293/456) of 64% with an average estimated 3 year survival of 58% (50-62%). The comparable figures for MOPP plus low-dose bleomycin are 99/118 84% complete response and

TABLE V. Worse Degree of Toxicity in MOPP 4 (SWOG 774)

Degree of toxicity	MOPP No. (%)	MOPP + low bleo No. (%)	MOPP + high bleo No. (%)	CPF No. (%)
None or mild	11 (23)	51 (40)	13 (28)	14 (29)
Moderate	24 (50)	49 (38)	24 (51)	7 (15)
Severe	11 (23)	23 (18)	6 (13)	6 (13)
Life threatening	1 (2)	5 (4)	1 (2)	0 (0)
Fatal	1 (2)	1 (1)	3 (6)	2 (4)

81% 3 year survival.

Table V demonstrates the cumulative worst degree of toxicity in the four limbs of the study. The most important toxicity was three fatal episodes which occurred on the MOPP plus high-dose bleomycin limb which were directly related to irreversible myelosuppression. One such episode was seen in the MOPP-alone limb and a single fatal toxicity in the MOPP plus low-dose bleomycin limb was related to overwhelming infection in a splenectomized patient who had adequate granulocytes. There was no life threatening or fatal pulmonary toxicity in this study.

There is no significant difference in survival when one compares those patients with mixed cellular Hodgkin's disease with those who had nodular sclerosis Hodgkin's disease ($p = 0.63$). Figure 4 demonstrates the survival curve of the mixed cellular Hodgkin's and nodular sclerosis patients lumped together and compared to the survival of patients with lymphocyte-predominant and lymphocyte-depleted Hodgkin's disease. There is suggestive evidence that the survival of patients with lymphocyte-depleted Hodgkin's disease was shorter than that of the combined mixed and nodular sclerosis group. There was no significant difference between the survival of the latter two and that of the patients with lymphocyte-predominant histology.

C. Consolidation

The consolidation limb of this study (SWOG 774–MOPP 4) was based principally on our experience from MOPP 1 and 2 (Frei *et al.*, 1973) in which it was clear that MOPP every other month administered for 18 months following 6 months of MOPP remission induction was advantageous in terms of disease-free survival ($p = 0.025$), an observation since disproven (Coltman *et al.*, 1976). A second result, which was important in the remission consolidation aspect of this study (SWOG 774-MOPP 4), was the observation, from the MOPP 1 and 2 study, that the area of major involvement prior to the institution of MOPP was the major area of relapse of Hodgkin's disease following MOPP remission induction. That is to say, the disease recurred in previously bulky lymph nodes rather than previously uninvolved sites. The first remission consolidation limb consisted of MOPP every other month for 18 months, followed by unmaintained remission. The second limb involved the administration, at the time of complete response, of 4000 rads of radiotherapy to the area of major

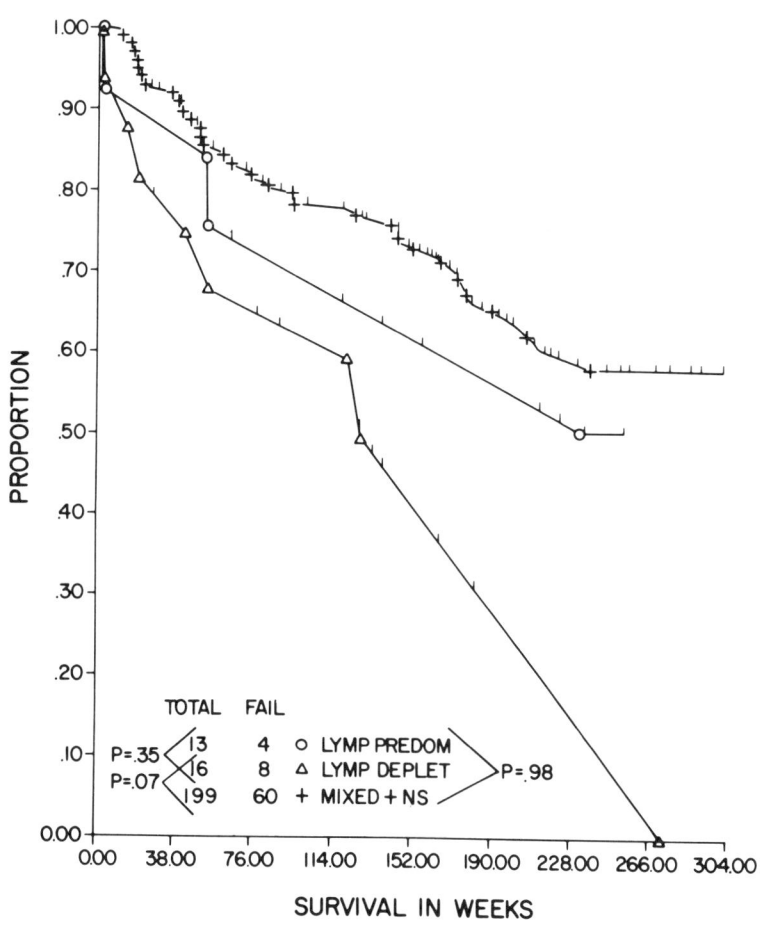

Fig. 4. MOPP 4 (SWOG 774) survival by cell type.

lymph node involvement prior to the institution of MOPP. This radiotherapy was followed by MOPP every other month for 18 months. The third and final limb of the study involved the administration of MOPP every month for a total of 18 months.

There is no evidence of a difference of length of remission between the three consolidation therapies (p = 0.80). Figure 5 shows the survival by consolidation regimen and there are no significant differences in the three regimens with follow-up to 5½ years.

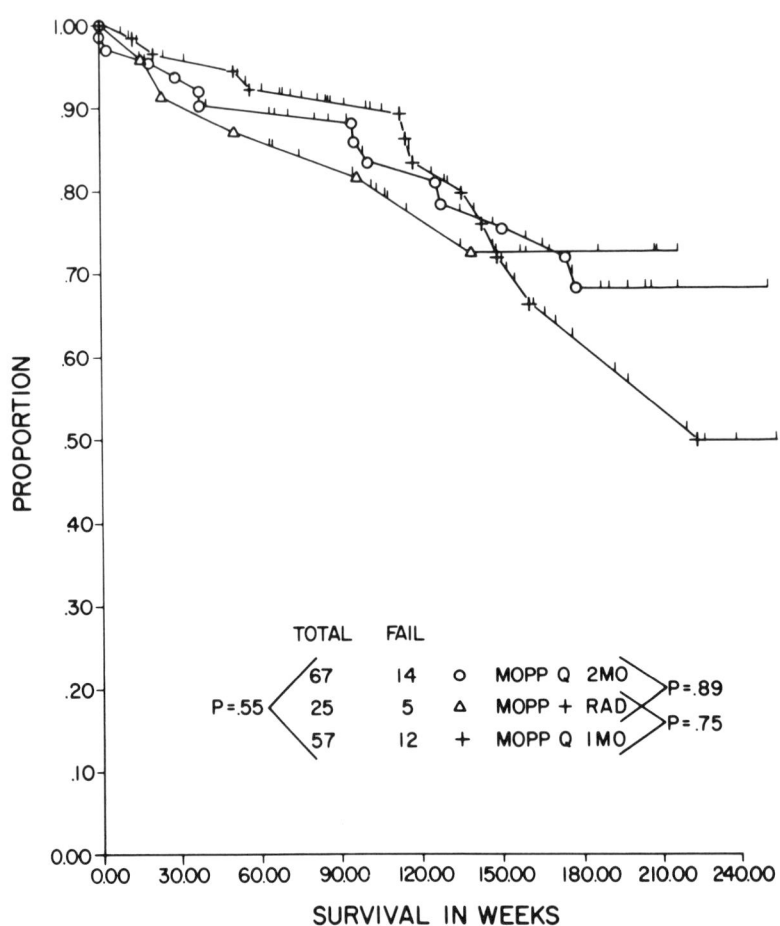

Fig. 5. MOPP 4 (SWOG 774) survival by consolidation regimen.

III. MOPP PLUS LOW-DOSE BLEOMYCIN
PLUS ADRIAMYCIN COMBINATIONS

Since MOPP plus low-dose bleomycin represented the best remission induction regimen yet developed by the Southwest Oncology Group, it was incorporated, as a control, in a three-limb remission induction program (Fig. 6) for patients with advanced Hodgkin's disease (MOPP 5–SWOG 7406) (Coltman, 1975). MOPP plus low-dose bleomycin was compared directly to MOP-BAP 1 in which adriamycin was added to MOPP plus low-dose bleomycin by substituting adriamycin in a dose of

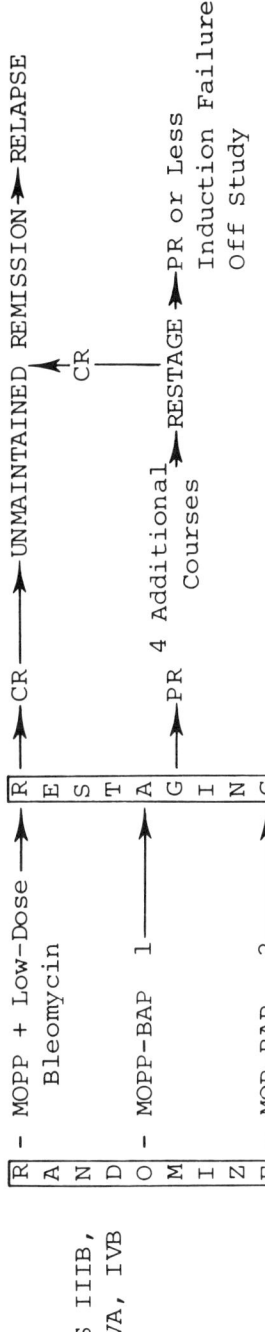

Fig. 6. MOPP 5 (SWOG 7406) schema.

TABLE VI. Response by Induction Regimen in MOPP 5 (SWOG 7406) [a]

Regimen	Total (%)	CR (%)	PR (%)
MOPP + LDB	61 (41)	33 (54)	20 (33)
MOP-BAP 1	54 (36)	41 (76)	10 (19)
MOP-BAP 2	35 (23)	27 (77)	8 (23)

[a] $p = 0.02$.

30 mg/m^2 on day 8 in place of the dose of nitrogen mustard. A third comparison was MOP-BAP 2, in which the dose of adriamycin was 15 mg/m^2 given on days 1 and 8 along with an attenuated dose of nitrogen mustard at a level of 3 mg/m^2 on days 1 and 8. The latter limb was closed early because it was similar in response and more difficult to give than MOP-BAP 1.

This study differed significantly from the previous one (SWOG 774–MOPP 4), in that systematic restaging was required in order to determine the completeness of the patient's response. In a preliminary analysis of this study (Herman and Jones, in press), occult Hodgkin's disease was identified in 12% of the patients thought to be in complete response clinically, who subsequently underwent systematic restaging. It further differed from all previous Southwest Oncology Group studies in that patients who were documented to have complete remission, based on systematic restaging, were followed in unmaintained remission until relapse.

The analysis of the MOPP 5 study is still quite preliminary but at this time the complete response rate for MOPP plus low-dose bleomycin is statistically significantly lower than the complete response rate of the other two limbs of the study (Table VI). The 54% complete response rate for MOPP plus low-dose bleomycin in this study was significantly lower than the complete response rate for the other two limbs of the study ($p = 0.02$), significantly lower than MOPP plus low-dose bleomycin in the MOPP 4 study (SWOG 774) ($p = 0.001$), and 10% lower than any complete response rate ever achieved by the Southwest Oncology Group using MOPP alone. Although the systematic restaging might have counted for differences between the complete response rate in this study and previous studies, it cannot account for the disparity between the complete response rate in the three limbs of the MOPP 5 (SWOG 7406) study.

An analysis of the pretreatment characteristics compared to response for bone-marrow status is shown in Table VII. It can be seen from this table that 35% of the

TABLE VII. Response by Pretreatment Characteristics in MOPP 5 (SWOG 7406)

Characteristic	MOPP + LDB		MOP-BAP 1		MOP-BAP 2	
	Total (%)	CR (%)	Total (%)	CR (%)	Total (%)	CR (%)
Marrow biopsy						
Not biopsied	4 (4)	1 (25)	4 (5)	2 (50)	1 (3)	1 (100)
Biopsied neg	56 (61)	33 (59)	71 (82)	45 (63)	25 (74)	19 (76)
Biopsied pos	32 (35)[a]	12 (38)[b]	12 (14)	6 (50)	8 (24)	7 (88)

[a] More Biopsy Pos in MOPP + LDB ($p < 0.01$).
[b] Lower CR Rate in MOPP + LDB ($p = 0.04$).

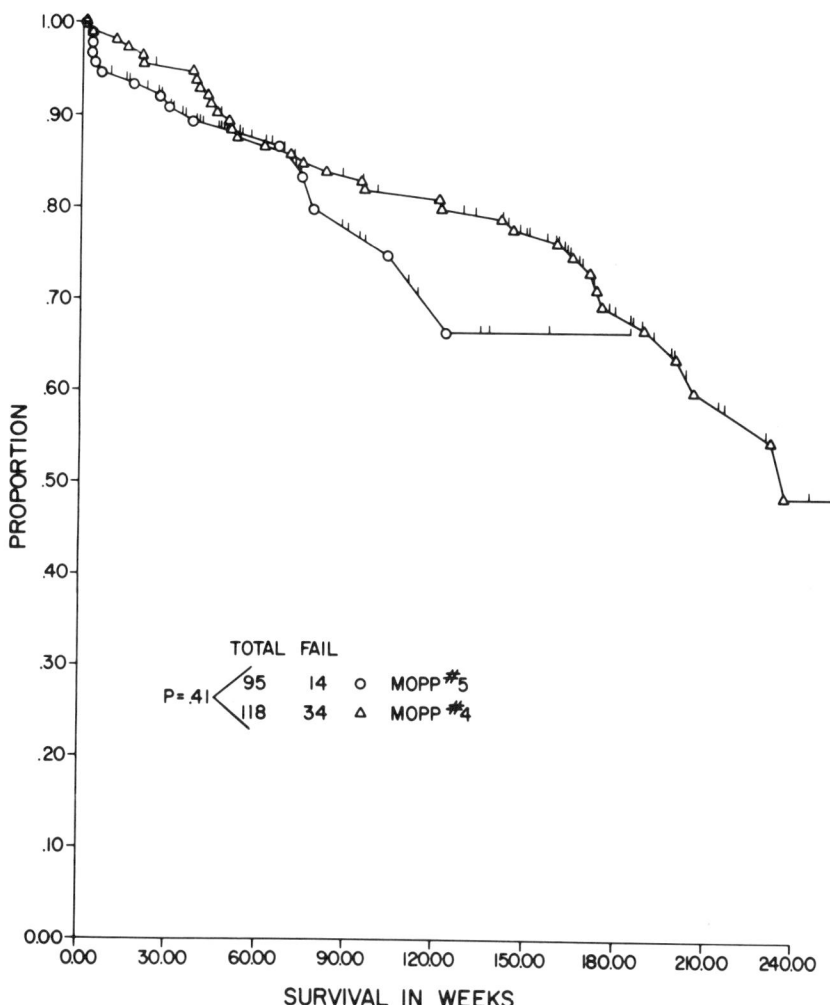

Fig. 7. Comparative survival of MOPP plus low-dose bleomycin in MOPP 4 (SWOG 774) and MOPP 5 (SWOG 7406).

patients on the MOPP plus low-dose bleomycin limb of MOPP 5 (SWOG 7406) had a positive bone-marrow biopsy, a figure which was statistically significantly higher than the MOP-BAP 1 limb of the study (p=0.027). Also patients receiving MOPP plus low-dose bleomycin on SWOG 7406 had a statistically significantly higher proportion of positive biopsy than those on the SWOG 774 (p < 0.01). The 38% complete response rate in MOPP plus low-dose bleomycin patients who had positive bone-marrow biopsies is statistically significantly lower than the complete response rate of the other limbs of the study (p = 0.04). In addition, the MOPP plus low-dose bleomycin limb of the MOPP 5 (SWOG 7406) study had a significantly larger percentage of patients who were symptomatic than the MOPP plus low-dose bleomycin limb of the MOPP 4 study (p < 0.01), a factor which adversely influenced complete response rate (p = 0.009). It is likely that the lack of comparability in these two prognostically important pretreatment characteristics significantly skewed the result of this randomized study against the MOPP plus low-dose bleomycin limb.

There is no statistically significant difference in the response duration in the MOPP plus low-dose bleomycin limbs of MOPP 4 when compared to MOPP 5 (p = 0.41), and Fig. 7 shows the comparative survival of the two limbs of these two studies in which there is no significant difference at this point in time (p = 0.41).

IV. MOPP PLUS BLEOMYCIN IN STAGE III HODGKIN'S DISEASE

The Southwest Oncology Group has recently completed a phase I (SWOG 160-CAR 1) study in stage III Hodkin's disease in which 144 patients with pathologically staged Hodgkin's disease were treated with MOPP followed by total nodal radiotherapy (Coltman et al., 1977). These data show that three cycles of MOPP, followed by total nodal radiotherapy, could be safely delivered to patients with intermediate stage Hodgkin's disease with an estimated 76% of those who achieved a complete response remaining free of disease, with the curve plateauing, with follow-up to 250 weeks. The Southwest Oncology Group study 7518 (CAR 2) was based on this phase I study (SWOG 160-CAR 1) as well as the MOPP 4 (SWOG 774) In CAR 2, patients with pathologic stage IIIA and B Hodgkin's disease were randomly assigned to treatment with MOPP plus low-dose bleomycin for three cycles followed by total nodal radiotherapy or MOPP plus low-dose bleomycin for 10 cycles, as in MOPP 5 (SWOG 7406). In both limbs of the study patients proven to have a complete response by systematic restaging were followed in unmaintained remission until relapse. In the very preliminary results of this study, the complete response rates in the two limbs are comparable at 76% (MOPP plus bleomycin plus radiotherapy) and 79% (MOPP plus bleomycin alone) and the complete plus partial response rates are 94% and 100%, respectively. The complete response rate for MOPP plus low-dose bleomycin in the CAR 2 study of 79% is comparable to the complete response rate of the stage IIIA and B patients treated on the MOPP plus low-dose bleomycin limb of MOPP 4 (SWOG 774) of 83%. Furthermore, the complete plus partial response rate for MOPP plus low-dose bleomycin in both studies (MOPP 4 and CAR 2) is 100%.

V. SUMMARY

The Southwest Oncology Group has firmly established the complete response rate for MOPP in advanced Hodgkin's disease in 456 patients at 64%. Furthermore, the 3 year survival estimate has been established at 58%. There seemed to be a great deal of logic in combining the relatively nonmyelosuppressive antibiotic bleomycin with the very myelosuppressive MOPP combination chemotherapy for advanced Hodgkin's disease in order to improve the complete and the partial response rate and survival of patients with advanced Hodgkin's disease. There is suggestive evidence from the Southwest Oncology Group study 774 (MOPP 4) that bleomycin, when added to MOPP in low dose, enhances complete response rate ($p = 0.076$) and survival ($p=0.06$) when compared to MOPP alone. It is of further interest that when bleomycin was added to the MOPP regimen at a dose of 10 u/m^2 on days 1 and 8 of MOPP that unacceptable myelosuppression became evident. Three patients died of irreversible myelosuppression and because of that unacceptable toxicity the high-dose bleomycin limb of the study was closed.

Patients with significant compromise of pulmonary function were excluded from the randomization in this study because of concern about bleomycin pulmonary toxicity. These patients were treated on an independent MOPP-alone limb in order to determine whether or not the study was significantly biased by the exclusion of patients who had a potentially adverse prognostic factor. It is quite clear that significant compromise of pulmonary function does not adversely influence the complete response rate ($p = 0.25$), response duration ($p = 0.44$), or survival ($p = 0.29$) in patients treated with MOPP alone when compared to patients without significant compromise of pulmonary function similarly treated.

The complete response rate of MOPP plus low-dose bleomycin in the MOPP 4 (SWOG 774) and the MOPP 5 (SWOG 7406) studies were significantly different ($p = 0.002$). This lower complete response rate is contributed to by a higher proportion of patients in the MOPP plus low-dose bleomycin limb of the study with adverse prognostic features, in spite of randomization. There is a higher proportion of marrow biopsy-positive patients ($p < 0.01$) and a lower proportion of asymptomatic and active patients ($p < 0.01$) in MOPP 5 than in MOPP 4, both of which adversely influenced complete response rate. It seems likely that this unbalanced randomization contributed significantly to the low response rate.

MOPP plus low-dose bleomycin has more recently been used in a fashion exactly similar to that of MOPP 5 in patients with stage IIIA and B Hodgkin's disease (SWOG 7518–CAR 2). The complete response rate of 79% in that group of patients is comparable to the complete response rate of stage IIIA and B patients treated on the MOPP low-dose bleomycin limb of MOPP 4 (83%).

The data from these three studies suggest that bleomycin added to MOPP, when compared to MOPP alone in a randomized prospective fashion, may have made a contribution in response and survival. On the other hand, this study reaffirms the observation that no regimen has *conclusively* been proven to be better than MOPP alone in the management of advanced Hodgkin's disease.

REFERENCES

Bonadonna, G., De Lena, M., Monfardini, S., Bartoli, C., Bajetta, E., Baretta, G., and Fossati-Bellani, F. (1972). *Eur. J. Cancer 8,* 205.

Coltman, C. A., Jr. (1975). *Cancer Chemother. Rep. 6,* 375.

Coltman, C. A., Jr., Frei, E., III, and Delaney, F. C. (1973). *Proc. Am. Soc. Clin. Oncol. 14,* 62.

Coltman, C. A., Jr., Frei, E., III, and Moon, T. E. (1976). *Proc. Am. Soc. Clin. Oncol. 17,* 289.

Coltman, C. A., Jr., Montague, E., and Moon, T. E. (1977). In *Adjuvant Therapy of Cancer,* Salmon, S. E., and Jones, S. E. (Eds.), Elsevier/North-Holland, Amsterdam, pp 529–536.

DeVita, V. T., Jr., Serpick, A., and Carbone, P. P. (1970). *Ann. Intern. Med. 73,* 881.

Frei, E., III, Luce, J. K., Gamble, J. F., Coltman, C. A., Jr., Constanzi, J. J., Talley, R. W., Monto, R. W., Wilson, H. E., Hewlett, J. S., Delaney, F. C., and Gehan, E. A. (1973). *Ann. Intern. Med. 79,* 376.

Haas, C. D., Coltman, C. A., Jr., Gottlieb, J. A., Haut, A., Luce, J. K., Talley, R. W., Samal, B., Wilson, H. E., and Hoogstraten, B. (1976). *Cancer 38,* 8.

Halnan, K. E., Bleehen, N. M., Brewin, T. B., Deeley, T. J., Harrison, D. F., Howland, C., Kunkler, P. B., Ritchie, G. L., Wiltshane, E., and Todd, I. D. (1972). *Br. Med. J. 4,* 635.

Herman, T. S., and Jones, S. E. *Ann. Intern. Med.* (in press).

Kimura, I., Onoshi, T., Kunimasa, I., and Takano, J. (1972). *Cancer 29,* 58.

Chapter 21

THE CURRENT ROLE OF BLEOMYCIN IN THE MANAGEMENT OF NON-HODGKIN'S LYMPHOMAS AND CUTANEOUS T-CELL LYMPHOMAS

Frederick P. Smith
Daniel Hoth
Philip Schein

I. INTRODUCTION

Bleomycin is an antineoplastic antibiotic isolated from the fermentation of *Streptomyces verticillus* by Umezawa in 1965. During the initial clinical trials, antitumor activity was demonstrated for squamous cell carcinomas (Ichikawa, 1968). Studies of drug distribution in animals had shown high concentrations in skin and lung and also in the lymphatic system (Umezawa, 1968). In 1969, Kimura *et al.* reported that bleomycin produced remissions in malignant lymphoma, an observation that was subsequently confirmed in clinical trials conducted in the United States and by the European Organization for Research on the Treatment of Cancer (E.O.R.T.C.) (Blum *et al.*, 1973).

Great emphasis has been placed on this agent's reduced myelosuppressive activity, relative to other active anticancer agents, which has facilitated the treatment of patients with impaired bone-marrow function resulting from involvement by tumor or the toxicity of prior therapy. In addition, there have been several attempts to exploit this property in the design of new combination chemotherapy regimens. In this review, we will briefly outline the evidence that bleomycin is an active therapy for non-Hodgkin's lymphoma, and describe the results of recently completed combination chemotherapy programs that have incorporated this agent.

II. SINGLE-AGENT THERAPY

Table I presents the results of seven phase II trials of bleomycin in non-Hodgkin's lymphoma, in addition to a previous review by Blum *et al.* (1973) on the cumulative results of trials conducted in the United States and by E.O.R.T.C. up to 1973. It should be emphasized that many of the reports were published prior to the current general use of the Rappaport histologic classification. Consequently the results are expressed in the generic terminology of "lymphosarcoma" and "reticulum cell sarcoma," without regard to the presence of nodular versus diffuse involvement of the lymph node architecture. We have taken the liberty of "normalizing" the data into the current nomenclature of lymphocytic and histiocytic lymphoma, respectively, for purposes of uniformity. Several of the reports did not provide sufficient detail as to magnitude of the reported responses, or used the less objective Karnofsky system, which prevents a full interpretation of the data. In this section we will emphasize those reports that allowed for an adequate assessment of the effects of treatment.

The majority of the patients had stage IV disease, and essentially all had received extensive prior treatment with combination chemotherapy, radiotherapy, or both. Nevertheless, bleomycin has consistently demonstrated activity for non-Hodgkin's lymphomas. Response rates of 30-45% have been reported for the lymphocytic lymphomas, and 15-73% (average 30%) for histiocytic lymphomas. Disappointingly, the remission durations have been quite short, averaging 2 to 4 months. This is not unexpected for a single-agent treatment, used as a second or fourth line therapy in a patient with widely metastatic disease.

In 1972 Rudders reported the results of his trial using the two dose schedules shown in Table I. Two of four patients with nodular histologies evidenced a complete remission. In addition, two of six cases with diffuse poorly differentiated lymphocytic lymphoma and one of five patients with diffuse histiocytic lymphoma achieved a partial remission. The median duration of response was 2 months, but one patient was maintained in a remission status for over 8 months. Pulmonary toxicity was encountered in 10% of the series at total doses of 210-295 mg, with one fatality at a total dose of 210 mg.

Haas *et al.* (1976) have reported the results of a large phase II trial conducted by the Southwest Oncology Group. A dose schedule of 10 mg/m² twice a week for 3 months was employed, following which the responding patients were placed on a weekly maintenance dose of 10 mg/m² if there was no evidence of pulmonary toxicity. Both intravenous and intramuscular routes were utilized. This trial included 28 patients with non-Hodgkin's lymphoma. For the 15 patients with lymphocytic lymphoma, one patient achieved a complete remission and five patients evidenced a partial response for a response rate of 40%. Thirteen patients with histiocytic lymphoma were also treated, and two (15%) demonstrated a partial remission. The median duration of response was 4 months with a range of 1-28 months. An analysis of the influence of route of administration demonstrated some provocative results in regard to both therapeutic efficacy and toxicity. When the lymphomas, Hodgkin's and non-Hodgkin's, were combined, the response rate for the intramuscular route

TABLE I. Single-Agent Activity of Bleomycin in Non-Hodgkin's Lymphoma

	Dosage	Histology	No. of patients	Overall response rate (%)	Duration (mo)
Shastri et al. (1971)	15 mg IV or IM × 30 mg BIW or TIW	Lymphocytic	5	20	
Kimura et al. (1972)	15 mg IV or BIW	Lymphocytic	1	100	Not available
		Histiocytic	5	60	Not available
Rudders (1972)	0.5 mg/kg/wk or 0.1 mg/kg/gd	Nodular	4	50	
		Diffuse well-differentiated lymphoma	3	0	2 (median)
		Diffuse poorly-differentiated lymphoma	6	33	
		Diffuse histiocytic	5	20	
Yagoda et al. (1972)	0.25 mg/kg IV g.d. until response—1 mg g.d.	Lymphocytic	17	83 ("adequate responses")	2–2.5
		Histiocytic	35	88 ("adequate responses")	1–2.5
Blum et al. (1973)	Variable IV 15 mg/m² BIW	Lymphocytic	43	35	3.1 (median)
		Histiocytic	59	29	1.8 (median)
Hubbard et al. (1975)	2 mg/m²/day × 5, of mo.	(Non-Hodgkin's)	10	30	1
Haas et al. (1976)	10 mg/m²/BIW IM or IV × 12 –10 mg/m² qwk × 12	Lymphocytic	15	40	4 (median)
		Histiocytic	13	15	1.25–28 (median)
Bonadonna et al. (1976)	Variable	Lymphocytic	6	66	2 (median)
		Histiocytic	11	73	1

was 46% compared to 29% for intravenous administration; this result was not statistically significant. However, a decrease in the severity of pulmonary toxicity was found for the patients receiving intramuscular bleomycin ($p < 0.05$), while the overall incidence (10%) was identical for the two regimens.

The efficacy of intensive courses of high-dose bleomycin has been evaluated at the National Cancer Institute (Hubbard et al., 1975). Patients received 25 mg/m^2 / day intravenously for 5 consecutive days with repeat courses at monthly intervals. Ten patients with non-Hodgkin's lymphoma refractory to combination chemotherapy were treated, and three demonstrated a transient response. Pulmonary toxicity was observed in two cases at total doses of 100 mg/m^2 (204 mg) and 125 mg/m^2 (245 mg). No therapeutic advantage could be found for this schedule when compared to results with conventional low-dose administration.

The results of these and subsequent trials are in basic agreement with the analysis of accumulated U.S. and E.O.R.T.C. data for bleomycin treatment reported in 1973 by Blum et al. They found a response rate of 31–41% for lymphocytic lymphomas and 24–36% for histiocytic lymphomas.

While the role of bleomycin in the treatment of cutaneous T-cell lymphoma "mycosis fungoides" has not received as much attention in the literature as the B-lymphocyte disorders, the cumulative results are nevertheless of great interest (E.O.R.T.C., 1972); Spiegel and Coltman, 1973. Takeda et al., 1970, Yagoda et al., 1972; and Haas et al., 1976). Table II presents the results reported from seven series; bleomycin has demonstrated consistent activity in this disease with all programs reporting response rates in excess of 50%, including complete responses. The remission durations are routinely short, 1–8 months; however, the patient population had in general received extensive prior therapy. It has been demonstrated that bleomycin concentrates in the skin, and further trials employing intramuscular or constant infusion for cutaneous T-cell lymphomas appear warranted.

The most serious and treatment-limiting toxicity of single-agent therapy has been pulmonary fibrosis, which has been observed in approximately 10% of patients. In the analysis of changes in pulmonary diffusion capacity and total lung capacity conducted by Yagoda and co-workers (1972), patients with lymphoma did not

TABLE II. Bleomycin Activity in Cutaneous T-Cell Lymphoma (Mycosis Fungoides)

Reference	No. of patients	Objective response	Duration of response (mo)
Takeda et al. (1970)	7	7 (1 CR)	Not available
E.O.R.T.C. (1972)	7	5 (1 CR)	3
Yagoda et al. (1972)	5	3	1–3.5
Spiegel et al. (1973)	1	1	8+
Haas et al. (1976)	2	2 (1 CR)	Not available

appear to be more sensitive to this toxic property of the drug when compared to those with solid tumors. However, as emphasized in the data from the trials reported by Rudders (1972) and the N.C.I. (Hubbard, 1975), clinically apparent toxicity and lethality have been observed at relatively low total doses.

III. COMBINATION CHEMOTHERAPY

Following the demonstration of single-agent activity for the non-Hodgkin's lymphoma and the evidence of reduced myelosuppression, a series of combination chemotherapeutic regimens were developed employing bleomycin during the remission induction (Table III: Schein et al., 1977; Skarin et al., 1977; McKelvey et al., 1976; Bonadonna et al., 1976; and Monfardini et al., in press), as well as in consolidation and maintenance phases of treatment (Diggs and Wiernick, 1977).

A program consisting of bleomycin, adriamycin, cyclophosphamide, vincristine, and prednisone (BACOP) was introduced by Schein and co-workers (1976) for the treatment of the advanced stages of diffuse histiocytic lymphoma (Table III). The design of this regimen took into account the relapse pattern in this disease; while partial responders demonstrated a deceptively favorable initial response, this was followed by rapid relapse between induction cycles during the bone-marrow recovery phases of combinations patterned after the MOPP regimen for Hodgkin's disease. The BACOP program utilized a standard myelosuppressive induction phase with cyclophosphamide and adriamycin; this was followed by continued treatment with two nonmyelosuppressive agents, bleomycin and prednisone, in an attempt to prevent tumor regrowth between cycles while allowing for full bone-marrow recovery. In the initial analysis of 25 patients with predominately stage IV diffuse histiocytic lymphoma, 12 (48%) achieved a pathologic complete remission documented by restaging 1 month following the completion of 6 months of treatment. The median duration of complete response was in excess of 1 year (range 5 to 30 months), and no patient had relapsed. Based on previous experience with this histology, it was anticipated that the majority of these patients would achieve an extended disease-free survival (Schein et al., 1974); this has been confirmed in a recently completed follow-up analysis. The use of bleomycin during the second 2 weeks of the regimen allowed for full or nearly complete recovery of bone-marrow function phase of therapy and 84% achieved a *clinical* complete remission during the 6 month period of treatment. However, six patients had only suppression of disease by the continuous exposure to chemotherapy, and the incompleteness of the remission could only be documented by restaging procedures 1 month after discontinuing treatment. Aside from the expected myelosuppression, the principal treatment-related toxicity was bleomycin pulmonary toxicity. With the original bleomycin dose of 15 u/m^2, four of 16 patients developed clinically severe respiratory embarrassment at relatively low total doses of 45, 45, 160, and 165 u/m^2. Progressive pulmonary toxicity contributed to the one treatment-related death in this series. No pulmonary toxicity had been observed in patients treated at the lower bleomycin dose of 5u/m^2.

TABLE III. Bleomycin in Combination

Author	Histology	No. of patients	Complete remission rate (%)	Median duration of response (range)
Schein et al. (1976) BACOP	Diffuse Histioclytic	25	12	17+ mo (5–30)
Skarin et al. (1977) BACOP	Nodular	9	89	
	Diffuse poorly differentiated lymphoma	15	80	
	Diffuse histiocytic	18	56	14 mo (projected)
	Diffuse mixed	6	67	(5–34)
McElvey et al. (1977) CHOP-Bleo	Nodular poorly differentiated lymphoma	13	62	4 yr (projected)
	Nodular mixed lymphocytic	3	67	52+, 64+ wk
	Diffuse poorly differentiated lymphoma	3	67	53+, 64+ wk
	Diffuse histiocytic	26	69	2 yr (projected)
Monfardini et al. (in press)	Lymphocytic Histiocytic	30 total	65 / 35	8+ mo / 11+ mo
Bonadonna et al. (1976) MABOP	Lymphocytic Histiocytic	58 total	56 / 55	20 mo / 9 mo

Recently Fisher *et al.* (1977) have retrospectively compared the efficacy of the C-MOPP regimen (cyclophosphamide, vincristine, procarbazine, and prednisone) and BACOP, and reported that by statistical analysis the regimens appeared to be comparable in response rates and in their potential for producing prolonged survival. However the BACOP patient population, when compared to C-MOPP, had a higher proportion of negative prognostic variables; this included a higher percentage of patients with stage IV disease (81% versus 67%) and a higher incidence of bone-marrow involvement (25% versus 17%), a particularly resistant site for chemotherapy, that predisposes to the subsequent development of leptomeningeal lymphoma (Table IV). A prospective randomized trial of BACOP and C-MOPP with appropriate stratification will be required to establish the relative efficacy of each regimen.

TABLE IV.   BACOP versus C-MOPP [a]

	BACOP	C-MOPP
No. of patients	32	24
Complete response rate (%)	46	41
Stage IV No. (%)	26 (81)	16(67)
Bone-marrow involvement (%)	8 (25)	4(17)

[a] From Fisher *et al.* (1977).

Skarin *et al.* (1977) have reported their results with a different dose schedule of the same five drugs, BACOP-Farber (Table III). The regimen consisted of a 7 week remission–induction period, followed by a consolidation phase for a total of 28 weeks of treatment. Bleomycin, administered at a dose of 15 mg/m^2 twice a week in the first 10 patients, was reduced to 4 mg/m^2 because of serious pulmonary toxicity. A total of 63 patients with non-Hodgkin's lymphoma were treated. Complete remission was documented in 56% of patients with diffuse histiocytic, and 80% of patients with diffuse poorly differentiated lymphocytic lymphomas. In nodular lymphoma the complete remission rate was 89%. The duration of complete remission was not as durable as with BACOP; the projected median duration was only 14 months. As expected, this correlated closely with survival; the median survival of all patients with diffuse histology was 14 months, with an estimated 42% of patients to survive beyond 20 months. Pulmonary infiltrates developed in 21/73 (29%) patients, but this was ascribed to bleomycin toxicity in eight (11%). In five patients the x-ray changes proved reversible, but three patients expired with pulmonary insufficiency, of which two had received high dose (15 mg/m^2) bleomycin. The average total dose in the reversible cases was 72 mg, compared to 93 mg in the fatal cases.

McKelvey *et al.* (1976) have reported on the regimen of cyclophosphamide, adriamycin, vincristine, prednisone, plus bleomycin (CHOP-Bleo). Forty-seven patients with advanced non-Hodgkin's lymphoma were treated, with an overall complete remission rate of 66%. For the 26 patients with diffuse histiocytic lymphoma, 18 (69%) achieved a complete remission. The results in smaller numbers of other histologic forms were comparably high. At the time of the report, three patients with diffuse histiocytic lymphoma had relapsed, but the projected median duration of response was in excess of 2 years. The survival curve becomes flat at 70 weeks and there is some expectation that the majority of these patients will remain disease free. Of particular interest is the finding that no evidence of bleomycin pulmonary toxicity was clinically evident in this group of patients; however the dose of bleomycin, 15 u/day x 5, was reduced to only 4 u on days 1 and 5 for patients older than 60 years.

We have compared the results of the original CHOP regimen (McKelvey et al., 1976) with this subsequent report using CHOP-Bleo (Table V). There appears to be no improvement in response rate with the addition of bleomycin. However, it should be emphasized that these represent two different trials, one conducted by the SWOG and the other at the M.D. Anderson Hospital only. The SWOG has also reported preliminary data from a program in which they have randomized patients with non-Hodgkin's lymphoma to CHOP plus "low-dose bleomycin", COP plus low-dose bleomycin and CHOP plus BCG immunotherapy. The response rate (58%) did not differ for any of the induction regimens, although survival for patients with nodular lymphoma appeared improved for patients treated with CHOP-BCG, (Jones et al., 1977).

TABLE V. Response to CHOP versus CHOP-Bleo in NHL

	CHOP		CHOP-Bleo	
No. of patients	204		47	
Overall response				
complete remission	92%		92%	
Partial remission	71%		66%	
	No.	CR (%)	No.	CR (%)
Nodular lymphomas				
Well differentiated lymphoma	23	83	–	–
Poorly differentiated lymphoma	34	76	13	62
Histiocytic	7	71	–	–
Mixed	9	78	3	67
Diffuse lymphoma				
Well differentiated lymphoma	23	61	–	–
Poorly differentiated lymphoma	38	68	3	67
Histiocytic	53	68	26	69
Mixed	14	71	–	–

Monfardini *et al.* (in press), have compared an adriamycin, bleomycin, and prednisone (ABP) regimen against the standard CVP regimen for previously untreated patients with non-Hodgkin's lymphoma. In 30 patients treated with the former regimen, a 46% complete response rate was obtained; 62% of lymphocytic and 35% of histiocytic lymphoma achieved CR. The complete remission rate with CVP was 44%, and there was no statistical difference in response rate for initial treatment in the two regimens. Moreover, after crossover for progression or relapse, no cross-resistance was detected, with 40–50% of patients achieving a complete or partial response. Because of the high efficacy and lack of cross-resistance, Bonadonna *et al.* (1977) have used CVP and ABP in sequential fashion. Preliminary findings failed to show an increase in response rate.

Pulmonary toxicity has been the dose-limiting factor in the use of bleomycin in combination chemotherapy with an overall incidence of 10% with 1% fatal toxicity. In initial reports, pulmonary toxicity appeared to be incrased with total dosage above 450 mg, and as a consequence most authors have recommended a bleomycin dose ceiling of 200–250 mg/m^2 (Blum *et al.*, 1973). There has, however, been the observation of serious and fatal toxicity with dosages as low as 90 mg total in single-agent therapy and at 45 mg/m^2 with bleomycin in combination treatment of NHL. In both Schein's (1976) and Skarin's (1977) variations of BACOP, a significant incidence of bleomycin pulmonary toxicity was noted.

IV. CONCLUSIONS

Bleomycin as a single agent has been demonstrated to induce a 30–40% response rate in previously treated advanced NHL. The responses occur early with relatively low cumulative dosage of bleomycin, but are short-lived, lasting on the average 2–4 months. Bleomycin in combination regimens has been used both in induction and maintenance phases. Although results with these combinations have been encouraging, the actual contribution of bleomycin cannot be assessed. This will ultimately require controlled trials of regimens with and without bleomycin with careful patient stratification. Pulmonary toxicity has appeared relatively early and at much lower cumulative dosage of bleomycin in at least two of these combinations, which suggests either an enhancement of toxicity by the combination, or perhaps a particular sensitivity to this toxic manifestation in patients with non-Hodgkin's lymphoma.

Further trials to discern the optimal dosage and mode of administration of this active bone-marrow sparing agent for both the B & T lymphocytic disorders appear warranted. Lower cumulative doses of bleomycin may suffice in achieving the desired response. The relative merit of intramuscular versus intravenous route of administration or the use of prolonged low-dose infusion should be further investigated in controlled trials. Particular emphasis should be given to the results of Haas *et al.* (1976) showing somewhat greater therapeutic efficacy with less severe pulmonary toxicity with the use of intramuscular administration.

REFERENCES

Blum, R. H., Carter, S. K., and Agre, K. (1973). *Cancer 31*, 903.

Bonadonna, G., Tancini, G., and Bajetta, E. (1976). *Prog. Biochem. Pharmacol. 11*, 172.

Bonadonna, G., Monfardini, S., and Villa, E. (1977). *Cancer Treatment Rep.*

Diggs, C. H., and Wiernick, P. H. (1977). *Proc. Am. Assoc. Clin. Oncol. 18*, 288.

E.O.R.T.C. (1972). *Br. Med. J. 1*, 285.

Fisher, R. I., DeVita, V. T., Johnson, B. L., Simon, R., and Young, R. C. (1977). *Am. J. Med. 63*, 177.

Haas, C. D., Coltman, C. A., Gottlieb, J. A., Haut, A., Luce, J. K., Talley, R. W., Samal, B., Wilson, H. E., and Hoogstraten, B. (1976). *Cancer 38*, 8.

Hubbard, S. P., Chabner, B. A., Canellos, G. P., Young, R. C., and DeVita, V. T. (1975). *Eur. J. Cancer 11*, 623.

Ichikawa, T. (1968). *Naika 22*, 630.

Jones, S. E., Salmon, S. E., Moon, T. E., and Butler, J. J. (1977). *Proc. Am. Soc. Clin. Oncol. 18*, 291.

Kimura, I., Onoshi, T., Kunimosa, I., and Tanako, J., (1972). *Cancer 29*, 58.

Kimura, K., *et al.* (1969). *Proc. Jpn. Cancer Assoc. 244.*

McKelvey, E. M., Gottlieb, J. A., Wilson, H. E., Haut, A., Talley, R. W., Stephens, R., Lane, M., Gamble, J. F., Jones, S. E., Grozea, P. N., Gutterman, J., Coltman, C., and Moon, T. E. (1976). *Cancer 38*, 1484.

Monfardini, S., Tancini, G., DeLena, M., and Bonadonna, G. *J. Med. Pediatr. Oncol* (in press).

Rudders, R. A. (1972). *Blood 40*, 317.

Schein, P. S., Chabner, B. A., Canellos, G. P., Young, R. C., Berard, C., and DeVita, V. T. (1974). *Blood 43*, 181.

Schein, P. S., DeVita, V. T., Hubbard, S., Chabner, B. A., Cannellos, G. P., Berard, C., and Young, R. C. (1976). *Ann. Intern. Med 85*, 417.

Shastri, S., Slayton, R. E., Wolter, J., Perlia, C. P., and Taylor, S. G (1971). *Cancer 28*, 1142.

Skarin, A. T., Rosenthal, D. S., Moloney, W. C., and Frei, E. (1977). *Blood 49*, 759.

Spiegel, S. C., and Coltman, C. A. (1973). *Cancer 32*, 767.

Takeda, K., Sagawa, Y., and Arakaw, T. (1970). *Gann 61*, 207.

Umezawa, H. (1965). *Antimicrob. Agents Chemother. 5*, 1079.

Umezawa, H. (1968). Speech at the 5th Meeting of the Bleomycin Study Society, January 10.

Yagoda, A., Mukherji, B., Young, C., Etcubanas, E., Lamonte, C., Smith, J. R., Tan, C. T. C., Krakoff, I. H. (1972). *Ann. Intern. Med. 77*, 861.

Chapter 22

BLEOMYCIN AND RADIOTHERAPY: AN OVERVIEW OF CLINICAL STUDIES IN THE UNITED STATES

Todd H. Wasserman

I. GENERAL CONSIDERATIONS OF COMBINED CHEMOTHERAPY AND RADIOTHERAPY CLINICAL TRIALS

The success of cancer chemotherapy in the palliation, remission, and occasional cure of certain hematologic and solid cancers has led to clinical trials of the integration of cancer chemotherapy into the primary treatment of solid tumors, traditionally treated by surgery and/or radiotherapy. The principles and overall strategy of such combined modality treatment of solid tumors are discussed by Carter and and Soper (1974). In general, the aims of combined radiotherapy and chemotherapy are either improved local "tumor cell kill" or the chemotherapeutic control of occult micrometastases outside the radiation field, or both. The local effects may be either the additive effect of the chemotherapy cell kill on that of the radiation or a potentiation of the radiation cell kill by the chemotherapy. The particular goal that prevails will depend on the specific cancer type, stage, histology, and knowledge of the failure patterns of such specific clinical cancer situations. Also, the therapeutic ratio should be such that the combined effects are greater in the tumor than the dose-limiting normal tissue. A more complete discussion of the principles, rationale, and future clinical and experimental goals of combined radiotherapy and chemotherapy is found in a recent review (Anonymous, 1976). Muggia *et al.* (1977) recently published a review of the current clinical trials in each solid tumor type, as well as an outline of the specific organ toxicity of each chemotherapy plus radiotherapy combination.

The clinical researcher approaches the design of combined modality trials with a myriad of possible choices. If we consider that in the integration of a single chemotherapy agent with radiotherapy some critical experimental variables are drug dose schedule, radiation dose schedule, dose ratio, and dose sequence, and that the number of possibilities for each variable is, respectively, 3, 3, 3, and 7, then the number of potential individual trials is 189 (the product of all the variables). Obviously, the limitations of clinical trials, such as time, money, availability of clinical researchers, availability of patients, and ethics, preclude testing all of the experimental possibilities. The clinical trials are thus largely empirical, based on the clinician's rational analysis of past clinical experience, his clinical interest, and his clinical intuition as to what might offer the best chance of success. The clinician looks to the experimentalist for aid and data in making his choices. However, too often the experimentalist and the clinician have not adequately communicated with each other. Further discussion on these points is found in the paper by Carter and Wasserman (1975).

The conduct of combined modality trials is difficult and time consuming, requiring that careful experimental design be used so that the data resulting from such trials can be reliably interpreted. After an initial pilot study of the feasibility of a particular radiotherapy and chemotherapy combination, it is usually necessary to initiate controlled, stratified, randomized trials because of the variability of the patient population and the results expected. Indeed, one cannot lump all head and neck cancers together, as natural history varies with the primary site and stage, just as the natural history of lung cancer varies with the stage and histologic type. Other prognostic factors also need to be controlled. The traditional study end points of tumor response may not be valid, as partial response is virtually always achieved by radiotherapy alone. Many tumors treated are not amenable to measurement, and a complete response is often difficult to assess. Thus, to be meaningful a trial may require that the end points be disease-free interval, relapse rate, and ultimately survival. These end points require studies of long-term follow-up and much expenditure of time and money. Also, to focus only on the effect of the therapy on the tumor without an analysis of the morbidity on normal tissue makes for an incomplete evaluation. Few combined modality trials adequately document such morbidity. Most studies do not provide for two dose schedules or either the chemotherapy, radiotherapy, or both, thus not allowing for an analysis of dose-effect curves for either the tumor or the normal tissues. It is for future investigators to develop the knowledge, techniques, and skills to conduct clinical trials which answer all the potential criticisms and yet which are practical.

II. PRECLINICAL AND CLINICAL RATIONALE FOR BLEOMYCIN AND RADIOTHERAPY CLINICAL TRIALS

The clinical evaluation of bleomycin has demonstrated anticancer activity both as a single agent and in combination with other chemotherapeutic agents in squamous cell carcinomas of various sites, Hodgkin's and non-Hodgkin's lymphomas, and testicular cancer (Crooke and Bradner, 1976; Blum *et al.*, 1973). Many of the patients treated in the studies that led to knowledge of this clinical activity had been previously treated with radiotherapy. The activity of the chemotherapy in such advanced patients led to therapeutic trials of said chemotherapy in "high risk" patients who also required local–regional therapy with radiation. The Japanese have reported over the last several years on a variety of such trials in head and neck cancers, lung cancers, esophageal cancer, and gynecologic cancers (Crooke and Bradner, 1976).

Preclinically, the effects of bleomycin and radiotherapy have been studied in bacterial and mammalian cell culture systems, and in tumor-bearing animal systems. Such studies have supported the preliminary conclusion of additive and somewhat synergistic antitumor activity of the combination (Crooke and Bradner, 1976). However, the refinements of the data as to time-dose effects, dose ratio effects, and other parameters await further preclinical evaluation. Such rational evaluation of chemotherapy and radiotherapy has recently been the subject of a large cancer research emphasis grant (CREG) from the National Cancer Institute. Phillips and Fu (1976, 1977) have developed some preclinical and clinical data on the normal tissue effects of combined radiation and chemotherapy. Specifically, they outline data on the dose-modifying effect of bleomycin on the tolerance of skin, mucous membranes, gastrointestinal mucosa, and lung tissue to radiation. In general, the effect of the bleomycin is mild to moderate.

The clinical trials of bleomyicn and radiotherapy in the United States are early in their evolution, and are in the following cancer types: head and neck cancers, lung cancers, esophageal cancer, and cervical cancer. Data on the trials will be reported below by the specific cancer type. In addition, trials by some other non-Japanese, non-United States investigators are presented. As the data are often preliminary, and as important parameters of the patient populations are often not analyzable, it is difficult to integrate the results of said trials into the general treatment knowledge of a specific cancer type and thus conclude when it is valuable to use such a chemotherapy–radiotherapy approach in a particular patient.

III. CLINICAL TRIAL RESULTS

A. Head and Neck Cancers

The integration of chemotherapy into a combined modality approach of therapy for the patient with primary head and neck cancers was recently reviewed by Gold-smith and Carter (1975). Most of the studies reported used intraarterial or systemic methotrexate as the adjuvant chemotherapy. The authors conluded that there had not yet been a clear delineation of the role of chemotherapy in combination with surgery and radiotherapy in the treatment of primary head and neck cancer of any site. Crooke and Bradner (1976) reviewed clinical trials of bleomycin and radio-therapy in head and neck cancers and concluded that it was difficult to assess the role of bleomycin in such situations, due to incomplete data on patient prognostic parameters and optimal dose schedules.

Table I lists a series of controlled and uncontrolled studies using bleomycin in conjunction with radiotherapy for head and neck cancers. The only U.S. study, by Silverberg *et al.* (1976), in advanced (stage III and IV) cancers of different sites, using high-dose radiation and two dose schedules of bleomycin, yielded good complete and partial response rates. The durations of the complete responses were quite long. More mucositis and secondary breaks in the radiotherapy were seen at the higher dose level of bleomycin. When this group sought to use bleomycin and other anticancer drugs together in a combination used in conjunction with radiotherapy, the toxicity (mucositis) was markedly increased without apparent increased efficacy (Silverberg *et al.*, 1978). Table I lists three other non-Japanese, non-United States studies which report increased response rates with bleomycin and radiotherapy. Table II reports on a study by Shanta and Krishnamurthi (1976) of India, in oral cancer, with a randomized comparison of radiotherapy +/- bleomycin. The radiotherapy dose schedule is a standard one (although no interstitial irradiation was used, as might be added in many treatment centers), with some dose reduction when the bleomycin was added. Only complete tumor clearance with no subsequent recurrence within the irradiated volume, whatever the length of follow-up, was recorded as a response. The data suggest a higher response rate to the bleomycin and radiation than to the radiation alone or with a placebo. Although the response rates for radiation alone are somewhat lower than expected from other treatment centers, the response rates with the combination of radiotherapy and bleomycin are the highest reported for such advanced stage patients. The route of administration of the bleomycin did not seem to affect the response rate. The higher response rate with the use of bleomycin was reflected in a longer median disease-free survival for those patients (Table II). The cause of failure and death in those patients who died was not given in the paper. Apparently, severe mucositis (not documented by any objective parameter) was seen in the bleomycin patients, but a newer trial of IM administration (30 u biw x 2½ wk) (for which no efficacy data are available) apparently shows reduced toxicity.

The overall data of bleomycin and radiotherapy in head and neck cancers, from several controlled and uncontrolled studies, show apparent increased tumor clearance, with moderate to severe mucositis. Further analysis of the existing data and any future data by primary site and stage is needed. Optimal dose schedules of either the bleomycin or the radiotherapy are not clearly established, although it appears that bleomycin doses of more than 10 u/wk throughout the course of radiotherapy (about 7 weeks) will cause delays in radiotherapy due to mucositis. There is need for further large-scale controlled clinical trials to answer these points. The Northern California Oncology Group has started a randomized trial of bleomycin and radiotherapy for stage III and IV head and neck cancer patients, who are inoperable.

B. Lung Cancers

The treatment of localized but unresectable lung cancers of the non-oat-cell type is primarily with local–regional radiotherapy. Such radiotherapy is of palliative value

TABLE I. Bleomycin + Radiotherapy—Head and Neck Cancer[a]

Investigator	Type	XRT	Chemo.	No. of patients	CR+PR	Response (%)	Comments
Silverberg et al. (1976) San Francisco	Oral cavity Larynx Pharynx Stages III and IV	6500 r/7 wk	Bleo 15 u IV biw or 5 u IV biw	19 18	9+9 12+6	94 100	Med. duration surv. CR—447+ days, PR—150 days. More mucositis and days break in XRT with higher dose schedule
Silverberg et al. (1978)	Same	Same	Bleo + Cyclo + VCR	15	4+6	67	Markedly increased mucositis without established increased efficacy.
Clifford et al. (1976) Royal Mardsen, London	All types	5500–6200 r /6–8 wk	Bleo+VCR +MTX +CF	30	–	80	Mostly stage III patients
Kapstad et al. (1977) Bergen, Norway	All types	1500 r /10 fx 1 wk break 1500 r /10 fx	Bleo-15 u IM tiw—wks 1, 2, 4, 5, (total 180 u) Placebo	15 14	4+5 1+3	60 29	All patients operable–preop. Rx. Randomized, double blind study. No increased toxicity with bleo
Berdal (1976)	Larynx Hypopharynx Oral cavity	Skin dose 350 r/6 fx wks 1, 3 (4200 r total) (T.D.∿2500 r)	Bleo-15u IM qd x 6, wk 1 tiw wk 3 tiw wk 3 (total 180 u)	90 21 33	66+18 8+12 18+11	93 95 88	Regression rates subdivided by TNM stage. Duration of follow-up good (1–3 yr) with 85% of larynx patients still in remission. Toxicity–moderate mucositis and skin changes. Only one case lung toxicity.
Other Total				$\frac{67}{212}$	$\frac{22+27}{115+68}$	$\frac{73}{86}$	

[a] Bleo = bleomycin; Cyclo = cyclophosphamide; CF = citrovorum factor; MTX = methotrexate; VCR = vincristine.

TABLE II. Bleomycin + Radiotherapy—Head and Neck Cancer[a,b]

Site	Therapy	No. of patients	No. of CR	% CR
Buccal mucosa	XRT	32	6	19 ⟍ 9/53 (17%)
	XRT + Bleo IA	42	33	79 ⟋
	XRT + placebo IV	21	3	14 ⟍ 51/64 (80%)
	XRT + Bleo IV	22	18	82 ⟋
Ant. tongue	XRT + placebo IV	10	2	
	XRT + Bleo IV	10	6	

Survival free of disease (total group):

	1 yr	2 yr	3 yr	4 yr
Bleomycin	57/74=77%	49/74=66%	16/27=59%	6/12=50%
Control	11/63=17%	7/63=11%	2/14=14%	1/11=9%

[a] Shanta and Krishnamurthi (1976), India.
[b] Comments: Most patients—Grade I and II tumors (87%) with T_3 or T_4 stages (93%). Toxicity—severe mucositis. Only one case of lung toxicity. XRT alone 6500 r/6.5–7 wk, XRT 5500 r/7 wk (200–250r/tiw) + Bleo 10–15 u IA or IV tiw (total 150–250 u).

with short durations of response and equivocal overall effects on survival. The use of chemotherapy in radiation failures usually meets with no significant success. Attempts have been made to combine the chemotherapy with radiotherapy in hopes both of improving local controls and preventing the development of disseminated disease. Crooke and Bradner (1976) reported on several uncontrolled studies of bleomycin and radiotherapy in lung cancers. The only controlled study, by Chan et al. (1976), is reported in Table III along with other recent studies. Chan et al. (1976), in patients with squamous cell lung cancer treated with split course radiotherapy, found a higher response rate and median survival in those randomized patients who received radiotherapy and bleomycin versus those who received radiotherapy alone. The incidence of local relapse was also reduced in the bleomycin-treated patients. They concluded that further clinical trials of the bleomycin and radiotherapy combination were indicated. The same authors (Chan et al., 1976, 1977) treated a variety of lung cancers with a combination of bleomycin and adriamycin in conjunction with radiotherapy. They had previously demonstrated good additive efficacy with adriamycin and radiotherapy. The response data are given in Table III by cell type with an apparent higher response rate for the squamous cell type than obtained in the previous study with bleomycin alone (although not directly compared). In neither of these studies was an abnormal degree of pulmonary toxicity observed. Data from Samuels et al. (1975), using a bleomycin combination chemotherapy in conjunction with radiation, with a good response rate in squamous cell type and with survival of responders increased over that of nonresponders, are also included in Table III. Again, no dramatically increased pulmonary toxicity was seen. However, in the two remaining studies in Table III, in which patients with oat-cell type lung cancer (who are presumed to have nonlocal, metastatic disease) were treated with combination chemotherapy including bleomycin, adriamycin, cyclophosphamide, and vincristine, in conjunction with both primary lung and whole-brain radiotherapy, a dramatic increase in pulmonary toxicity was observed. This diffuse interstitial fibrosis resulted in several deaths. Einhorn et al. (1976) did not see such pulmonary toxicity in patients treated with the same chemotherapy without radiotherapy or in patients treated with the radiotherapy and a chemotherapy combination without the bleomycin. Both groups of investigators have eliminated the bleomycin in the therapy of subsequent patients, because of this pulmonary toxicity. Why this group of patients is uniquely sensitive to the pulmonary toxicity of combined bleomycin and radiation is not known. This may represent a peculiarity of the histologic type, the combination of cyclophosphamide and bleomycin with radiation, or some other unknown factor. The efficacy of the above studies in oat-cell type, as measured by response rate, complete response rate, or survival, is not clearly greater than that in other studies of radiotherapy and combination chemotherapy (without bleomycin) (Holoye et al., 1977; Kent et al., 1977).

C. Esophageal Cancer

Crooke and Bradner (1976) reported on several Japanese studies of bleomycin in conjunction with radiotherapy either as definitive therapy or as preoperative therapy.

TABLE III. Bleomycin + Radiotherapy–Lung Cancer [a]

Investigator	XRT	Chemo	Type	No. of patients	CR+PR	Response (%)	Comments
Chan et al. (1976)	2000 r/5 d ⎰ 3 wk split ⎱ 2000 r/5 d	None Bleo 10 u/m² IV biw x 6 wk	Squamous	15 15	2+2 0+7	26 46	Med. serv. increased with Bleo (13 vs 6 mo). Surv. of responders > nonresponders only for XRT + bleo (4 patients alive at 2 yr). No increased lung or esophageal toxicity.
Chan et al. (1976, 1977)	Same	Bleo 15 u biw with XRT + Adria 40 mg/m² q 3 wk	Squamous Large Small Adeno Total	19 7 7 7 40	2+9 2+2 3+2 1+2 8+15	58 — — — 57	Med. surv. = 9 mo
Samuels et al. (1975)	3000 r/10 d 4 wk split 3000 r/10 d	Bleo 15 u IM biw x 3 wk + VCR 2.0 mg IV q wk x 3 + MTX 25–30 mg p.o. biw x 3 wk	Squamous Adeno	21 6	5+4 0+0	43 —	Med. surv. 13+ mo–squamous, 10.5 mo–overall. Survival of responders (16 mo) nonresponders (6.5 mo)

Einhorn et al. (1976)	2000 r/5 d 3 wk split + 2000 r/5 d (primary and brain)	Bleo 15 u IV q wk x 6 + Adria 50 mg/m^2 IV q 3 wk x 9 + Cyclo 750 mg/m^2 IV q 3 wk + VCR 1.0 mg/m^2 IV q wk x 6	Oat cell	13	4+7	85	5 patients (3 deaths) with diffuse interstitial fibrosis not seen in any of 29 patients treated with same chemotherapy alone (no XRT) or in 20 patients treated with same XRT and same chemotherapy excluding Bleo
Skarin et al. (1975)	6000 r – split course + 3000 r/whole brain	Bleo 4 u/m^2 IV biw x 6 wk + Adria 45 mg/m^2 IV q 3 wk + Cyclo 600 mg/m^2 IV q 3 wk + VCR 1.2 mg/m^2 IV q wk x 6 + Pred 40 mg/m^2 qd x 4 wk	Oat cell	10	4+3	70	Lung toxicity in 3 patients (2 deaths)

[a] Bleo = bleomycin; Adria = adriamycin; VCR = vincristine; Cyclo = cyclophosphamide; MTX = methotrexate; Pred = prednisone.

These studies reported some apparent efficacy. These reports prompted the Eastern Cooperative Oncology Group to start a randomized study of radiotherapy +/- bleomycin. The radiotherapy dose schedule is 5000-6000 rads/5-6 weeks, and the bleomycin dose schedule is 15 u/day x 14 days. Since January 1974, 67 patients have been entered in the study. The end points of the study are symptomatic improvement and survival. The study is both ongoing and coded (C. G. Moertel, 1977, personal communication).

D. Cervical Cancer

The integration of chemotherapy into a combined modality approach for the treatment of cervical cancer has been recently reviewed by Wasserman and Carter (1977). They concluded that there was a need to define those patients who had a poor chance of cure with local-regional therapy of radiation and surgery, and to conduct clinical trials of adjuvant chemotherapy in such patients.

Two pilot studies of radiotherapy and bleomycin in patients with stage IIIB and IV cervical cancer are reported below. Byfield *et al.* (1976) reported on 10 patients treated with pelvic radiotherapy and radium therapy in conjunction with bleomycin (10 u/m² each week), with seemingly increased local control without markedly increased toxicity. J. E. Torres and J. V. Schlosser (1977, personal communication) have treated 30 patients in a randomized study of radiotherapy (pelvic and radium) with or without bleomycin (10 u/m² biw). Again, seemingly increased local control has been seen without undue toxicity. Crooke and Bradner (1976) report on a randomized Japanese study in which a higher 3 year survival rate is seen in those patients treated with radiotherapy and bleomycin versus those treated with radiotherapy alone.

These pilot studies suggest the feasibility of considering a large randomized clinical trial of bleomycin and radiotherapy in advanced localized cervical cancer.

E.   Normal Tissue Toxicity

1.   Skin and Mucous Membranes

The usual and expected mucocutaneous toxicity of radiation is somewhat enhanced by bleomycin in both animal and clinical studies. This includes esophageal and gut mucosa. In particular, those studies in head and neck cancers have shown moderately to markedly increased radiation mucositis. It is well known that bleomycin has a preferential tissue distribution to skin and mucous membranes. Mucocutaneous toxicity is seen with bleomycin used alone without radiotherapy. The enhancement of these toxicities by bleomycin is not as marked as seen with combinations of actinomycin-D and radiation or adriamycin and radiation.

2. Lung

As discussed in Section III,B, studies in oat-cell lung cancer of bleomycin in combination chemotherapy in conjunction with radiotherapy have yielded a higher

TABLE IV. Bleomycin + Radiotherapy: Lung Toxicity [a]

Investigator	Type	Therapy	No. patients with lung toxicity/ No. patients treated	Comments
Chan et al. (1976)	Lung—squamous	XRT + Bleo	1/15 (7%)	
Samuels et al. (1975)	Lung—mixed	XRT + Bleo + VCR + MTX	1/27 (4%)	
Einhorn et al. (1976)	Lung—oat cell	XRT + Cyclo + Adria + Bleo + VCR	5/13	Three deaths, all in wks 11–15 p̄ Rx.
Skarin et al. (1975)	Lung—oat cell	XRT + Adrea + Cyclo + VCR + Bleo + Pred	3/10	Two deaths
SWOG—Haas et al. (1976)	Mixed	Bleo IM vs. IV	79/382 (21%)	No correlation with prior XRT—22% in toxic and nontoxic group had prior XRT. More frequent and more severe toxicity–IV
Samuels et al. (1976)	Testis	Bleo + VLB or Bleo + COMF	9/101 ⎰ 5/12 prior XRT ⎱ 4/89 (4%) no prior XRT	3/4 prior whole-lung XRT + 2/8 prior mediastinal XRT. High median total dose of bleo—600 u

[a] Bleo = bleomycin; VCR = vincristine; MTX = methotrexate; Cyclo = cyclophosphamide; Adria = adreamycin; Pred = prednisone; VLB = velban; COMF = cyclophosphamide + vincristine + methotrexate + 5-fluorouracil.

than expected rate of severe and often fatal pulmonary toxicity. The explanation for this is not clear (Section III, B). These data are reported again in Table IV. Also in this table are two other lung cancer studies of bleomycin in conjunction with radiotherapy in which no apparent increased pulmonary toxicity was seen. The Southwest Oncology Group (SWOG) conducted a broad phase II study of bleomycin via two routes (IM and IV) in a large number of patients and found an overall 21% incidence of pulmonary toxicity (using a broad clinical definition of such toxicity) with no correlation as to whether the patient had prior lung radiation. The last study listed in Table IV is that of Samuels *et al.* (1976), who found a higher incidence of pulmonary toxicity in those testicular cancer patients who had received prior radiotherapy, with most of those patients having had prior whole-lung radiotherapy in the treatment of metastatic testicular cancer in the lung. Also, his patients received a high median dose of bleomycin (600 u).

From the above data no definite conclusion can be drawn as to the role of radiotherapy in enhancing bleomycin pulmonary toxicity. Clinical studies of bleomycin pulmonary toxicity show that although the overt manifestations are related to total cumulative dose of bleomycin and to the age of the patient, subclinical toxicity can be detected using measurements of pulmonary reserve at lower doses. To the extent that any prior radiotherapy induces radiation fibrosis of the lung and secondarily decreases pulmonary reserve, such a patient is likely to have a higher chance of overt clinical toxicity from bleomycin. As animal models of bleomycin pulmonary toxicity are developed it will be important to study the role of radiotherapy. Similar experimental studies of the effect of bleomycin on a radiation lung toxicity animal model are under way (Phillips and Fu, 1977).

IV. SUMMARY

The clinical use of bleomycin in conjunction with radiotherapy has just begun its research evolution. Several interesting pilot studies and small randomized studies have reported improved efficacy in head and neck cancers (particularly oral cavity, larynx, and pharynx), squamous cell lung cancer, and cervical cancer. Such efficacy has been shown in advanced stage patients by improved tumor clearance, by improved survival of responders versus nonresponders, and in certain studies by overall improved survival. It is anticipated that these early results will be put to further clinical testing in large, multiinstitutional, stratified, randomized clinical trials. Only after such more detailed evaluation can decisions on the value of such combined modality therapy be made for clinical practice.

The clinical use of combined bleomycin and radiotherapy has been accompanied by a moderate increase of mucocutaneous toxicity. However, the therapeutic ratio is such that further clinical evaluation is not prohibitive.

For the clinician to be successful in the design of combined therapy with radiation and drugs (including bleomycin) he must be able to look to the experimentalist for some help in answering the many questions that arise in developing combined modality therapies. Hopefully, the experimentalists will develop systems to answer the questions he hears the clinicians asking.

REFERENCES

Anonymous. (1976). *Cancer 37*, Suppl., 2093.

Berdal, P. (1976). *Gann Monogr. Cancer Res. 19*, 133.

Blum, R. H., Carter, S. K., and Agre, K. (1973). *Cancer 31*, 903.

Byfield, J. E., Seagren, S. L., and Weintraub, I. (1976). *Am. Soc. Clin. Oncol. Abstr. 17*, 244.

Carter, S. K., and Soper, W. T. (1974). *Cancer Treatment Rev. 1*, 1.

Carter, S. K., and Wasserman, T. H. (1975). *Cancer Chemotherapy Rep. 5*, 235.

Chan, P. Y. M., Byfield, J. E., Kagan, A. R., and Aronstam, E. M. (1976). *Cancer 37*, 2671.

Chan, P. Y. M., Byfield, J. E., Aronstam, E., and Kagan, A. R. (1977). *Am. Soc. Clin. Oncol. Abstr. 18*, 347.

Clifford, P., Dalley, V., O'Connor, D., and Dearden-Smith, J. (1976). *Am. Soc. Clin. Oncol. Abstr. 17*, 264.

Crooke, S. T., and Bradner, W. T. (1976). *J. Med. 7*, 333.

Einhorn, L., Krause, M., Hornback, H., and Furnas, B. (1976). *Cancer 37*, 2414.

Goldsmith, M. A., and Carter, S. K. (1975). *Cancer Treatment Rev. 2*, 137.

Haas, C. D., Coltman, C. A., Gottlieb, J. A., Haut, A., Luce, J. K., Talley, R. W., Samal, B., Wilson, H. E., and Hoogstraten, B. (1976). *Cancer 38*, 8.

Holoye, P. Y., Samuels, M. L., Lanzotti, V. J., Smith, T., and Barkley, H. T. (1977). *J. Am. Med. Assoc. 237*, 1221.

Jorgensen, S. J. (1972). *Eur. J. Cancer 8*, 531.

Kapstad, B., Bang, G., Rennas, S., and Dahler, A. (1977). *Proceedings of the Second London International Symposium on Bleomycin in the Treatment of Malignant Disease*. Heffer, Cambridge, pp. 2–9.

Kent, C. H., Brereton, H. D., and Johnson, R. E. (1977). *Int. J. Radiat. Oncol. Biol. Phys. 2*, 427.

Muggia, F. M., Cortes-Funes, H., and Wasserman, T. H. (1977). *Int. J. Radiat. Oncol. Biol. Phys.*

Phillips, T. L., and Fu, K. K. (1976). *Cancer 37*, 1186.

Phillips, T. L., and Fu, K. K. (1977). *Cancer 40*, 489.

Samuels, M. L., Barkley, H. T., Holoye, P. Y., Rosenberg, P. J., and Smith, P. L. (1975). *Cancer Chemother. Rep. 59*, 377.

Samuels, M. L., Johnson, D. E., Holoye, P. Y., and Lanzotti, V. J. (1976). *J. Am. Med. Assoc. 235*, 1117.

Shanta, V., and Krishnamurthi, S. (1976). *Gann Monogr. Cancer Res. 19*, 159.

Silverberg, I. J., Phillips, T. L., Fu, K. K., and Chan, P. Y. M. (1976). *Am. Soc. Clin. Oncol. Abstr. 17*, 279.

Silverberg, I. J., Phillips, T. L., Fu, K. K., and Friedman, M. (1978). *Am. Soc. Clin. Oncol. Abstr. 18*, 345.

Skarin, A., Lokich, J., Goodman, R., Chaffey, J., and Frei, E. (1975). *Am. Soc. Clin. Oncol. Abstr. 16*, 264.

Wasserman, T. H., and Carter, S. K. (1977). *Cancer Treatment Rev. 4*, 25.

Chapter 23

BLEOMYCIN TREATMENT OF HEAD AND NECK CARCINOMA IN JAPAN

Yukio Inuyama

I. INTRODUCTION

Since 1963 we have incorporated chemotherapy in our cancer therapy system as the third treatment next to surgery and radiotherapy. Our method of cancer chemotherapy has undergone several changes in the past. Between 1963 and 1967 we used Endoxan or cyclophosphamide (EX), Toyomycin or chromomycin A_3 (TM), mitomycin-C (MMC) and 5-fluorouracil (5-FU). In 1967, we began to use bleomycin (BLM). We have reported several studies of cancer chemotherapy (Inuyama, 1967; Suzuki *et al.*, 1969; Inuyama *et al.*, 1975).

In this paper we report the results of bleomycin treatment at our department.

II. PATIENTS AND METHODS

We have administered BLM to a total of 275 patients. Administration was done by intraarterial infusion in 230 cases (84%) and by intravenous injection in 43 cases (15%). The daily dose of BLM was 15 mg by intraarterial infusion and 30 mg by intravenous injection, to a total dosage of 300 mg.

Sometimes we used chemotherapy alone, but mostly we combined it with surgery

TABLE I.   Mode of Administration

Treatment	No. of cases
IA alone	12
IA → Surg.	85
IA ∓ Rad.	80
IA ∓ Rad. → Surg.	53
IV alone	5
IV → Surg.	3
IV ∓ Rad.	24
IV ∓ Rad. → Surg.	11
IM → Rad.	2
Total	275

or radiation. Radiotherapy comprised supervoltage radiation using either ^{60}Co or linear accelerator (Linac).

The most favored mode of treatment was intraarterial infusion followed by surgery; 85 patients received such treatment. Next to that, a combination of intraarterial infusion and irradiation was most frequently adopted; 80 patients received such treatment. Combined intraarterial infusion and irradiation was followed by surgery in 53 cases, and intravenous injection was combined with irradiation in 24 cases (Table I).

III.   RESULTS

A.   Effect of BLM

To see the effect of chemotherapy, we examined 178 patients, who received intraarterial infusion of some drug before surgical operation or irradiation. The result was excellent in 71%, or five of seven cases with adriamycin, 65% or 55 of 84 cases with BLM, 60% or three of five cases with 5-FU, 33% or 14 of 42 cases with TM, and 14% or four of 29 cases with MMC (Table II).

B.   Five Year Survival Rate

Table III shows the results of chemotherapy combined with radiation or surgery. The 5 year survival rate was 40% or 43/107 in the BLM group, and 39% or 17/44 in the 5-FU group. It was almost the same in these two groups. The values were lower with the other drugs. It was 27% or 6/22 in the MMC group, and 24% or 10/42 in the TM group.

We will deal separately with specific cancers that are relatively frequent and well suited to the intraarterial infusion. These are malignant tumors of the maxillary sinus, nasopharynx, tonsil, and tongue.

TABLE II. Effect of Intraarterial Chemotherapy

Drugs used	No. of cases	Excellent	Good	Unchanged
EX	11	0 (0%)	6	5
TM	42	14 (33%)	17	11
MMC	29	4 (14%)	13	12
5-FU	5	3 (60%)	1	1
BLM	84 [a]	55 (65%)	24	5
ADM	7	5 (71%)	1	1
Total	178	81 (46%)	62	35

[a] 1967–1972.

1. Maxillary Sinus

We treated 195 patients with malignant tumor of the maxillary sinus between 1957 and 1976. The tumor was carcinoma in 184 cases and sarcoma in 11 cases. It was identified as squamous cell carcinoma in 178 cases (91%). The 5 year survival rate in 165 patients with malignant tumor of the maxillary sinus treated in 1957 through 1972 was 30%. Table IV shows 5 year survival rates in a total of 127 patients treated between 1957 and 1966, when BLM was still not being used. In all, 32 patients (25%) survived 5 years. Surgery alone produced the best result, affording 5 year survival of 31%. Next to surgery, combined intraarterial infusion and radiation followed by surgery was the most effective; the 5 year survival rate in this group was 27%, which approximated that in the surgery group. The 5 year survival rate in patients who received TM or MMC by intraarterial infusion and then underwent operation was 22%. It was relatively high (38%) in patients treated by combined intraarterial infusion and radiation; this treatment was performed largely for reticulum cell sarcoma. The 5 year survival rate in patients treated between 1967 and

TABLE III. Survival Rates by Cancer Chemotherapy Combined with Radiation or Surgery

Drugs used	Survival			
	3 years		5 years	
	No.	%	No.	%
EX	2/11	18	2/11	18
TM	17/42	41	10/42	24
MMC	7/22	32	6/22	27
5-FU	17/44	39	17/44	39
BLM	72/142	51	43/107	40

TABLE IV. Five Year Survival Rate in Malignant Tumors of
the Maxillary Sinus (1957–1966)

Treatment	Five year survival	
	No.	%
Surgery alone	14/45	31
Radiation→ surgery	3/19	16
Infusion → surgery	6/27	22
Infusion + radiation→surgery	6/22	27
Radiation alone	0/6	0
Infusion + radiation	3/8	38
Total	32/127	25

TABLE V. Five Year Survival Rate in Malignant Tumors
of the Maxillary Sinus (1967–1972)

Treatment	Five year survival	
	No.	%
BLM (IA)→ surgery	16/31	52
BLM (IA) + radiation → surgery	1/4	25
BLM (IA) + radiation	0/1	0
BLM alone	1/2	50
Total	18/38	47

1972, when BLM was used, is shown in Table V. Of a total of 38 patients in this period, 18 survived 5 years, which makes the survival rate 47%. Compared with the results between 1957 and 1966, this is a marked improvement. The most effective treatment was intraarterial infusion of BLM followed by surgery, which afforded 5 year survival of 52%.

In addition to the clinical trials of the combined treatment, a pathological study was designed to evaluate the efficacy of the preoperative treatment on tumor tissue in patients of each group. Tumor tissue extirpated *en bloc* during surgery from 57 patients was submitted to pathological studies. The removed tissue was processed into large serial sections and examined under a light microscope. In evaluating the effect of various preoperative treatments the tumor tissue response was classified according to the method proposed by Shimosato (1971) (Table VI). On analysis of the results, the degree III response, which is indicative of regional regression of tumor proliferation, was found in two out of nine cases (22%) in the preoperative radiotherapy group, in one out of 24 (4.1%) in the preoperative infusion (excluding BLM) groups, in two out of 12 (16%) in the preoperative combined radiation and chemotherapy group, and in two out of 12 (16%) in the BLM-treated group. There

TABLE VI. Efficacy of Preoperative Treatment on Tumor Tissue in 57 Maxillary Cancers (Squamous Cell Carcinoma)

Degree	Tumor tissue response	Irradiation 4500–5000 rads (nine cases)	Mitomycin-C, Toyomycin infusion 25–35 vials (24 cases)	5-FU infusion, 250 mg x 30. Irradiation, 6000 rads (12 cases)	BLM infusion 300 mg (12 cases)
IV	Complete arrest of tumor proliferation				
III	Low probability of recurrence of tumor proliferation	○○	x	□□	△△
IIb	Moderate probability of recurrence of tumor proliferation	○○○○	xx	□□□□□ □□□	△△△△
IIa	High probability of recurrence of tumor proliferation	○	xxxx	□□	△△△△△
I		○○	xxxxxx xxxxx		△
0			xxxxx xx		

TABLE VII. Five Year Survival Rate in Malignant Tumors of
the Nasopharynx (1963–1968)

Treatment	Five year survival	
	No.	%
Radiation alone	2/9	22
Infusion ∓ radiation	10/21	48
Total	12/30	40

was no significant difference in the results among these groups. The degree IV response, indicative of complete arrest of tumor cell proliferation, was not detected in the tumor tissues in any of the patients. The degree IIb response, where a possibility exists of reproliferation of tumor cells was achieved in four out of nine cases (44.4%) in the preoperative radiotherapy group, two out of 24 (8.3%) in the preoperative infusion (excluding BLM) group, eight out of 12 (66.6%) in the preoperative radiation and chemotherapy group, and four out of 12 (33.3%) in the preoperative BLM infusion group. Analysis of the overall results has demonstrated an inhibitory effect on tumor growth in decreasing order of the combined radiation and chemotherapy, radiotherapy, BLM infusion treatment, and other infusion treatments (Suzuki et al., 1976).

2. Nasopharynx

We treated 71 patients with nasopharyngeal tumor between 1963 and 1976. The histologic type was carcinoma in 60 cases and sarcoma in 11 cases. Of these patients, 43 had poorly differentiated squamous cell carcinoma, and 15 had undifferentiated carcinoma. These two types of tumor accounted for 82% of the cases. Recently, many researchers have pointed out that EB virus is closely associated with nasopharyngeal carcinoma. Therefore, we evaluated anti-VCA antibody titers in 51 patients with nasopharyngeal carcinoma, and found that geometric mean titer (GMT) in these patients was a high as 1:794. The geometric mean titer in carcinoma of the maxillary sinus, on the other hand, was as low as 1:163, and those in carcinoma of the larynx and carcinoma of the tongue were, respectively, 1:214 and 1:219. Ridit analysis also revealed that anti-VCA titers in patients with nasopharyngeal carcinoma were significantly higher than in those with carcinoma of some other site. The 5 year survival rate in a total of 45 patients treated between 1963 and 1972 was 38%. The 5 year survival rate was 40% in patients treated between 1963 and 1968, when BLM was still not used: That is, 12 of 30 patients in that period survived 5 years (Table VII). It was a relatively high 48% in patients treated by combined 5-FU intraarterial infusion and radiation. The 5 year survival rate in patients treated between 1968 and 1972, when BLM was used, is shown in Table VIII. Of 15 patients in this period, five survived 5 years, which makes the rate 33%. This result is slightly poorer as compared with the result between 1963 and 1968. If the

TABLE VIII. Five Year Survival Rate in Malignant Tumors of
the Nasopharynx (1968–1972)

| Treatment | Five year survival | |
	No.	%
BLM (IA) + radiation	5/11	45
BLM (IV) + radiation	0/2	0
BLM alone	0/2	0
Total	5/15	33

results of particular modes of treatment are observed, it will be found that combined BLM intraarterial infusion and radiation treatment yielded a 5 year survival rate of 45%, or 5/11. This is roughly the same as the result produced by combined 5-FU intraarterial infusion and radiation treatment.

3. Tonsil

There were 59 patients with malignant tumors of the tonsil treated by us between 1963 and 1976. The histologic type was carcinoma in 24 cases, and sarcoma in 35 cases. Of these patients, 33 (56%) had reticulum cell sarcoma. The 5 year survival rate was 39% or 16/41 of the patients treated between 1963 and 1972. The 5 year survival rate was 45% in patients treated between 1963 and 1968, when bleomycin was not being used; nine of 20 patients in that period survived 5 years. The 5 year survival rate by combined irradiation and surgery was 67%, and that by combined 5-FU intraarterial infusion and radiation treatment was 50% (Table IX). Table X shows the 5 year survival rate in patients treated between 1968 and 1972, when BLM was used. Of 21 patients in that period, seven were alive as of 5 years after treatment, which makes the rate 33%. This result is inferior to that of 1963 through 1968. From the results classified by the mode of treatment, however, it will be found that combined BLM intraarterial infusion and radiation treatment produced a 5 year survival rate of 57% or 4/7. This is better than the result produced by combined 5-FU intraarterial infusion and radiation treatment. The result was not so good in patients treated by combined BLM intraarterial infusion and surgery; the rate was 30% or 3/10.

4. Tongue

There were 68 patients with malignant tumor of the tongue treated by us between 1963 and 1976. The histologic type was squamous cell carcinoma in all the cases. The 5 year survival rate was 41% or 15/37 of patients treated between 1963 and 1972. The 5 year survival rate was 31% or 5/16 in the period between 1963 and 1968, when BLM was not being used. It was 50% in patients treated by surgery alone (Table XI). The 5 year survival rate in patients treated between 1968 and 1972, when BLM was used, is shown in Table XII. It was 48% or 10/21, which was

TABLE IX. Five Year Survival Rate in Malignant Tumors
of the Tonsil (1963–1968)

	Five year survival	
Treatment	No.	%
Infusion ∓radiation	7/14	50
Radiation alone	0/2	0
Radiation → surgery	2/3	67
Infusion + radiation → surgery	0/1	0
Total	9/20	45

TABLE X. Five Year Survival Rate in Malignant Tumors
of the Tonsil (1968–1972)

	Five year survival	
Treatment	No.	%
BLM (IA) + radiation	4/7	57
BLM (IA) → surgery	3/10	30
BLM alone	0/4	0
Total	7/21	33

TABLE XI. Five Year Survival Rate in Carcinoma of
the Tongue (1963–1968)

	Five year survival	
Treatment	No.	%
Surgery alone	3/6	50
Infusion →surgery	0/2	0
Infusion + radiation → surgery	1/3	33
Infusion + radiation	1/5	20
Total	5/16	31

TABLE XII. Five Year Survival Rate in Carcinoma of
the Tongue (1968–1972)

	Five year survival	
Treatment	No.	%
BLM (IA) →surgery	10/14	71
BLM (IA) + radiation → surgery	0/2	0
BLM (IV) + radiation	0/3	0
BLM alone	0/2	0
Total	10/21	48

better than the result between 1963 and 1968. Of various modes of treatments, combined BLM intraarterial infusion and surgery produced an excellent result of 71% or 10/14.

In short, the 5 year survival rate afforded by BLM treatment was as high as 47% in patients with carcinoma of the maxillary sinus and 48% in those with carcinoma of the tongue, while it was an unsatisfactory 33% in patients with carcinoma of the tonsil or the nasopharynx. When BLM was combined with radiation, however, the result was much better. In patients with tumor of the tonsil and those with tumor of the nasopharynx treated by combined BLM intraarterial infusion and radiation, the 5 year survival rate was, respectively, 45% and 50%. These results were as good as those produced by combined 5-FU and radiation treatment. The 5 year survival rate in patients with laryngeal tumor was as high as 75%, but BLM treatment has been tried on only a few patients with this tumor, so that it is difficult to make any comment in this respect. As a whole, BLM treatment afforded 5 year survival in 43 of 107 patients, or 40%.

The 5 year survival rates in different histologic groups produced by BLM treatment were as follows: In squamous cell carcinoma, which was most frequent, the rate was 39%, that is, 33 of 85 patients survived 5 years. In undifferentiated carcinoma, on the other hand, none of the four patients achieved 5 year survival, though we must take into account the small number of patients in this category. BLM produced the best result of 56% or 9/16 in reticulum cell sarcoma.

The 5 year survival rates in patients treated with BLM, classified by the mode of treatment, are shown in Table XIII. Treatment by BLM intraarterial infusion combined with subsequent surgery produced the best result: It afforded 5 year survival in 51% or 29 of 57 patients. Treatment by BLM intravenous injection combined with subsequent surgery was almost as effective, though it was done only in four cases; the rate was 50% in this group. Combined BLM intraarterial infusion and radiation also produced a good result of 47%. Combined BLM intraarterial infusion and radiation followed by surgery, however, produced a poor result; it afforded 5 year survival only in 17% or one of six cases. We may attribute such a poor result to the fact that this mode of treatment was used mainly for tumors that spread widely, and that patients were given overdoses both of BLM and radiation. Combined BLM intravenous injection and radiation also produced a poor result; it afforded 5 year survival in none of the five patients.

TABLE XIII. Five Year Survival Rate According to Mode of Treatment

Treatment	Five year survival	
	No.	%
BLM (IA) → surgery	29/57	31
BLM (IA) + radiation → surgery	1/6	17
BLM (IV) → surgery	3/6	50
BLM (IA) ∓ radiation	9/19	47
BLM (IV) + radiation	0/5	0
BLM alone	1/14	7
Total	43/107	40

TABLE XIV. BLM Treatment Combined with Radiotherapy

BLM (mg) \ Radiation (rads)	No. of patients treated				
	2000	2001– 4000	4001– 6000	6001	Total
100	3	7	7	1	18
101–200	1	14	4	1	20
201–300	1	13	7	3	24
301–	1	5	3	1	10
Total	6	39	21	6	72

We then examined the incidence of recurrence in patients treated with BLM. In a total of 107 patients recurrence followed BLM treatment in 48 patients or 45% and metastasis was observed in nine patients or 8%. The incidence of recurrence was as high as 60% in patients treated by combined BLM intravenous injection and radiation. It was 42% both in patients treated by BLM intraarterial infusion followed by surgery and in those treated by combined BLM intraarterial infusion and radiation. In patients treated by combined BLM intraarterial infusion and radiation followed by surgery or in those treated by BLM intravenous injection and surgery, the incidence was 33%. Among 17 patients treated with BLM who died of other diseases, one patient died from pulmonary fibrosis caused by BLM.

C. Dosage in Combined BLM and Radiation

Among 72 patients treated with combined BLM and radiation, 14 patients or the largest proportion received 101–200 mg BLM and 2001–4000 rads each. The second largest group, containing 13 patients, had 201–300 mg BLM and 2001–4000 rads each (Table XIV).

Chronologically speaking, patients received an average of 298 mg BLM and 4700 rads each in 1967 through 1973, and an average of 147 mg BLM and 3600 rads in 1974 through 1976. It seems that the amount of BLM was too great for a combination treatment in early days. Recently, we began to try a combination treatment proposed by Miyamoto et al. (1977); this consists of sequential combination of BLM and MMC (B–M therapy) and radiotherapy.

D. A Sequential Combination of BLM and MMC (B-M Therapy)

In this treatment, we administered 5 mg BLM daily for 1 week by intramuscular injection, then injected 10 mg MMC intravenously on the following day. This makes up one course. Table XV shows the effect of B–M therapy. In previously untreated cases the excellent result was not obtained in any of the cases, because only one course was given before radiotherapy, but the result was evaluated as "good" in

TABLE XV. Effect of B-M Therapy

Effect	Previously untreated	Treated	Response rate (%)
Excellent		8	26 ⎫ 48
Good	4	3	23 ⎭
Unchanged	4	12	
Total	8	23	

four cases. In recurrent cases the result was excellent in eight cases and good in three cases. In all, the result was favorable in 48% of the cases.

IV. CONCLUSION

The results of BLM treatment for malignant tumors of the head and neck have been outlined. In carcinoma of the tongue or the maxillary sinus, which almost invariably or predominantly is well-differentiated squamous cell carcinoma, we obtained good results from BLM intraarterial infusion followed by surgery. In malignant tumors of the nasopharynx or tonsil, on the other hand, combination of BLM-intraarterial infusion and radiation was roughly as effective as combination of 5-FU intraarterial infusion and radiation with respect to 5 year survival rate. I expect that the results of BLM treatment will be much improved in the future, for example, with adoption of B-M therapy or a newly developed derivative of BLM named NK-631.

REFERENCES

Inuyama, Y. (1967). *Jpn. J. Otol., Tokyo, 70*, 612 (in Japanese).

Inuyama, Y., Ozu, R., Horiuchi, M., Asaoka, K., Sakamoto, Y., Matsukawa, J., Honmura, Y., and Shinkawa, A. (1975). *Jpn. J. Cancer Clin. 21*, 1301 (in Japanese).

Miyamoto, T., Takabe, Y., Watanabe, M., and Terashima, T. (1977). *Cancer and Chemother. 4*, 273 (in Japanese).

Shimosato, Y. (1971). *Jpn. J. Clin. Oncol. 1*, 19.

Suzuki, Y., Miyake, H., Sakai, M., Inuyama, Y., Matsukawa, J., and Fujii, K. (1969). *Keio J. Med. 18*, 153.

Suzuki, Y., Miyake, H., and Sakai, M. (1976). *Gann Monogr. Cancer Res. 19*, 151.

Chapter 24

BLEOMYCIN PULMONARY TOXICITY

Robert L. Comis

I. INTRODUCTION

Bleomycin is being increasingly employed in aggressive combination chemotherapy programs because of its lack of significant myelotoxicity and demonstrated antitumor activity in lymphomas, testicular carcinomas, and squamous cell carcinoma of the head and neck. The well known dose-limiting toxicity of bleomycin is pulmonary fibrosis. Bleomycin is unlike most other pulmonary toxins in that the pulmonary toxicity of most other drugs tends to be sporadic, idiosyncratic, and not dose limiting. This is true of the antineoplastic agents which have been associated with pulmonary toxicity such as busulfan, methotrexate, and cyclophosphamide. In addition, it is a relatively unique pulmonary toxin because of its encompassing pulmonary toxicity within mammalian species. Pulmonary toxicity has been noted in rodents, dogs, rabbits, monkeys, and man. The purpose of this paper is to review the pertinent preclinical, pathologic, and clinical data on the pulmonary effects of bleomycin.

II. PRECLINICAL DATA

Early pharmacologic studies in rodents indicated that the lung, as well as the skin, was a site of preferential drug distribution relative to plasma (Ishizuka *et al.*, 1967). Pulmonary and dermal toxicities were first noted in these early studies employing the drug administered on chronic schedules. Umezawa *et al.* (1972) subsequently showed that most organs were capable of rapidly inactivating the microbiologic activity of bleomycin. This inactivating activity was lower in skin and lungs when compared to other tissues, particularly liver. Inactivation appears to be due to an enzyme present in the supernatant of the 150,000g centrifugation fraction of mouse liver homogenates. This enzyme has been termed bleomycin hydrolase. Muller and Zahn (1976), employing an assay for DNA dependent-DNA polymerase activity, have also demonstrated bleomycin inactivating activity which is highest in liver and significantly lower in lung and skin.

In addition to the organ specificity of bleomycin hydrolase, Umezawa *et al.* (1972) have reported that in mice this activity is age related. Young mice (3 weeks old) had significantly higher levels of bleomycin hydrolase activity than older (28-week-old) mice.

Although these preclinical observations fit well with clinical human toxicology, to date similar studies indicating the preferential distribution of bleomycin in the lungs and the inability of lung to inactivate bleomycin have not been reported in man. Furthermore, although bleomycin pulmonary toxicity appears to be more common over age 70 (see below), a relationship between age-related pulmonary toxicity and bleomycin inactivating activity has not been demonstrated in man.

There is a tendency for the severity of pulmonary toxicity to be related to the total dose of bleomycin administered. Adamson and Bowden (1974), studying mice, found that histopathologic changes in the lungs tended to be more severe with increasing total doses of bleomycin. Also, the severity of pulmonary lesions was noted to be progressive when animals surviving bleomycin therapy were sacrificed at increasing intervals after the cessation of therapy (Fleishman *et al.*, 1974).

Pulmonary function studies have been performed in anesthetized dogs and correlated with x-ray changes. Valicenti *et al.* have shown that changes in pulmonary function tests including the static lung compliance, total lung capacity, vital capacity, and diffusion capacity occur prior to demonstrable x-ray changes (1972). In another study, changes in pulmonary function tests were noted prior to changes in x-ray findings, although when x-ray changes occurred the severity of the changes correlated with the severity of the histopathologic lesions (Schaeppi *et al.*, 1972).

In summary, preclinical data indicated that bleomycin was a drug which was preferentially distributed in the lung, an organ rather deficient in inactivating capacity, particularly in older animals. Pulmonary toxicity occurred in a variety of mammalian species, and tended to be total dose- and time-dependent. In addition, x-ray changes tended to occur later than changes in pulmonary function tests, but they did correlate well with the severity of histopathologic change.

III. PATHOLOGY

Pulmonary fibrosis appears to be the final common expression of lung injury. Pulmonary fibrosis associated with severe bleomycin pulmonary toxicity cannot be readily distinguished from other injury associated with most other pulmonary toxins or idiopathic pulmonary fibrosis.

Because of the difficulty in obtaining serial pulmonary tissue samples in man, the majority of the data on the morphologic sequence of injury derive from animal experimental observations. Table I lists a proposed sequence of toxic pulmonary events which occur with increasing degrees of pulmonary damage, leading to pulmonary fibrosis. These observations are derived from both light and electron microscopy studies in rodents, dogs, and man.

Endothelial "blebs" have been demonstrated in mouse alveolar capillary endothelium soon after bleomycin administration (Adamson, 1976). Although these changes have not been consistently found in all experiments or species, if, in fact, they are the first to occur, the lack of consistency may be more a function of experimental design than species specificity. Interstitial and fibrinous edema within alveolar sacs have been described, as well as the development of hyaline membranes. Both electron microscopic and light microscopy studies have led to certain conclusions relating the response of Type I and Type II alveolar macrophages to bleomycin effects. Electron microscopic studies have shown a decrease in Type I alveolar pneumocytes (Aso *et al.*, 1976; Bedrossian *et al.*, 1972; DeLena *et al.*, 1972). It has been suggested that these observations imply an early destruction of these cells as a response to bleomycin injury. Type II alveolar macrophages have been noted to proliferate, change morphologically, delamellate, and "migrate" into the alveolar spaces. The alveolar septa become thickened, and collagen fibers adjacent to fibroblasts are noted. Finally, a dense proliferation of fibrous tissue and a decrease in the alveolar septae occur. None of these changes appears to be specific to bleomycin effects.

The *in vitro* and *in vivo* morphologic effects of bleomycin on Novikoff hepatoma cells have been described. These changes, apparent in transmission electron microscopy, include an increase in nucleolar fibrillar center formation, fragmentation of nucleolar fibrillar elements, the development of nucleolar microspherules, and the formation of nuclear and cytoplasmic bodies (Daskal *et al.*, 1975). Similar changes

TABLE I.   Pathological Changes Induced by Bleomycin: Nonspecific

? Endothelial damage
Increased interstitial fluid
Intraalveolar fibrinous edema
Destruction of Type I pneumocytes
Type II pneumocytes ⟨ Proliferation / Migration / Delamellation
Fibrous proliferation

TABLE II. Bleomycin Pulmonary Toxicity: Symptoms and Signs

Cough
Exertional dyspnea
Dyspnea at rest
Tachypnea
Fever
Cyanosis

have recently been described in electron microscopic studies of lung tissue obtained by pulmonary biopsy and at autopsy in patients treated with bleomycin. The nucleoplasm of Type II cells has been noted to contain a large number of nucleolar bodies when compared to control tissues, or type I pneumocytes. Additionally, fibrillar centers were noted in the nucleoli of Type I and II pneumocytes (Daskal *et al.*, 1978).

In summary, although most studies have not described changes specific to bleomycin effects, evidence is developing to indicate that specific ultrastructural changes related to bleomycin can be detected in human lung exposed to the drug.

IV. CLINICAL FEATURES OF BLEOMYCIN PULMONARY TOXICITY

A. Symptoms and Signs

Table II lists the major symptoms and signs of bleomycin pulmonary toxicity. A dry, hacking cough and exertional dyspnea are the earliest symptoms of bleomycin pulmonary toxicity. As the lesion progresses, dyspnea at rest, tachypnea, fever, and cyanosis ensue. The latter signs and symptoms are manifestations of more severe pulmonary toxicity.

B. Physical Findings

Table III lists the physical findings which are associated with progressive pulmonary toxicity. DeLena *et al.* (1972) have extensively detailed the physical findings considered to be manifestations of bleomycin pulmonary toxicity. Initially,

TABLE III. Bleomycin Pulmonary Toxicity: Physical Findings

Fine bibasilar râles
Coarse râles—lower 1/3 lung fields
Rhonchi
Pleural friction rub
Intercostal retraction

TABLE IV.   Bleomycin Pulmonary Toxicity: Radiographic Findings

Fine reticular bibasilar infiltrate
Alveolar interstitial bibasilar infiltrate
Progressive lower lobe involvement
Lobar consolidation

fine crepitant râles are heard at one or both lung bases. With more severe involvement, these findings progress with the development of coarse bilateral râles, rhonchi and occasionally the development of a pleural friction rub. As patients progress to respiratory failure, intercostal retractions occur.

C.   Radiographic Findings

Table IV lists the radiographic findings seen with progressive pulmonary involvement. The earliest radiographic manifestation of bleomycin pulmonary toxicity is the development of a fine bibasilar reticular infiltrate. This lesion may resolve if bleomycin is discontinued, or progress with the development of bibasilar alveolar-interstitial infiltrates, progressive lower lobe involvement, and finally lobar consolidation. A significant pleural effusion is generally not seen.

Samuels *et al.* (1976) have described two types of pulmonary involvement termed "minimal disease" and "advanced disease." The "minimal disease" presentation consists of exertional dyspnea, without dyspnea at rest, "fine crackling râles" at both bases, and minimal bibasilar interstitial or alveolar infiltrates. Abnormal arterial pO_2 at rest, temperature elevation, sputum production, and leukocytosis are absent. This complex may resolve with cessation of bleomycin. The more advanced disease is associated with severe dyspnea and hypoxemia ($pO_2 \leq 55$ mm Hg) at rest, prominent radiographic and physical findings, with the radiograph progressing from bibasilar lower lobe infiltrates to frank consolidation. This presentation is generally irreversible.

D.   Pulmonary Function Tests

Several studies are available evaluating the relationship between bleomycin therapy and changes in pulmonary function tests. Most studies have employed measurements of the forced vital capacity (FVC), forced expiratory volume in one second (FEV_1), 1 minute single breath or steady-state carbon monoxide diffusion capacity (DL_{CO}), total lung capacity (TLC), or maximum breathing capacity (MBC). Few studies have employed systematic serial determinations or clearly defined the exact timing of pulmonary function testing relative to the total bleomycin dose or the cessation of bleomycin therapy. Within these constraints, there have been definite changes in TLC, FVC, and DL_{CO} seen with bleomycin therapy, but there have been no consistent relationships noted between total bleomycin dose and changes in pulmonary function (Pascual *et al.*, 1975; Yagoda *et al.*, 1972; Rudders, 1973).

Recently, Samuels *et al.* (1976) have stated that in a retrospective analysis patients exhibiting the advanced form of bleomycin pulmonary toxicity have shown a greater decrement and more rapid decrease in FVC than "controls" or patients with "minimal" bleomycin lung toxicity.

Perez-Guerra *et al.* (1973) have reported a single case study of a patient receiving bleomycin (15 u twice weekly) with serial FVC and DL_{CO} determinations performed at 30 u increments. A pulmonary biopsy was performed when the patient was totally asymptomatic with no physical or radiographic findings (bleomycin total dose, 240 u). The DL_{CO} and FVC had decreased approximately 50 and 13%, respectively. The patient had histologically documented interstitial fibrosis.

Recently Izbicki *et al.* (1977) and Comis *et al.* (1977) have reported the results of serial studies of volumetric measurements (FVC and FEV_1) and DL_{CO}. The former study was performed in patients with a variety of malignancies and the latter performed in young testicular carcinoma patients. The preliminary results of both studies show a linear fall in DL_{CO} with increasing total doses of bleomycin. Neither study showed a consistent relationship between FVC or FEV_1 determinations and bleomycin dose.

Presently, there is no pulmonary function test which is clearly predictive of significant bleomycin pulmonary toxicity, although systematic serial determinations of DL_{CO} may be a sensitive indicator of subclinical bleomycin pulmonary toxicity. Whether the DL_{CO} will predict when bleomycin should be discontinued in order to avert clinically significant bleomycin pulmonary toxicity remains to be established by further studies.

V. INCIDENCE

The reported incidence of bleomycin "pulmonary toxicity" has ranged between 0–40%. This large range is a function of the number of patients treated in each study and the criteria used for defining pulmonary toxicity. The problems in defining the incidence of bleomycin pulmonary toxicity are illustrated in Fig. 1, which is an adaptation of data presented by DeLena (1972). Depending upon the definition employed, the incidence of bleomycin pulmonary toxicity ranged from 0.5 to 40% within this single study.

Recently Crooke and Bradner (1976) have tabulated the results of 14 studies. Excluding the data reported in the review by Blum *et al.* (1973), which may overlap with some of the more recently reported studies, published data on 1890 patients were reviewed. Overall, "morbidity" from bleomycin therapy occurred in 11% of the reported cases. Deaths due to bleomycin-induced pulmonary toxicity occurred in 0–6% of these cases.

Several large series from throughout the world indicate that fatal bleomycin pulmonary toxicity occurs in about 1–2% of cases, whereas nonlethal pulmonary fibrosis occurs in an additional 2–3% (Ichikawa, 1976; E.O.R.T.C., 1970; Halnan *et al.*, 1972; Yagoda *et al.*, 1972). The greatest range in the incidence figures occurs within groups termed "questionable," "mild to moderate" toxicity, or those cases in which purely clinical criteria are used for diagnosis.

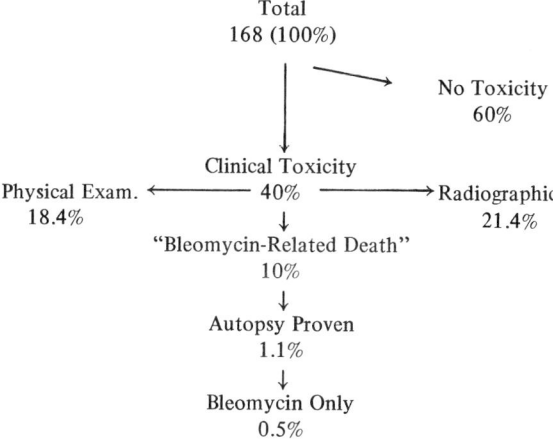

Fig. 1. Breakdown of 168 patients with bleomycin pulmonary toxicity. Adapted from Delena *et al.*, (1972).

The data reported by Blum *et al.* (1973) were based upon case reports on 808 patients reviewed at the time of the submission of the bleomycin new drug application (NDA) in 1972. The results of these data are provided in Table V. A similar review, employing the same criteria, was performed in 1974.

Definite toxicity refers to those cases in which bleomycin-related interstitial fibrosis was the cause of death and autopsy proven; *probable toxicity* was that in which the clinical setting was that of bleomycin-related pulmonary fibrosis with most cases being documented at autopsy, but with some cases having concomitant pulmonary processes such as metastases; *questionable cases* were those with mainly clinical criteria and generally moderate to severe pulmonary involvement with metastatic disease, with little autopsy verification; *unexpected autopsy findings* were those cases in which interstitial fibrosis was present at post mortem without any clinical indication of bleomycin-related pulmonary damage.

TABLE V. Bleomycin Pulmonary Toxicity in 808 patients [a]

Toxicity category	No.	%
Definite	9	1.1
Probable	15	1.9
Unexpected autopsy findings	16	2.0
Questionable	46	5.1
Overall	85	10.7

[a] Adapted from Blum *et al.* (1973).

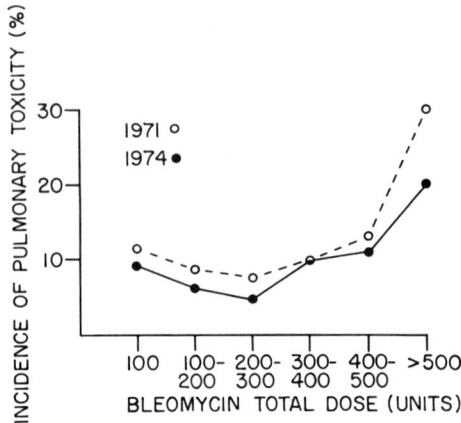

Fig. 2. Incidence of all categories of bleomycin pulmonary toxicity related to total dose.

Figure 2 shows the incidence of all categories of bleomycin pulmonary toxicity, i.e., definite, probable, questionable, and unexpected autopsy findings, for both NDA reviews. The definitions, as described above, were the same for the 808 patients reviewed in 1971 and the 600 patients reviewed in 1974. For neither analysis is there a clear-cut dose-response relationship. Rather, there does appear to be a significant increase in toxicity when total doses of greater than 500 u are employed.

Figure 3 present the data on all categories of pulmonary toxicity plus a breakdown of those cases in which there was good evidence for bleomycin pulmonary

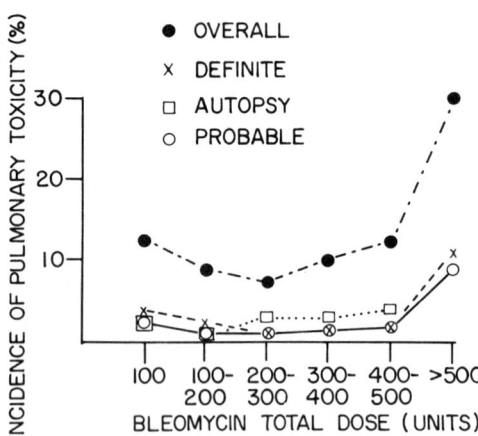

Fig. 3. Incidence of bleomycin pulmonary toxicity for all categories and patients with definite probable, and unexpected autopsy findings related to total dose (*NDA Review*, 1971, 808 patients).

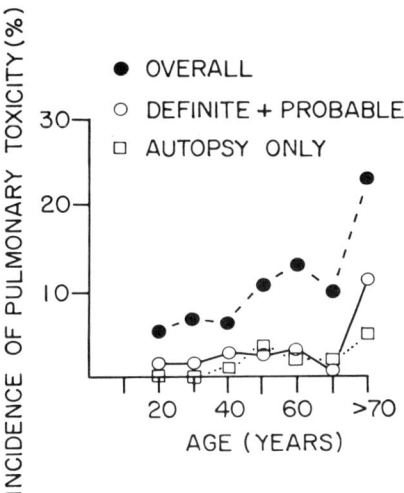

Fig. 4. Incidence of bleomycin pulmonary toxicity related to age (*NDA Review*, 1971, 808 patients).

toxicity, i.e., definite, probable, and unexpected autopsy findings. The incidence of bleomycin pulmonary toxicity is low and consistent with doses of 100–500 u of bleomycin. There does appear to be significant increase in well defined toxicity with doses greater than 500 u. In addition, the incidence of unexpected autopsy findings parallels the definite and probable cases throughout the dose ranges for which there is adequate data.

These data indicate that pulmonary toxicity occurs in a relatively constant small proportion of cases receiving from 100–500 total dose units of bleomycin. There is *no* classic dose-response relationship throughout this range. There does appear to be a threshold dose (>500 u) after which the incidence of bleomycin pulmonary toxicity significantly increases. Stated differently, the pulmonary toxicity associated with bleomycin is unpredictable and *not* dose-related with total doses ranging from 100 to 500 units of bleomycin.

These findings imply that there may be a certain subset of patients who are particularly susceptible to the pulmonary toxicity of bleomycin. The nature of this predisposition, i.e., genetic, pharmacogenetic, or disease-related, is currently unknown. The findings of a comparable proportion of patients with unexpected autopsy findings indicates that subclinical pulmonary toxicity, which can be documented histopathologically, occurs with *at least* the same frequency as clinically significant toxicity. In fact, the incidence of subclinical pulmonary toxicity may be significantly underrepresented, since a more appropriate denominator would be the number of cases treated at each dose level who were autopsied, rather than the entire patient population. The number of patients autopsied at each dose level is not available for this determination. Although there does not appear to be a dose-toxicity

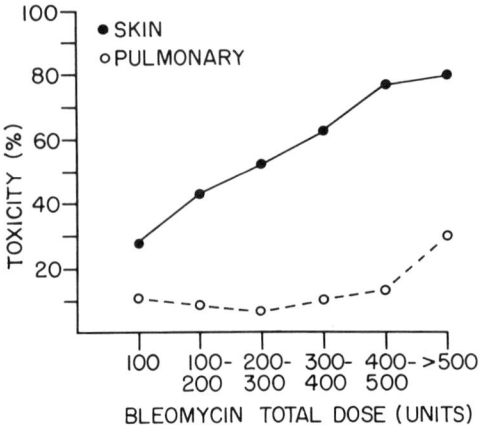

Fig. 5. Incidence of pulmonary and skin toxicity related to total dose (*NDA Review*, 1971, 808 patients).

relationship for significant bleomycin pulmonary toxicity, this does not obviate the possibility that there may be a dose-toxicity relationship which could be detected by a sensitive indicator of subclinical bleomycin pulmonary toxicity.

The relationship between age and bleomycin pulmonary toxicity is presented in Fig. 4. When definite and probable cases of bleomycin pulmonary toxicity, as well as unexpected autopsy cases, are considered there is no significant increase in the relatively low incidence of bleomycin pulmonary toxicity until patients over 70 years of age are considered. Again, the incidence of subclinical, histopathologically documented cases parallels the clinically documented cases.

Figure 5 shows the total dose relationship between patients with skin toxicity versus those with pulmonary toxicity. All categories of pulmonary toxicity are considered. As opposed to pulmonary toxicity, there does appear to be a significant dose-reponse relationship for skin toxicity. This observation may be a function of reporting since clinical observations of the skin are more readily obtained and more sensitive than those derived from a visceral organ. Alternatively, the skin may be more uniformly susceptible to bleomycin than pulmonary tissue.

VI. FACTORS THAT MAY ALTER THE INCIDENCE OF BLEOMYCIN PULMONARY TOXICITY

A. Radiotherapy

Studies by Einhorn *et al.* (1976), Skarin *et al.* (1975), Yagoda *et al.* (1972), and Samuels *et al.* (1976) indicate that prior or concomitant irradiation to the chest increases the incidence of significant bleomycin pulmonary toxicity.

Pulmonary fibrosis was documented in five of 13 patients with small-cell ana-plastic carcinoma treated with combination chemotherapy (bleomcyin, adriamycin, cyclophosphamide, and vincristine) plus concomitant radiotherapy (4000 r) to the primary lesion and mediastinal lymph nodes (Einhorn *et al.*, 1976). Three of the five patients succumbed to the pulmonary toxicity. No patient received more than 90 u of bleomcyin. Similar effects were noted by Skarin *et al.* (1975) in a compar-able treatment program for small-cell anaplastic carcinoma.

Samuels *et al.* (1976) have reported that 5/9 patients who developed pulmonary toxicity after treatment with vinblastine and bleomycin had prior radiotherapy. In all, five of 12 patients with prior radiotherapy developed significant bleomcyin pulmonary toxicity versus four of 89 without prior chest irradiation.

Although chest irradiation can cause a radiation pneumonitis with subsequent fibrosis, it is significant that most cases of bleomycin pulmonary toxicity which have occurred in conjunction with chest irradiation involve the entire lung and not just the radiation portal.

B. Route of Administration

A large comparative study of intravenous versus intramuscular bleomycin has recently been reported (Haas *et al.*, 1976). The overall incidence of bleomycin pulmonary toxicity was 23% versus 15% for intravenous and intramuscular admin-istration, respectively. This difference was reported to be statistically signficant. No clear-cut definition of the grades of pulmonary toxicity was given, but toxicity was graded from mild to life-threatening. There was no significant difference in severe and life-threatening toxicities, 4 and 3% for the intravenous versus intramuscular route, respectively. The major differences occurred in patients with "mild" or "moderate" toxicity. It is therefore not clear from this study that intravenous bleo-mycin administration definitely increases the risk of developing pulmonary toxicity.

C. Combination Chemotherapy of Non-Hodgkin's Lymphomas

Several combination chemotherapy studies including bleomycin in the treatment of non-Hodgkin's lymphoma have been published. Most studies have included bleo-mycin combined with cyclophosphamide, vincristine, and prednisone and adriamy-cin. Schein *et al.* (1976) reported that significant pulmonary toxicity occurred in patients receiving bleomycin, 15 mg/m^2, twice monthly. Five of the first 16 pa-tients (31%) treated at this dose developed "severe respiratory embarrassment" at relatively low total doses of bleomycin, 45, 45, 160, and 165 u/m^2, respectively. The dose of bleomycin was decreased to 5 mg/m^2 on the same schedule and signifi-cant pulmonary toxicity was not seen in nine subsequent patients. Similarly, Skarin *et al.* (1977) and Coltman *et al.* (1977) have reported that dose reductions of bleo-mycin were necessary in the BACOP and COP-Bleo regimens, respectively. BACOP, as employed by Skarin, included a projected bleomycin dose of 15 u/m^2 2x/week for 12 doses. This was decreased to 4 mg/m^2 on days 1 and 5 of therapy, monthly.

In the COP-Bleo study, severe pulmonary toxicity was noted in 9% of patients treated with 10 u/m^2 daily for 4 days every month. As a result, this bleomycin dose was reduced to 4 u/m^2 on days 1 and 8 of therapy monthly. The regimens noted above all included cyclophosphamide, which has been associated with the sporadic occurrence of pulmonary toxicity. Bonadonna et al. (1977), employing bleomycin combined with adriamycin and prednisone (15 u/m^2, on days 1 and 8, q 3 weeks) reported a 12% incidence of reversible interstitial pneumonitis at a mean total bleomycin dose of 142 u/m^2 (range 60–240 u/m^2).

In summary, there appears to be suggestive evidence that patients with non-Hodgkin's lymphoma on combination chemotherapy display an increased sensitivity to bleomycin. This may be more striking in patients treated with combinations including cyclophosphamide than in those combinations in which cyclophosphamide has not been employed. On the other hand, lymphoma patients have been noted to be particularly prone to the "acute fulminant reaction" to bleomycin described by Blum et al. (1973). It remains to be determined whether these initial reports truly represent an increased sensitivity to bleomycin, and, if so, whether this is a disease-related phenomenon or a result of significant drug interactions.

D. Age

As noted above, bleomycin pulmonary toxicity is more frequent in patients over 70 years of age. Samuels et al. (1976) have recently reported that young patients with testicular carcinoma tolerate high total doses of bleomycin. Ninety patients treated with vinblastine and bleomycin received a median total dose of bleomycin of 600 u, with a range of 120–1212 u; nine patients (10%) developed significant pulmonary toxicity, with four (4.4%) developing fatal bleomycin pulmonary toxicity. The median total dose at which toxicity developed was 530 u (range 120–1100). Einhorn and Donohue (1977) have recently reported data on 50 patients treated with vinblastine, bleomycin, and cis-diamminedichloroplatinum. The median age was 26 years. One of 50 patients (2%) developed lethal pulmonary toxicity. The total dose limit of bleomycin was 360 u. As mentioned previously, the incidence of significant bleomycin pulmonary toxicity occurs more frequently with total bleomycin doses of over 500 u. With lower doses the toxicity occurs at a relatively low rate independent of total dose. The data of Samuels and Einhorn are in keeping with these observations and do not necessarily imply that younger patients, because of an increased ability to inactivate bleomycin, have a decreased incidence of pulmonary toxicity, as proposed (Samuels et al., 1976).

VII. SUMMARY

The major dose-limiting toxicity of bleomycin is pulmonary fibrosis. The exact pathogenesis of pulmonary toxicity and its alteration by various disease and host-related factors are currently poorly understood. Further investigation of structure-toxicity relationships and the basic mechanisms involved in the genesis of the pathologic pulmonary process may lead to the attenuation of this dose-limiting process, either by leading to the development of new analogs or by defining patients particularly susceptible to developing pulmonary toxicity.

REFERENCES

Adamson, I. Y. R. (1976). *Ex. Health Perspect. 16*, 119.

Adamson, I. Y. R., and Bowden, D. H. (1974). *Am. J. Pathol. 77*, 185–197.

Aso, Y., Yoneda, K., and Kikkawa, Y. (1976). *Lab. Invest. 35*, 558.

Bedrossian, C. W. M., Luna, M. A., Mackay, B., and Lightfuiger, B. (1973). *Cancer 32*, 44.

Blum, R. H., Carter, S. K., and Agre, K. (1973). *Cancer 31*, 903.

Bonadonna, G., Monfardini, S., and Villa, E. (1977). *Cancer Treatment Rep. 61*, 117.

Coltman, C. A., Luce, J. K., McKelvey, Z. M., Jones, S. E., and Moon, T. E. (1977). *Cancer Treatment Rep. 61*, 1067.

Comis, R. L., Ginsberg, S. J., Prestayko, A. W., Auchincloss, J. H., and Crooke, S. T. (1977). Proceedings of the 10th International Congress on Chemotherapy, p. 585.

Crooke, S. T., and Bradner, W. T. (1976). *J. Med. 7*, 333.

Daskal, Y., Crooke, S. T., Smetana, K., and Busch, H. (1975). *Cancer Res. 35*, 374.

Daskal, Y., Gyorkey, F., Gyorkey, P., and Busch, H. (1978). *Cancer Res.* (1978).

DeLena, M., Guzzon, A., Monfardini, S., and Bonadonna, G. (1972). *Cancer Chemother. Rep. 56*, 343.

Einhorn, L. H., and Donohue, J. (1977). *Ann. Intern. Med. 87*, 293.

Einhorn, L. H., Krause, M., Hornback, N., and Furnas, B. (1976). *Cancer 37*, 2414.

E.O.R.T.C. (1970). *Br. Med. J. 2*, 643.

Fleishman, R. W., Baker, J. R., Thompson, G. R., *et al.* (1974). *Thorax 26*, 675.

Haas, C. D., Coltman, C. A., Gottlieb, J. A., *et al.* (1976). *Cancer 38*, 8.

Halnan, K. E., Bleehen, N. M., Brewin, T. B., *et al.* (1972). *Br. Med. J. 4*, 635.

Ichikawa, T. (1976). In *Gann Monogr. Cancer Res. 19*, 99.

Ishizuka, M., Takayama, H., Takeuchi, T., and Umezawa, H. (1967). *J. Antibiot. 20*, 15.

Izbicki, R. M., and Baker, L. H. (1977). *Proc. Am. Soc. Clin. Oncol. 18*, 345.

Muller, W. E. G., and Zahn, R. K. (1976). In *Progress in Biochemical Pharmacology: Biological Basis of Clinical Effect of Bleomycin*, Caputo, A. (Ed.). Karger, Basel, p. 199.

Pascual, R. S., Mosher, M. B., Rajiner, S. S., *et al.* (1975). *Am. Rev. Respir. Dis. 108*, 211.

Perez-Guerra, F., Harkleroad, L. E., Walsh, R. L., Costanzi, J. J. (1973). *Am. Rev. Respir. Dis. 108*, 211.

Rudders, R. A. (1973). *Ann. Intern. Med. 78*, 618.

Samuels, M. L., Johnson, D. E., Holoye, P. Y., and Lanzotti, V. J. (1976). *J. Am. Med. Assoc. 15*, 1117.

Schaeppi, U. H., Fleishman, R. W., Rosenkrantz, H., *et al.* (1972). U.S. Nat. Tech. Inform. Serv. P. B., Rep. No. 207943.

Schein, P. D., DeVita, V. T., Hubbard, S., *et al.* (1976). *Ann Intern. Med. 85*, 417.

Skarin, A., Lokich, J., Goodman, R., *et al.* (1975). *Proc. Am. Soc. Clin. Oncol. 16*(3), 264.

Skarin, A. T., Rosenthal, D. S., Maloney, W. C., and Frei, E, III. (1977). *Blood 49*, 759.

Umezawa, H., Takeuchi, T., Hori, S., *et al.* (1972). *J. Antibiot. 25*, 409.

Valicenti, J. F., Redding, R. A., and Stein, M. (1972). *Physiologist 15*, 292.

Yagoda, A., Mukerji, B., Young, C. *et al.* (1972). *Ann. Intern. Med. 77*, 861.

Chapter 25

DEVELOPMENT OF QUANTIFIABLE PARAMETERS OF BLEOMYCIN TOXICITY IN THE MOUSE LUNG

Branimir Ivan Sikic
Edward G. Mimnaugh
Theodore E. Gram

I. INTRODUCTION

Pulmonary toxicity due to bleomycin has been described in several mammalian species, including the mouse (Adamson and Bowden, 1974; Sikic *et al.*, 1978). A major difficulty in approaching this problem in both animals and man has been the lack of reproducible, sensitive, and quantifiable measures of lung toxicity. We have been interested in deriving such parameters in a mouse model, utilizing both biochemical and histopathologic methods.

II. HYDROXYPROLINE LEVELS

NIH/Swiss mice were treated with three doses of bleomycin, subcutaneously, twice weekly, for up to 6 weeks. The highest dose, 40 mg/kg, produced 100% lethality before the end of the treatment period. The intermediate dose, 20 mg/kg, produced 35% mortality; and the low dose, 1 mg/kg, resulted in no deaths. The two higher-dose groups also developed progressive losses of body weight and increases in wet weight of the lungs. A parallel control group was treated with 0.9% NaCl.

Hydroxyproline content of the whole right lungs was measured as an index of collagen (Crystal, 1974). Significant increases of 130–150% were observed in whole-lung collagen content 6 and 8 weeks after initiation of treatment with 20 mg/kg of

TABLE I. Whole-Lung Hydroxyproline Content after Initiation of
Treatment wth Various Doses of Bleomycin

	Weeks			
	2	4	6	8
Controls [a]	106 ± 14 [b]	97 ± 14	109 ± 16	123 ± 9
1 mg/kg bleomycin	110 ± 9	88 ± 7	103 ± 10	118 ± 11
20 mg/kg bleomycin	117 ± 18	113 ± 16	157 ± 33 [c]	156 ± 33[c]

[a] Animals were injected twice weekly, subcutaneously, for up to 6 weeks. Controls received 0.9% NaCl.

[b] Data expressed as micrograms of hydroxyproline per whole right lung. Mean ± SD, N = 6.

[c] Significantly different from controls ($p < 0.05$)

bleomycin (Table I). All animals in the 40 mg/kg group had died 3 to 5 weeks after initiation of treatment, and did not demonstrate increases in hydroxyproline content.

III. MORPHOMETRY

The left lung of each animal was perfused *in situ* with a modified Karnovsky's fixative at 30 cm fluid pressure, and serially sectioned for light microscopic measurements. We considered it desirable to be able to correlate biochemical with histopathologic measurements in each animal, and applied morphometric analysis to statistically compare indices of histopathologic damage between treatment groups (Weibel, 1963). Thus, one might systematically examine effects of other drugs, putative antidotes, new analogs, or changes in schedule of administration of bleomycin on the development of chronic pulmonary toxicity. The following features were selected for morphometric analysis: number of intraalveolar macrophages and leukocytes per square millimeter of lung area, total pulmonary cell count per square millimeter, mean alveolar wall thickness, and percent consolidation of lung parenchyma. These methods have been described in detail (Sikic *et al.*, 1978).

TABLE II. Number of Intraalveolar Macrophages and Leukocytes per Square
Millimeter of Lung Area at Various Times after Initiation of Treatment with Bleomycin

	Weeks			
	2	4	6	8
Controls [a]	232 ± 72 [b]	240 ± 97	295 ± 83	300 ± 91
1 mg/kg bleomycin	280 ± 98	295 ± 95	315 ± 95	262 ± 126
20 mg/kg bleomycin	268 ± 83	360 ± 77 [c]	567 ± 267 [c]	630 ± 533
40 mg/kg bleomycin	352 ± 209	800 ± 577 [c]	—	—

[a] Animals were injected subcutaneously twice-weekly for up to 6 weeks. Controls received 0.9% NaCl.

[b] Mean ± SD, N = 6.

[c] Significantly different from controls ($p < 0.05$).

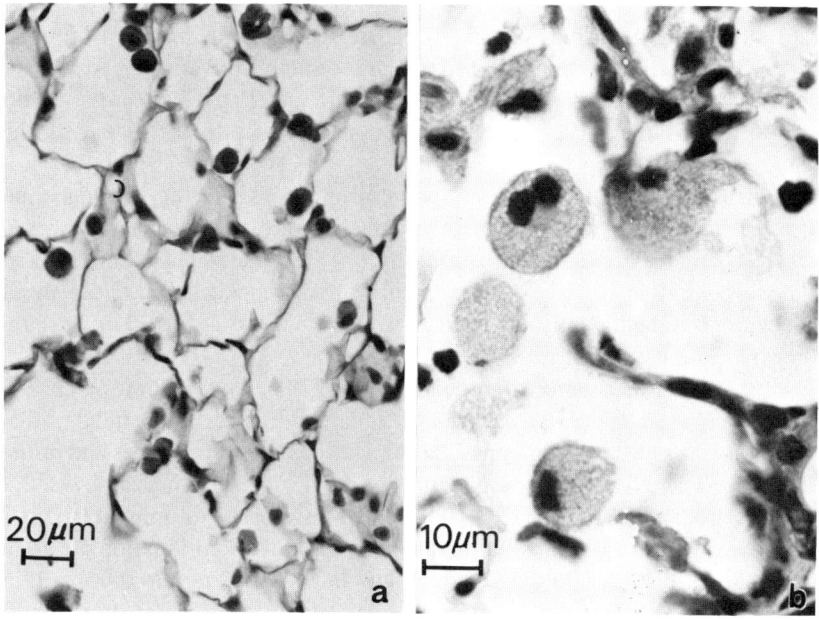

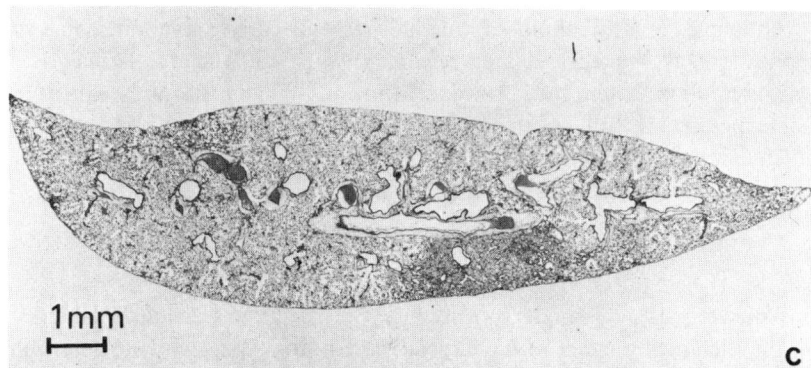

Fig. 1. (a) Increase in number of intraalveolar macrophages 6 weeks after initiation of treatment with bleomycin, 20 mg/kg SC twice weekly. H and E stain, x 350; (b) large, foamy intraalveolar macrophages from an animal receiving 20 mg/kg of bleomycin twice weekly for 6 weeks. H and E stain, x 880; (c) cross section of the left anterior lobe of a mouse treated with 40 mg/kg bleomycin twice weekly for 4 weeks, showing 9% consolidation as measured by projection on a point-counting grid. H and E stain, x 8.

Significant increases in the number of intraalveolar macrophages and leukocytes per square millimeter of lung area were observed on light microscopy by 4 weeks in the 20 and 40 mg/kg groups (Table II). These macrophages were not only more numerous, but also frequently contained the large amounts of vesicular, foamy cytoplasm associated with active phagocytosis (Figs. 1a and 1b). This increase in intraalveolar cells was the most sensitive morphometric indicator of bleomycin lung toxicity.

An increase in total pulmonary cell count also occurred in the two higher-dose groups, but to a lesser degree than the number of intraalveolar macrophages and leukocytes. Total cell count was significantly ($p < 0.05$) elevated to 134% of controls at 8 weeks after initiation of treatment in the 20 mg/kg group. Mean alveolar wall thickness was significantly increased to 1.9 μ at 8 weeks in the 20 mg/kg group, as compared to 1.1 μ in controls.

Finally, we measured percent consolidation, defined as area of lung parenchyma in which alveolar air space was replaced by cellular infiltrate, fluid exudate, and/or connective tissue (Fig. 1c). No consolidation was observed in controls and in the 1 mg/kg group. There was 36% consolidation in the 40 mg/kg groups at 4 weeks, by which time the animals appeared moribund and histological examination revealed large amounts of intraalveolar fluid and cellular exudate. Consolidation did not appear until week 6 in the 20 mg/kg group, and included numerous fibroblasts and collagen bundles demonstrated by Masson's and van Gieson's stains. In this group there was 25% consolidation at 6 weeks and 37% consolidation at 8 weeks.

The lowest dose of bleomycin, 1 mg/kg twice weekly for 6 weeks, produced no pulmonary toxicity as measured by hydroxyproline levels and the four morphometric indices.

Although these morphometric methods are currently too cumbersome for such applications as large-scale analog screening, when combined with analysis of lung hydroxyproline content they provide sensitive and reliable measurements of bleomycin pulmonary toxicity. Use of computerized image analyzers may facilitate handling of larger numbers of samples for other experiments or for screening purposes.

IV. FURTHER STUDIES

We have applied this model to a study of the effects of schedule of administration on the therapeutic index of bleomycin. Mice bearing subcutaneous Lewis lung carcinoma were treated with 10 mg/kg of bleomycin twice weekly, resulting in a 20% increase in life-span (ILS), not significantly different from controls. An equivalent total weekly dose given in smaller increments, 2 mg/kg 10 times weekly, produced a significant 34% ILS. Both schedules of administration produced moderate pulmonary toxicity. Thus, more frequent administration of smaller doses led to an increase in the therapeutic index of bleomycin. It has been suggested that the pulmonary toxicity is related to low levels of bleomycin hydrolase in lung (Umezawa, 1977). If so, it may be possible to select doses or schedules of administration of bleomycin which avoid a threshold of pulmonary toxicity but are still therapeutically effective.

Continuous infusion of the drug, as already used in some patients, may be a means of achieving this lowered toxicity. We are currently testing this hypothesis by treating mice bearing Lewis lung carcinoma with continuous bleomycin infusion via sub-cutaneously-implanted osmotic pumps, and comparing them to twice-weekly or 10-times weekly "bolus" injections of equivalent total doses of drug.

REFERENCES

Adamson, I. Y. R., and Bowden, D. H. (1974). *Am. J. Pathol.* 77, 185.
Crystal, R. G. (1974). *Fed. Pro. 33,* 2248.
Sikic, B. I., Young, D. M., Mimnaugh, E. G., and Gram, T. E. (1978). *Cancer Res. 38,* 787.
Umezawa, H. (1977). *Lloydia. 40,* 67.
Weibel, E. R. (1963). *Morphometry of the Human Lung.* Academic Press, New York.

Chapter 26

THE SEARCH FOR NEW BLEOMYCINS

Akira Matsuda
Osamu Yoshioka
Kazuo Ebihara
Hisao Ekimoto
Takumi Yamashita
Hamao Umezawa

I. INTRODUCTION

In the last 10 years great progress has been made in basic and clinical studies on bleomycin (BLM) (Umezawa, 1976; Ichikawa, 1976). Professor Umezawa (1967), in his early study on BLM, has suggested that results on the distribution of anti-tumor substances among various organs should be useful in estimating the sensitive tumor and toxic target organ. This principle has been extensively supported by the selective effect of BLM on squamous cell carcinoma and characteristic toxic effects in animals and patients.

If we could find a compound which has the same or a stronger antitumor activity and lower pulmonary toxicity compared with the present BLM, it might allow physicians to safely increase the total doses in cancer treatment.

In this paper we present data on antitumor activity and organ distribution, with special focus on pulmonary toxicity of the new BLMs.

II. EFFECT OF THE NEW BLEOMYCINS
ON TRANSPLANTED TUMORS

As previously reported (Matsuda *et al.*, 1977), the first step in the selection of new BLMs was to test for anti-HeLa cell activity. About 150 new BLMs were thus selected. In the second step, BLMs selected by anti-HeLa cell activity were tested on Ehrlich ascites carcinoma and the therapeutic indices were tested by inoculation as follows. Mice of ICR/JCL (male, 5 weeks old, five in each group) were inoculated with 2×10^6 Ehrlich ascites cells per mouse. BLM ranging from 25 to 0.19 mg/kg was administered intraperitoneally once a day for 10 days starting from 2 hours after the inoculation. Deaths were observed every day up to 50 days after the inoculation and body weight was measured every 5 days. LD_{50} was calculated by the Behrens–Kärber method from the group intoxicated at high dose levels. The survival percentage at each dose level was obtained assuming the average number of survival days observed with the control group administered with physiological saline solution of 100%, and doses producing survival for periods such as 200% of that of the control or longer were regarded as effective. The maximum dose level at which the mice survived for a period such as 100–200% of the survival period for the controls was signified by ED_{50}.

In general, the higher the therapeutic indices (LD_{50}/ED_{50}), the less toxic and the more effective is the tested sample.

In the third step, 100 new BLMs which had shown therapeutic indices not less than 16 were further tested on Ehrlich solid carcinoma. Mice of ICR/JCL (male, 5 weeks old, five per group) were inoculated in the axillary region with 2×10^6 Ehrlich ascites carcinoma cells per mouse. BLM ranging from 8.1 to 0.03 mg/kg was administered intraperitoneally once a day for 10 days starting from 24 hours after the inoculation. Animals were sacrificed on the 15th day after inoculation. The weight of tumor in the test animals was compared with that of control animals. Results were expressed as percentage of control growth, and ID_{50} (mg/kg) was calculated. Those BLMs for which ID_{50} was smaller than 1 mg/kg were selected.

III. DISTRIBUTION OF THE NEW BLEOMYCINS
IN VARIOUS ORGANS OF MICE

In the fourth step, the organ distribution in brain, lung, stomach, liver, spleen, kidney, skin, and tumor (Ehrlich solid) 1 hour after subcutaneous injection of 100 mg/kg of 75 new BLMs selected as above was tested by the microbiological method. A summary of results on interesting BLMs is shown in Tables I and II. Some of the BLMs, such as BLM-BAPP, BLM-PEP, BLM-A5196, and BLM-M5196, showed higher ID_{50} for HeLa cells compared with the present BLM. In the case of ID_{50} for Ehrlich solid carcinoma, BLM-DMPP, BLM-PEP, BLM-A5033, and BLM-M5196 were superior to the present BLM. BLM-PEP, BLM-A5196, adn BLM-M5196 were highly distributed in skin, lung, and stomach compared with the present BLM.

TABLE I. Biological Properties of New Bleomycins (Antitumor Activity)

	Code No.	Cu	$\dfrac{M.607}{B.\text{Sub}}$ (u/mg)	HeLa ID_{50} (μg/ml)	Ehrlich Ascites Index $\dfrac{LD_{50}}{ED_{50}}$ (mg/kg)	Ehrlich solid ID_{50} (mg/kg)
	BLM	–	$\dfrac{1234}{886}$	3.2	$\dfrac{13.1}{0.19}=68.9$	0.49
	BAPP	–	$\dfrac{8470}{19180}$	1.2	$\dfrac{8.44}{0.39}=21.6$	0.72
P	DMPP	–	$\dfrac{1670}{9600}$	3.6	$\dfrac{10.3}{0.19}=54.3$	0.045
	PEP	–	$\dfrac{7847}{1476}$	0.82	$\dfrac{9.38}{0.39}=24.1$	0.35
	A5033	–	$\dfrac{122}{52}$	8.0	$\dfrac{>25.0}{3.12}=>8.0$	0.38
D	A5196	–	$\dfrac{17588}{14367}$	1.6	$\dfrac{9.40}{0.19}=49.5$	0.74
	M5196	–	$\dfrac{19639}{12735}$	0.95	$\dfrac{6.1}{0.19}=32.1$	0.41
S	E4065	+	$\dfrac{1335}{1150}$	9.2	$\dfrac{>25.0}{3.12}=>8.0$	0.4

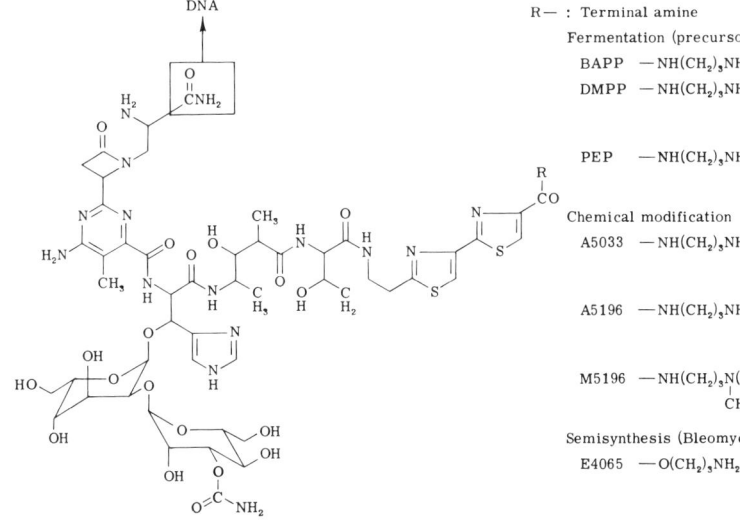

R— : Terminal amine

Fermentation (precursor)

BAPP —$NH(CH_2)_3NH(CH_2)_3NH(CH_2)_3CH_3$

DMPP —$NH(CH_2)_3NH(CH_2)_3N(CH_3)_2$

PEP —$NH(CH_2)_3NHCH$—⬡
$\qquad\qquad\qquad |$
$\qquad\qquad\quad CH_3$

Chemical modification

A5033 —$NH(CH_2)_3NH(CH_2)_4NHCO(CH_2)_2COOH$

A5196 —$NH(CH_2)_3NH(CH_2)_4NH\overset{NH}{\overset{\|}{C}}CH_2$—⬡—Cl

M5196 —$NH(CH_2)_3\underset{CH_3}{\overset{\;}{N}}(CH_2)_3NH\overset{NH}{\overset{\|}{C}}CH_2$—⬡—Cl

Semisynthesis (Bleomycinic acid : R = —OH)

E4065 —$O(CH_2)_3NH_2$

TABLE II. Biological Properties of New Bleomycins (Organ Distribution)

	Code No.	Cu	Serum	Lung	Skin	Liver	Kidney	Spleen	Stomach	Brain	Solid
							Distribution (100 mg/kg S.C., 1 hr)				
	BLM	−	38.0	9.7	18.5	0	23.3	0	2.6	0	12.9
P	BAPP	−	33	0.5	13.7	0	>100	0	0.32	0	3.1
	DMPP	−	19	0.35	0	0	0.3	0	0	0	
	PEP	−	83	14.1	26.6	1.2	57	0	7.5	2.8	22.1
D	A5033	−	25	0	18.5	0	7.2	0	0	0	0
	A5196	−	93.3	15.3	25.5	4.2	61.3	0.9	13.2	1.0	18.9
	M5196	−	85	23.5	21.0	3.4	122	2.4	4.1	1.7	21.8
S	E4065	+	4.2	0.6	4.2	0	67.3	0	0	0	0

IV. EFFECT OF THE NEW BLEOMYCINS ON
CHEMICALLY INDUCED CARCINOMA

Among BLMs, BLM-BAPP, BLM-PEP, and BLM-A5196 exhibited the same activity as the present BLM in squamous cell carcinoma of mice. Female dd/Y-S 10-week-old mice were used. Each group consisted of 12 mice. The hair in the application area was cut and saturated 20-methylcholanthrene (20-MC) solution in acetone was applied twice a week for 18 weeks. The doses of BLM were 62.5 and 250 μg/ mouse and were injected intraperitoneally twice a week for 15 weeks after the start of the first painting of 20-MC. Evaluation of the results was performed 1 week after the last injection of compound. The cancerous lesion was examined histologically for the presence of squamous cell carcinoma in each specimen. For a dose of 62.5 μg/mouse the results of cancerization for the various BLMs were as follows: BLM-BAPP–50%, BLM-PEP–45.8%, BLM-A5196–54.5%, and present BLM–50%. These compounds also exhibited inhibition against gastric adenocarcinoma of rats induced with N-methyl-N'-nitrosoguanidine (MNNG) (Matsuda *et al.*, 1977).

The experimental schedule is shown in Fig. 1. In the 18-19 weeks after cessation of administration of MNNG all rats were operated on and their stomachs examined for number, size, and localization of tumor. After the surgical observation, all rats were divided equally for tumor appearance in each group.

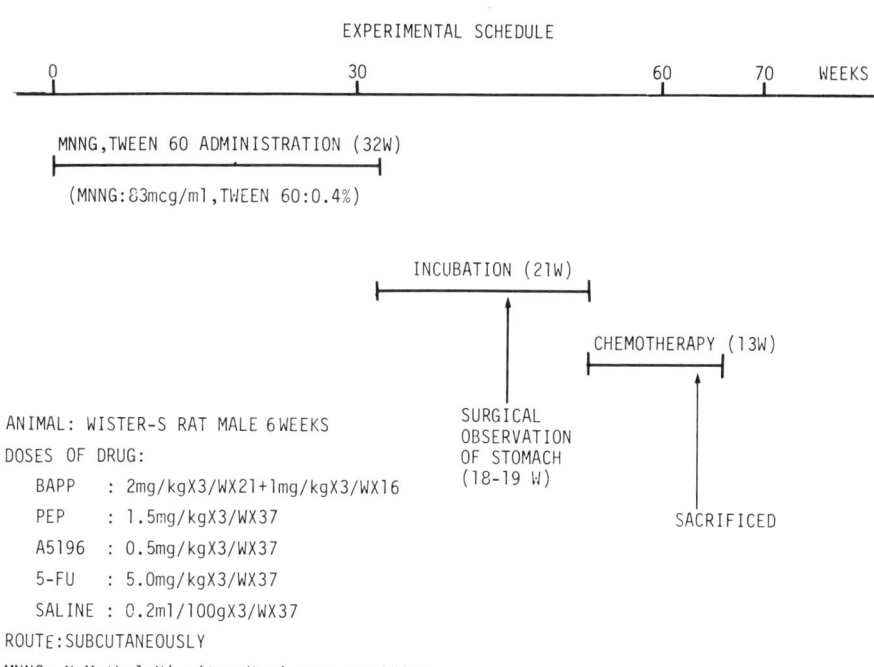

Fig. 1. Effect of bleomycins and 5-FU on chemically induced gastric cancer of rats.

The test compounds were given three time a week to a total of 37 times. The doses of each compound are shown in Fig. 1. 5-fluorouracil (5-FU) was used as a positive control drug. At the end of treatment, all rats in each group were sacrificed and their stomachs examined by macroscopic and microscopic methods. The number of rats with a persistant tumor and the number of rats with the appearance of tumor at the end of treatment are shown in Table III. The tumor persistence ratio in the BLM-BAPP and BLM-PEP groups were significantly lower than that of the control and 5-FU groups. This macroscopic observation has been confirmed by histopathological observation.

V. EXAMINATION OF PULMONARY TOXICITY OF THE NEW BLEOMYCINS

It is well known that BLM exhibits a significant therapeutic effect against squamous cell carcinoma, Hodgkin's disease, etc. The other characteristics of this antibiotic are its lack of bone-marrow depression and its adverse effect on skin and lungs. It seems that the effect on lungs limits the safe maximum administration of this antibiotic. If pulmonary toxicity, which is the most pronounced side effect, could be induced in experimental animals, this model system would be useful in the screening of new BLMs with lower toxicity and the development of a method for preventing this kind of toxicity. We therefore endeavored to establish a pulmonary toxicity test method using small experimental animals.

Umezawa (1974) had previously reported that the ability of the lung and the skin to inactivate BLMs was much weaker in old (28 weeks) than in young (3 weeks) mice. Based on these results, after the completion of various examinations on selection of suitable age of mice, doses of BLM, and time-course observation, we succeeded in the development of a test method for pulmonary toxicity.

Male ICR-SLC mice 15 weeks old (S.P.F.) were used. The test was carried out in a conventional animal room. Each group consisted of 10-20 mice which were injected with 5mg/kg of test BLM intraperitoneally, daily for 10 days. The control group received physiological saline solution injections. In order to examine the development of pulmonary fibrosis all surviving mice were sacrificed 5 weeks after the last injection. The lungs were fixed with neutral formalin solution and histological specimens were prepared. Sections were stained with hematoxylin and Eosin and Mallory trichrome. Usually the whole left lung, and the superior and inferior lobes of the right lung were examined by light microscopy. Mice that had infectious bronchitis and bronchopneumonia were excluded from the test.

The examination focused on the presence of fibrosis, although interstitial pneumonitis and pleural inflammations were also examined. In addition, the degree of congestion and interstitial and intraalveolar edema, the number of alveolar macrophage, and morphological changes in bronchial and alveolar epithelial cells and in blood vessel walls were examined.

The degrees of pulmonary fibrosis were divided into five classes rated as follows:

-     (0) indicating the absence of fibrosis
±   (1) the presence of areas with questionable fibrosis in alveolar septae
+   (2) a few foci of fibrosis, often in subpleural area
++   (4) scattered foci of fibrosis
+++   (6) diffuse fibrosis

The data were expressed as follows:

$$\text{Incidence } (\%) = \frac{\text{Number of mice with fibrosis in group}}{\text{Number of mice tested in group}} \times 100$$

$$\text{Grade (mean score)} = \frac{\text{Total score of specimens in group}}{\text{Number of specimens in group}}$$

For the evaluation of pulmonary toxicity of the new BLMs, the present BLM was taken as the control and the data were expressed as the relative toxicity value compared to BLM. A dose-response relationship as shown in Fig. 2 was observed in the dose range from 2.5 to 10 mg/kg of the present BLM.

The experimental results on the new BLMs are shown in Fig. 3. The compounds are different in degree of pulmonary toxicity. Among various BLMs, in terms of Index on Grade, BLM-M5196 was the lowest (0.05, 1/20 of present BLM) and BLM-HPE was the highest (3.68, 3.7 times the present BLM). As shown in Table I, BLM-M5196 which contained [(N-3-aminopropyl)-3-methylaminopropy]-p-chlorbenzyl-amidine in the terminal amine had the lowest index of pulmonary toxicity but a strong renal toxicity.

BLM which contains an amidine group in terminal amine has been found to have a strong renal toxicity in the same way as the guanidine group.

The index of BLM-A5033 which contained 1-N-succinyl-3-N-aminopropyl-diamino propane was 0.21. It showed a much weaker activity in Ehrlich ascites carcinoma, although it showed a similar activity against Ehrlich solid carcinoma and chemically induced squamous cell carcinoma as compared with the present BLM. Based on these results, Homma and his colleagues (1976) tested BLM-A5033 for pulmonary toxicity in 17 cases of cancer patients using various pulmonary function tests such as determination of DLco, DLco/Va, VC, and PaO_2. All patients except three who had had lung operations had no abnormality in the pulmonary function tests before the treatment with BLM-A5033. 10-20 mg/man, 2-3 times/week of BLM-A5033 in 13 cases, and 10-15 mg/man, 2-3 times/week of the present BLM in four cases were administered, respectively. Total doses varied from 60 to 300 mg/man. The test results indicate that BLM-A5033 showed less pulmonary toxicity than the present BLM, as shown in Table IV.

The index of pulmonary toxicity of BLM-PEP which contained 3-[(s)-1-phenyl-ethylamino] -propylamine was 0.25. In the phase I study of BLM-PEP on 32 cancer patients, abnormal shadows were found radiographically in two cases, so medication was discontinued, though the change was very slight.

We are proceeding to the phase II clinical study with some expectation of decrease of pulmonary toxicity as seen with BLM-A5033.

TABLE III. Effect of Bleomycins and 5-FU on Chemically Induced Gastric Cancer of Rats

Drug	Number of rats	Number of survivors[a]	Survivors — Number of rats with persistent tumors[o,c]	Survivors — Number of rats with appearance of tumors[d]	Dead — Number of rats with persistent tumors	Dead — Number of rats with appearance of tumors[d]	His. finding. AD.C + S.AD.C No. of rats[e]
BAPP	30	15/30 (50)	2/9 (22) ▲▲	1/6 (17) ▲ ■	5/11 (45)	0/4 (0)	6/24 (25)
PEP	29	25/29 (86)	5/16 (31) ▲▲■■	0/9 (0) ■	0/3 (0)	0/1 (0)	8/27 (30)
A5196	29	26/29 (90)	11/19 (58) ▲▲	4/7 (57)	1/1 (100)	0/2 (0)	10/28 (36)
5-FU	29	26/29 (90)	14/16 (88)	5/10 (50)	0/2 (0)	0/1 (0)	14/27 (52)
Saline	30	27/29 (90)	17/17 (100)	5/10 (50)	2/2 (100)	1/1 (100)	22/28 (79)

[a] Percentages in parentheses in all columns.
[b] Significantly different from control: ▲ $-p<0.05$; ▲▲ $-p<0.01$. Significantly different from 5-FU: ■ $-p<0.05$; ■■ $-p<0.01$.
[c] Rats which had tumors before treatment.
[d] Rats which had no tumors before treatment.
[e] AD.C = adenocarcinoma; S.AD.C = suspicious adenocarcinoma.

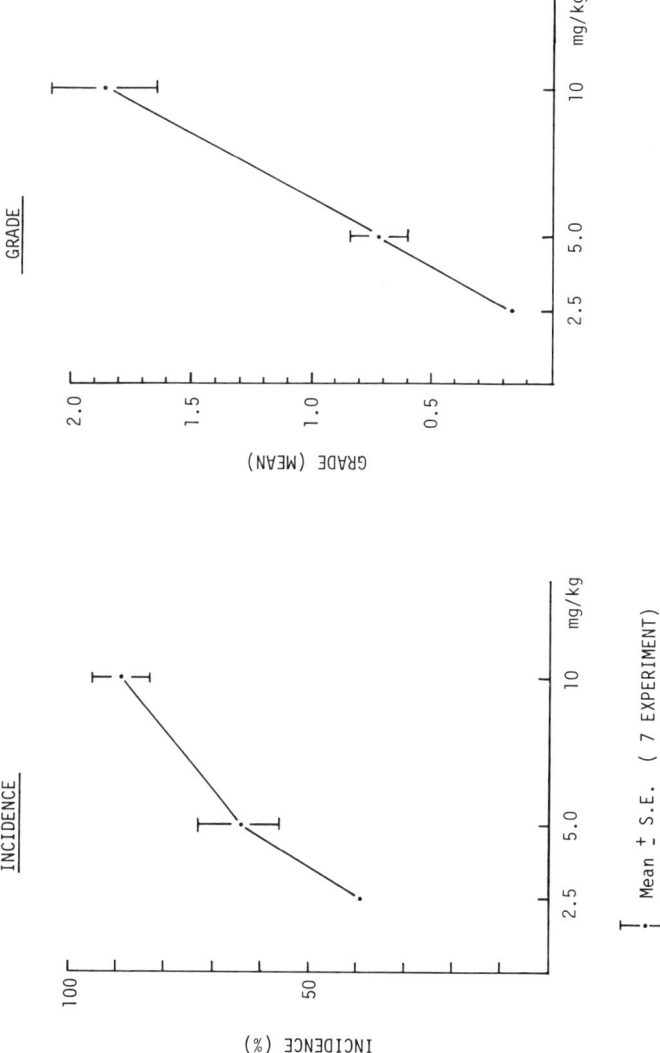

Fig. 2. Bleomycin: dose-response curve of lung fibrosis in mice.

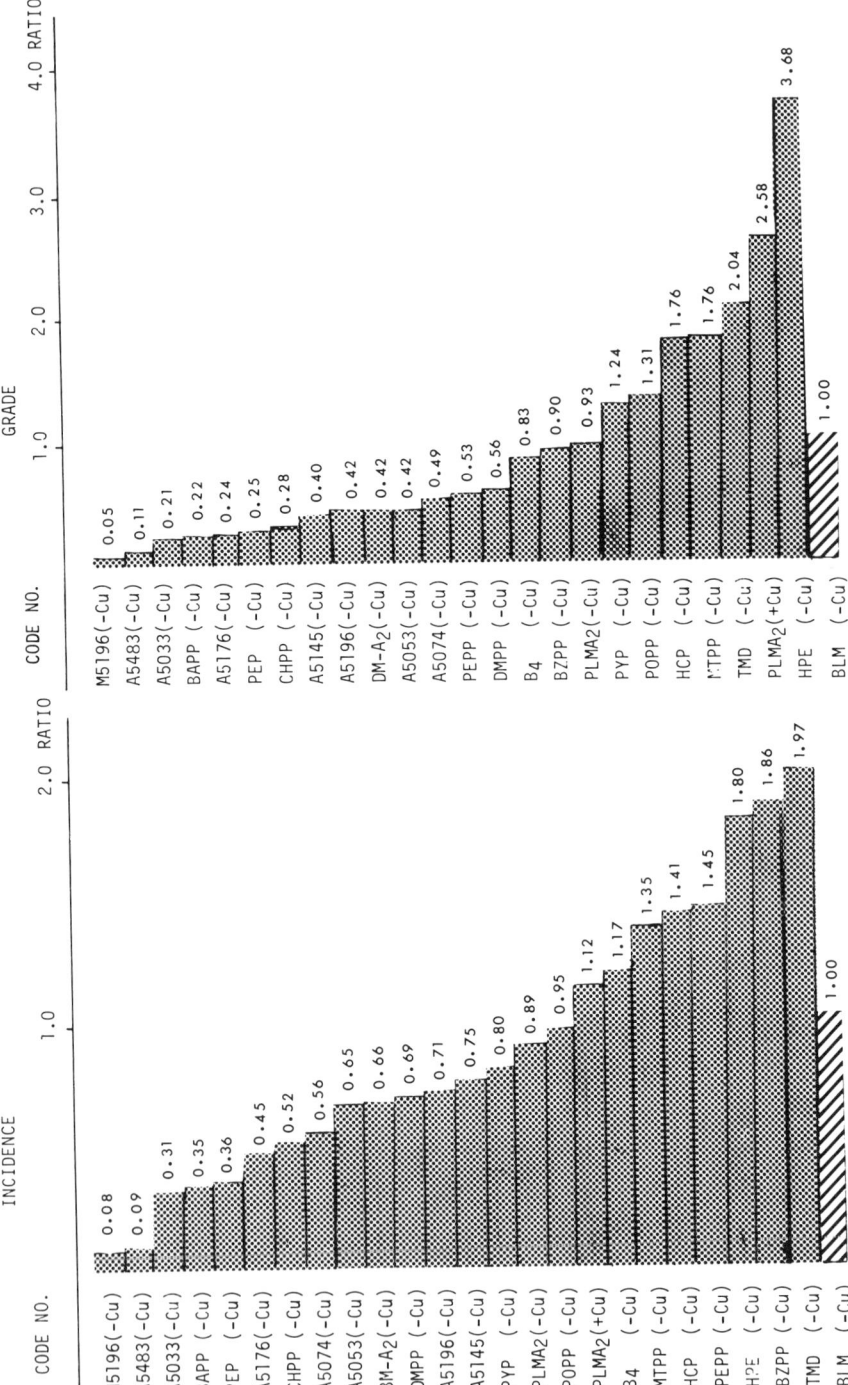

Fig. 3. Magnitude of pulmonary fibrosis of new bleomycins (compared with bleomycin–5 mg/kg).

TABLE IV. Comparison of Pulmonary Toxicity of BLM-A5033 and Present BLM
in Cancer Patients[a]

Pulmonary toxicity [b]	A 5033	BLM	
A	4 (30.8%)	1 (25%)	
B	8 (61.5%)	0	
C	1 (7.7%)	3 (75%)	
Total	13	4	17

[a] From Homma et al. (1976).
[b] A: No abnormal changes in subjective and objective symptoms, chest radiography, and pulmonary function tests; B: impairment in pulmonary function tests only; C: abnormal change in all test items.

The fact that there are encouraging coincidences between experimental and clinical results on the pulmonary toxicity of BLM-A5033 suggests that this model system in small experimental animals may be useful for the prediction of this type of toxicity in the BLMs in clinical use.

VI. CONCLUSION

The antitumor activities and pulmonary toxicity of new BLMs were reported. BLM-BAPP, BLM-PEP, BLM, BLM-DMPP, BLM-A5196, and BLM-M5196 showed higher antitumor activity in transplanted tumor systems than the present BLM. BLM-BAPP, BLM-PEP, and BLM-A5196 showed effects similar to those of the present BLM on chemically induced squamous cell carcinoma, and furthermore, marked effects were exhibited on chemically induced gastric carcinoma, which has been shown to be insensitive to the present BLM.

For the study of pulmonary fibrosis of new BLMs, a model system using small experimental animals was established, and was used to test the degree of pulmonary fibrosis of the new BLMs.

BLM-M5196, BLM-A5033, BLM-PEP, and BLM-BAPP showed lower pulmonary toxicity than the present BLM. BLM-A5196 showed the lowest pulmonary toxicity, while it showed a strong renal toxicity.

The results on BLM-A5033 in the model system were confirmed by various pulmonary function tests in cancer patients. Most of the patients treated with BLM-A5033 showed abnormality in one of the pulmonary function tests. However, the incidence of advanced pulmonary fibrosis decreased markedly.

It may be suggested that data on the new BLMs which were obtained in the model system may be useful for prediction of clinical utility in addition to antitumor activity and general toxicity.

From the results as described in this paper, BLM-PEP was selected for clinical trial because of the following results: (1) higher antitumor activity; (2) lower pulmonary toxicity, (3) stronger effect on chemically induced squamous cell carcinoma and gastric carcinoma. The details of preclinical properties of this compound will be in a future paper.

Further studies of new analogs and/or derivatives that change not only the terminal amine moiety but also the mother molecule will yield more useful cancer chemotherapeutic agents in the near future.

ACKNOWLEDGMENT

We are pleased to acknowledge the considerable assistance of Miss Y. Ichoda and S. Aoyagi.

REFERENCES

Homma, H., *et al*. (1976). *J. Thorac. Dis. 14*, 14 (Extra No.) (in Japanese).
Ichikawa, T. (1976). *Gann Monogr. Cancer Res. 19*, 99–45.
Matsuda, A., *et al*. (1977). *Recent Results Cancer Res. 63*.
Umezawa, H. (1967). *Gann Monogr. Cancer Res. 2*, 197–203.
Umezawa, H. (1974). *J. Antibiot. 25*, 409–420.
Umezawa, H. (1976). *Gann Monogr. Cancer Res. 19*, 3–36.

Chapter 27

PRECLINICAL STUDIES ON
BLEOMYCIN-PEP (NK-631)

Akira Matsuda
Osamu Yoshioka
Katsutoshi Takahashi
Takumi Yamashita
Kazuo Ebihara
Hisao Ekimoto
Fuminori Abe
Yoshimasa Hashimoto
Hamao Umezawa

I. INTRODUCTION

As already reported in our previous paper, (this volume) BLM-PEP was selected for further preclinical tests based on the screening results in antitumor activity, organ distribution, and pulmonary toxicity. In this paper, we will report on the outline of preclinical characteristics of BLM-PEP compared with the present BLM.

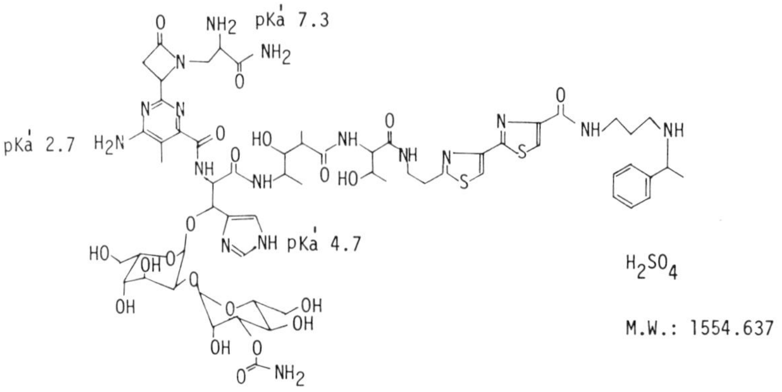

3-[(s)-1'-phenylethylamino]-propylaminobleomycin sulfate

Fig. 1. Chemical Structure of BLM-PEP.

II. CHEMICAL STRUCTURE

The chemical structure of BLM-PEP is shown in Fig. 1. The drug is prepared by precursor-fed fermentation. The terminal amine moiety of BLM-PEP is 3-[(s)-1'-phenylethylamino] -propylamine.

III. ANTIMICROBIAL ACTIVITY

The antimicrobial activity examined by the agar-medium dilution method of BLM-PEP is shown in Table I. *Bacillus subtilis* was the most sensitive test organism as with the present BLM. Antimicrobial activity of BLM-PEP was about twice as great as that of the present BLM in various species of bacteria. The biopotency against *Mycobacterium* 607 and *Bacillus subtilis* was 7847 u/mg and 1476 u/mg, respectively, compared with BLM-A$_2$ as the standard substance (1000 u/mg).

IV. ANTITUMOR ACTIVITY

A. Action on HeLa S$_3$ Cells in Culture

The anti-HeLa-cell activity of BLM-PEP compared with the present BLM is shown in Table II. The activity of BLM-PEP was about twice as great as that of the present BLM.

TABLE I. Antimicrobial Activity

	M.I.C. (μg/ml)	
Test organisms	BLM-PEP	BLM
Gram positive		
Staphylococcus aureus	25.0	50.0
S. aureus 209P	25.0	50.0
S. epidermidis	25.0	50.0
Sarcina lutea PCI 1001	25.0	100.0
Bacillus subtillis PCI 219	0.1	0.39
B. anthracis	6.25	3.13
Gram negative		
Escherchia coli NIHJ	0.39	0.78
E. coli K12W3630S	50.0	100.0
Shigella flexneri EW8	3.13	0.78
Shi. sonnei	3.13	3.13
Salmonella typhimurium H901	0.39	0.78
S. typhimurium LT22	0.78	3.13
Klebsiella SP	6.25	12.5
Proteus mirabilis	>100.0	>100.0
Enterobactor aerogenes	6.25	6.25
Pseudomonas aeruginosa	>100.0	>100.0

	BLM-PEP	BLM	BLM-A$_2$
M.607 (μ/mg)	7847	1234	1000
B. Sub (μ/mg)	1476	886	1000

TABLE II. Antitumor Activity: HeLa S$_3$ Cell

	ID$_{50}$ (μg/ml)
BLM-PEP	0.82
BLM	1.70

$$\text{Inhibition } \% = 100 - \frac{A-C}{B-C} \times 100 \;^a$$

^{a} A: cell number 72 hours after treatment with drug;
B: cell number 72 hours after treatment without drug;
C: cell number at drug addition time.

TABLE III.   Ehrlich Solid Carcinoma in Mice [a]

Dose (mg/kg x 10)	BLM-PEP		BLM	
	Tumor weight (mg)	Inhibition (%)	Tumor weight (mg)	Inhibition (%)
2.7	310 ± 70 [a]	84	790 ± 170	67
0.9	640 ± 130	68	1090 ± 170	55
0.3	1220 ± 130	39	1230 ± 260	49
0.1	1510 ± 290	24	1840 ± 310	24
0.03	1620 ± 110	19	1920 ± 260	21
0	1990 ± 210	0	2420 ± 120	0
ID_{50}	0.35		0.49	

[a] Mean ± SE.

B. Action on Ehrlich Solid Carcinoma in Mice

ID_{50} of BLM-PEP compared with the present BLM is shown in Table III. The activity of BLM-PEP was slightly stronger than that of the present BLM.

C. Action on Ehrlich Ascites Carcinoma in Mice

The chemotherapeutic index of BLM-PEP compared with the present BLM is shown in Table IV. The activity of BLM-PEP was different from the case of solid form, that is, about half as great as that of the present BLM.

TABLE IV.   Ehrlich Ascites Carcinoma in Mice.

Dose (mg/kg x 10)	Mean survival days: ratio (%)	
	BLM-PEP	BLM
25.0	50 (−)	89 (−)
12.5	96 (−)	125 (±)
6.25	286 (+)	312 (++)
3.12	299 (+)	336 (++)
1.56	231 (+)	333 (+)
0.78	216 (+)	243 (+)
0.39	175 (±)	271 (+)
0.19	134 (±)	112 (±)
0	100 (−)	100 (−)
Index $= \dfrac{LD_{50}}{ED_{50}}$	$24.1 = \dfrac{9.38}{0.39}$	$44.2 = \dfrac{8.4}{0.19}$

TABLE V. AH66-Ascites Hepatoma in Rats

Dose	Mean survival days: ratio	
(mg/kg x 10)	BLM-PEP	BLM
3.12	296	241
1.56	269	257
0.78	216	145
0.39	163	116
0.19	116	110
0	100	100

D. Action on AH66-Ascites Hepatoma in Rats

Donryu rats (male 7 weeks old, five in each group) were inoculated with 1×10^6 AH66 cells. BLM ranging from 3.12–0.19 mg/kg was administered intraperitoneally once a day for 10 days starting from 24 hours after the inoculation. Survival was observed every day up to the 30th day after inoculation. The longevity percentage at each dose level was obtained on the base of the average number of survival days observed with the control group administered saline solution. The ratio of mean survival days of BLM-PEP compared with the present BLM is shown in Table V. The activity of BLM-PEP was slightly greater than that of the present BLM.

E. Action on 20-Methylcholanthrene-Induced Squamous Cell Carcinoma in Mice

Inhibition percent of BLM-PEP compared with the present BLM is shown in Table VI. The activity of BLM-PEP was similar to that of the present BLM.

F. Action on N-Methyl-N-Nitro-N'-Nitrosoguanidine-Induced Gastric Carcinoma in Rats

After the surgical observation of the stomachs of rats treated with MNNG, all rats were divided equally on the basis of tumor appearance in each group. Each

TABLE VI. 20-Methylcholanthrene-Induced Squamous Cell Carcinoma in Mice.

	Dose (μg/mouse)	Mortality	Cancerization (ratio, %)	Inhibition (%)
BLM-PEP	62.5	1/12	5/11 (45.4)	47.8
Bleomycin	62.5	2/12	5/10 (50.0)	42.5
Control	0	1/24	20/23 (86.9)	0

TABLE VII. MNNG-Induced Gastric Cancer in Rats (1)[a]

			Survivor		Dead	
Drug	Number of rats	Number of survivors	Number of rats with persistent tumors[b]	Number of rats with appearance of tumors[c]	Number of rats with persistent tumors[b]	Number of rats with appearance of tumors[c]
BLM-PEP	29	25/29 (86)	5/16 (31) ▲▲■■[d]	0/9 (0) ▲■[d]	0/3 (0)	0/1 (0)
5-FU	29	26/29 (90)	14/16 (99)	5/10 (50)	0/2 (0)	0/1 (0)
Saline	30	27/30 (90)	17/17 (100)	5/10 (50)	2/2 (100)	1/1 (100)

[a] MNNG: N-Methyl-N'-nitro-N-nitrosoguanidine.
[b] Rats which had tumors before treatment.
[c] Rats which had no tumors before treatment.
[d] Significantly different from control: $p < 0.05$– ▲; $p < 0.01$– ▲▲ ;Significantly different from 5-FU: $p < 0.05$– ■; $p < 0.01$– ■■ .

TABLE VIII. MNNG-Induced Gastric Cancer in Rats (2)

Drug	Total number of rats	Chemotherapy	Number of rats with tumors Macro	His[a]	Total number of tumors Macro	His[a]	Total tumor size (mm²) Macro	His[a]	Mean tumor size (mm²)[b] Macro	His[a]
BLM-PEP	29	Before	19	5	24	5	316 } −201[c,d]		13±5.2	
		After	5	5	5	5	115 }	111	23±10.8	22.2±11.1
5-FU	29	Before	18	16	24	22	365 } +628		15± 4.0	
		After	19		35		993 }	821	28± 6.0	37.3±8.8
Saline	30	Before	19	22	30	30	328 } +1547		11± 3.5	
		After	25		40		1870 }	1733	46±11.7	57.8±14.9

[a] Malignant and suspected malignant tumors which were confirmed by histological analysis were counted.
[b] Mean ± SE.
[c] Significantly different from control ($p < 0.01$).
[d] Significantly different from 5-FU ($p < 0.05$).

TABLE IX. MNNG-Induced Gastric Cancer in Rats (3)

Histological observation of stomach	BLM-PEP	5-FU	Saline
Number of rats examined	27	27	28
Group[a] V. Adenocarcinoma	7 (26%)	14 (52%)	19 (68%)
IV. Lesion suspected of adenocarcinoma	1 (4)	0 (0)	3 (11)
III. Lesion between benign and malignant	3 (11)	3 (11)	0 (0)
II. Benign lesion with slight atypism	4 (15)	4 (15)	1 (4)
Sarcoma	0 (0)	0 (0)	1 (4)
Gastritis	12 (44)	5 (19)	4 (14)
Normal	0 (0)	1 (4)	0 (0)

[a] From "The General Rules for Gastric Cancer Study in Surgery and Pathology," Part III, 1974 (9th ed.), Japanese Research Society for Gastric Cancer.

group consisted of 20 rats with tumor and 10 rats without tumor macroscopically. The test compounds were given three times a week to a total of 37 times. The dose of each compound was as follows: 1.5 mg/kg for BLM-PEP and 5.0 mg/kg for 5-fluorouracil (5-FU) as positive control drug. After the end of treatment all rats in each group were sacrificed and their stomachs examined by macroscopic and microscopic observation. A summary of the number of rats with a persistent tumor and the number of rats with the appearance of tumor at the end of treatment is shown in Table VII. The tumor persistence ratio in each group was as follows: BLM-PEP: 5/16 (31%), 5-FU: 14/16 (88%), and saline 17/17 (100%). The tumor appearance ratio in each group was as follows: BLM-PEP: 0/9 (0%), 5-FU: 5/10 (50%), and saline: 5/10 (50%).

The tumor persistence and appearance ratios of BLM-PEP were significantly lower than those of the saline. A summary of number and size of tumors before and after treatment is shown in Table VIII. The total number of tumors in the BLM-PEP group decreased from 24 to 5, but in the 5-FU and saline groups the total increased from 24 to 35 and from 30 to 40 respectively. Conforming with these results, the total size of tumors decreased in the BLM-PEP group, but increased in 5-FU and saline groups. The effectiveness of BLM-PEP treatment in tumor size was also confirmed statistically.

The summary of histopathological findings is shown in Table IX. The stomachs of all rats which survived at the end of treatment or which died were examined histologically, but two in each of the groups of BLM-PEP, 5-FU, and saline which underwent strong autolysis were not examined.[1] The criteria of diagnosis were based on "The General Rules for Gastric Cancer Study in Surgery and Pathology, Part III" 1974, Japanese Research Society for Gastric Cancer.

[1] This examination was done by Prof. M. Enomoto, Department of Pathology, School of Medicine, St. Marianna University.

TABLE X. Dog and Human Gastric Cancer Heterotransplanted in Nude Mice

	mg/kg/day x 10	Tumor growth (mm^2) [a]	
		Dog	Human (G/W)
Control	0	2.21 (1.00) [b]	2.36 (1.00)
BLM	3	1.64 (0.74)	1.56 (0.66)
BLM-PEP	3	1.58 (0.71)	1.54 (0.65)
5-FU	15	1.95 (0.88)	2.06 (0.87)

[a] Mean of 4 mice/group.
[b] ( ): Ratio to control.

For the evaluation of the chemotherapeutic effects of the drugs, special attention has been given to the change of incidence of adenocarcinoma and suspicious
adenocarcinoma. Rats which had adenocarcinoma together with suspicious adenocarcinoma were counted as those bearing adenocarcinoma, and those which had
malignant and less malignant changes together were counted as bearers of malignant
ones.

The incidence of adenocarcinoma in each group was as follows: BLM-PEP: 30%,
5-FU: 52%, and saline: 79%.

Conforming to the decrease of adenocarcinoma and suspicious adenocarcinoma
in groups, the incidence of gastritis, which is an evidence of tumor healing, was
increased as follows: BLM-PEP: 44%, 5-FU: 19%, and saline: 14%. Thus, the effectiveness of treatment with BLM-PEP shown macroscopically was confirmed by
histopathological examination.

G. Action on Dog and Human Gastric Cancer
Heterotransplanted in Nude Mice

A solid tumor block of about 1 x 2 x 2 mm^3 was excised and implanted subcutaneously to the bilateral axillary regions of nude mice. Following inoculation,
tumors were measured in two dimensions with a slide caliper. The treatment with
drugs was started when tumor grafts had been accepted and measured about 30
mm^2. The drug was injected intraperitoneally daily for 10 days. One day after the
last treatment animals were sacrificed and tumors were weighed.

The summary of results on BLM-PEP, the present BLM, and 5-FU is shown in
Table X and Fig. 2. The growth inhibition ratio at the end of treatment and the
growth curves of tumor in the BLM-PEP and present BLM groups showed a clear
regression, whereas in 5-FU it showed only slight retardation in both dog and
human gastric cancer transplanted in nude mice. The cause of this unexpected
effectiveness of the present BLM against human gastric cancer may be preferential
distribution of the present BLM in the skin of nude mice.

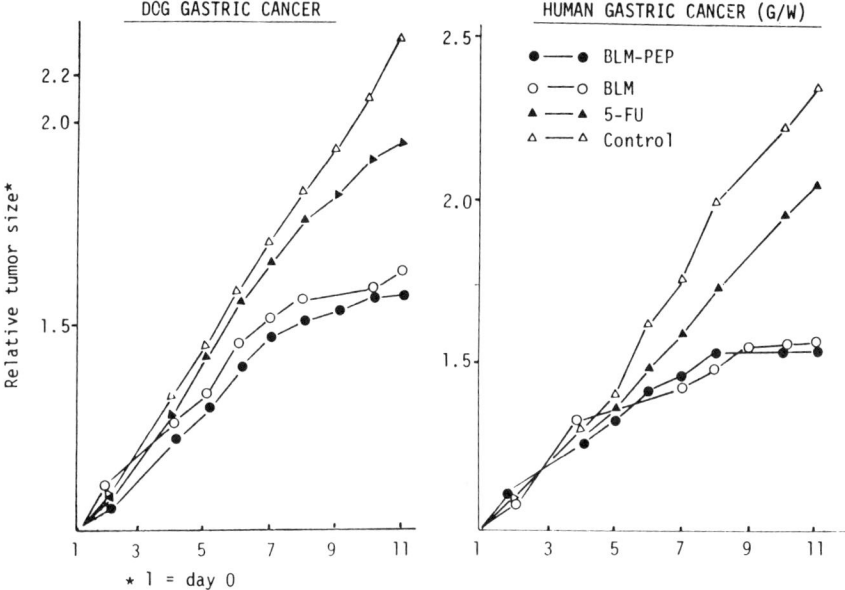

Fig. 2. Dog and Human Gastric Cancer Heterotransplanted in Nude Mice.

H.   Action on Spontaneously Grown
Sticker Sarcoma in Dogs

A mongrel (about 4–5 years old) with Sticker Sarcoma grown in the vaginal mucous membrane was treated with 0.6 mg/kg of BLM-PEP, twice a week intravenously to a total of 23 times. The dimensions of the sarcoma decreased from 3.8 x 2.5 cm^2 to 2.0 x 0.4 cm^2 after 17 treatments. Results are shown in Table XI.

V.   ORGAN DISTRIBUTION

One hour after intraperitoneal injection of 100 mg/kg of drug the concentration of drugs in each organ was determined by a microbiological method. The results on BLM-PEP compared with the present BLM are shown in Table XII. BLM-PEP was distributed in higher concentration than the present BLM in all of the tested organs except spleen.

TABLE XI.   Spontaneously Grown Sticker Sarcoma in Dog

Mongrel (about 4–5 years old)
Diagnosis: Sticker sarcoma in vagina
Treatment: BLM-PEP 0.6 mg/kg, 2 times/week, 23 times.
Reduction of tumor size: Before–3.8 x 2.5 cm; After–2.0 x 0.4 cm.

TABLE XII. Organ Distribution in Mice [a]

	Organ Distribution [b] ($\mu g/ml$ or $\mu g/g$)							
	Serum	Lung	Skin	Liver	Spleen	Stomach	Brain	Solid
BLM-PEP	83.0	14.1	26.6	1.2	0	7.5	2.8	22.1
BLM	38.0	9.7	18.5	0	0	2.6	0	12.9

[a] ICR male, 7 weeks old; dose: 100 mg/kg; route: subcutaneously.
[b] One hour after injection.

TABLE XIII. Acute Toxicity: LD_{50} (mg/kg) in Mice [a] and Rats [b] (Intraperitoneal Route)

	BLM-PEP	BLM
Mice, male	81.5 (102.1–65.0) [c]	256.9 (322.3–204.7)
Rats, male	155.0 (179.8–133.6)	168.0 (217.0–130.0)

[a] Mice: ddN, 6 weeks old.
[b] Rats: Donryu, 10 weeks old.
[c] 95% confidence limit.

TABLE XIV. Acute Toxicity in Dog [a]

	Body Weight (kg)	G.P.T.	G.O.T.	Al-p.	U-N	Clinical symptoms
Before treatment	11.5	19	20	5	17	
After treatment						
3 days	10.8 (6% ↓)	34 ↑	23	11 ↑	10	Appetite loss
7 days	10.0 (13% ↓)	122 ↑	39 ↓	14 ↑	20	
9 days	9.5 (17% ↓)	186 ↑	60 ↓	14 →	27 ↑	Slimy feces
12 days	9.0 (22% ↓)	185 →	50 ↓	22 ↑	40 ↑	Muco bloody feces (slight)
15 days	8.4 (27% ↓)	154 ↓	46 →	24 →	42 →	
34 days	7.5 (35% ↓)	120 ↓	38 ↓	19 ↓	25 ↓	
51 days	8.0 (30.4% ↓)	69 ↓	42 →	12 ↓	25 →	
108 days	9.7 (16% ↓)	34 ↓	24 ↓	7 ↓	25 →	

[a] Beagle, male, 12 months old, 11.5 kg; dosage: 50 mg/kg; route: IV; total dose: 575 mg.

TABLE XV. Pulmonary Toxicity in Mice [a]

	No. of animals	Body weight change (g)		Lung–body weight ratio (mean±SE)	Incidence of fibrosis	Incidence ratio to BLM	Total score No. of spec.	Grade ratio to BLM
		After drug treatment	After 5 weeks					
BLM-PEP [b]	12	-3.6	-1.4	0.50±0.02	4/12	0.36	6/36=0.167	0.25
BLM [b]	12	-6.6	-1.7	0.53±0.02	11/12	1.0	24/36=0.667	1.0
Control	6	+0.9	+3.6	0.46±0.02	0/6		0/18=0	

[a] ICR-SLC mice, 15 weeks old, S.P.F.
[b] Dose: 5 mg/kg.

VI. ACUTE TOXICITY

A. LD$_{50}$ in Mice and Rats

The LD$_{50}$ of BLM-PEP compared with the present BLM when given intra-peritoneally in mice and rats is shown in Table XIII. The LD$_{50}$ of BLM-PEP in male mice was 1/3 that of the present BLM, but in male rats was not different from that of the present BLM.

B. Acute Toxicity in Dogs

A beagle dog (male, 12 months old, 11.5 kg) was injected intravenously with BLM-PEP in a large dose (50 mg/kg). Summarized results on the acute toxicity of BLM in the dog are shown in Table XIV. On the third day after injection the dog showed a slight elevation of SGPT and alkaline phosphatase, accompanied by a loss of appetite and body weight; SGOT and BUN remained normal. On the seventh day, SGPT, SGOT, and alkaline phosphatase were elevated. Blood urea remained normal. After the ninth day, in addition to the other parameters, BUN elevated slightly and progressed until the 15th day with slimy and/or mucobloody feces. But these values gradually returned to normal by the 51st day. Finally, all toxic symptoms except body weight loss recovered by the 108th day.

VII. PULMONARY TOXICITY IN MICE

A test was carried out using the same method described in our previous paper. Pulmonary toxicity of BLM-PEP compared with the present BLM is shown in Table XV. The incidence and grade of pulmonary fibrosis of BLM-PEP were 0.36 and 0.25, respectively. The magnitude of pulmonary fibrosis of BLM-PEP was 1/2-1/4 that of the present BLM in this system.

VIII. MAXIMAL TOXICITY IN DOGS TREATED INTRAVENOUSLY EVERY FOURTH DAY

Studies were performed on 10 conditioned pure-bred beagle dogs 13-15 months old weighing 8-11 kg, obtained from Research Laboratories for Applied Toxicology, Nippon Kayaku Co. Ltd. The dogs were individually housed in cages with water available *ad libitum*. The dogs were fed once per day with dog pellets (CD-1, Nippon Clea Co.). Two dogs per group were injected intravenously with BLM-PEP and the present BLM in doses of 5.0 and 2.5 mg/kg body weight every fourth day for 11 treatments.

Two dogs served as controls and were injected with saline solution. Doses were adjusted weekly according to the weight of the animals. During the course of treatment physical examinations were performed daily, while body weight and urine

TABLE XVI. Summary of the BLM-PEP and BLM Experimental Protocol and Maximum Drug-Induced Toxicity [a]

	Drug									
	BLM-PEP				BLM				Saline	
Dog	77-1	77-2	77-5	77-6	77-7	77-8	77-9	77-10	77-3	77-4
Sex	♂	♂	♂	♂	♂	♂	♂	♂	♂	♂
Age (months)	14	14	14	15	13	13	13	14	14	15
Dosage (mg/kg)	5.0	5.0	2.5	2.5	5.0	5.0	2.5	2.5	0.0	0.0
Number of treatments	10	8	11	11	11	11	11	11	11	11
Total dose (mg)	458	340	270.8	262.8	478	420.5	237	276.8	0.0	0.0
Body weight										
Initial	10.0	10.5	10.6	9.3	10.6	9.3	8.8	11.7	9.4	10.0
Final	7.4	6.3	7.8	8.5	7.1	5.6	7.9	8.5	9.4	10.2
Necropsy day	37	33	43	48	43	47	48	47	48	49
Condition	Moribund	Died	Fair	Good	Poor	Poor	Good	Fair	Good	Good
Dermal toxicity[b]	++	+	+	±	++	+++	+	+++	–	–
Hepato toxicity										
(GOT)	+	±	–	–	–	–	–	–	–	–
(GPT)	++	++	–	–	–	–	–	–	–	–
(ALP)	+	–	–	–	–	–	–	–	–	–
Renal toxicity										
(BUN)	+	++	–	–	–	–	–	–	–	–
Pulmonary toxicity										
(Macro)	+	+	+	+	+	±	+	±	–	–
(Micro)	+	+	+	+	+	+	±	±	–	–

[a] Legend: (±) slight; (+) moderate; (++) marked; (+++) severe.

[b] Dermal toxicity contains foot pad ulceration and onychoptosis.

TABLE XVII. Summary of Maximum Toxicity for Dogs Treated with BLM-PEP and BLM [a]

	Drug									
	BLM-PEP				BLM				Saline	
Clinical observation										
Dog: number	77-1	77-2	77-5	77-6	77-7	77-8	77-9	77-10	77-3	77-4
Dose	5.0	5.0	2.5	2.5	5.0	5.0	2.5	2.5	0.0	0.0
Total dose (mg)	458	340	270.8	262.8	478	420.5	237	276.5	0.0	0.0
Number of treatments	10	8	11	11	11	11	11	11	11	11
Autopsy day	37	33	43	48	43	47	48	47	48	49
General condition	Moribund	Died	Fair	Good	Poor	Poor	Good	Fair	Good	Good
Weight loss	++	+++	++	±	++	+++	±	+	–	–
Anorexia	++	+++	±	±	++	+++	–	+	–	–
Foot pad ulcers	++	+	+	±	+++	+++	+	++	–	–
Toenail loss	++	++	+	+	++	+++	+	+++	–	–
Ocular discharge	–	+	–	–	–	+	–	–	–	–
Tongue ulceration	++	–	++	+	++	++	++	+++	–	–
Emesis	–	+	–	–	–	–	–	–	–	–
Alopecia	–	–	–	–	+	+	–	+	–	–
Hematology										
Hct		↑↑	↑		↑	←	←			
Hb		↑↑	↑			←	←			
RBC			↑	↑		←	←			
WBC		↑								

324

Chemistry								
Cl	→							
Na	→	→		→			→	→
K	↑↑	↑↑	↓	→	→	→	↑/↓	↑/↓
GPT	↓	↓						
ALP	↓	↑↑	→	→	→			
BUN	↓	↑↑						
Glucose	↓	↓	↑↑		↑	↑	→	↑
Total protein			↓		↑			
Albumin	↑/↓	↑/↓						
GOT	↓	↑↑	↑/↓	↑	↑			
LAP	↓	↑	↑					
Creatine		↑↑		←	←	→	→	←
Cholesterol		↑	←	←	←			
Urine								
Glucose	+++	+++	++	–	–	–	–	–
Protein	+	++	+	–	+	–	–	–
Occult blood	++	–	–	–	–	–	–	–

Legend: ± slight; ↑ moderate; ↑↑ marked; ↑↑↑ severe.

325

samplings were performed weekly. In addition, before and during treatment complete hematological and blood chemical analyses were performed. All dogs except those moribund or dead were necropsied at the termination of treatment. Organs were fixed in 4% neutral buffered formaline solution and stained with hematoxylin and eosin for pathological examination. For the staining of lung, Mallory trichrome stain was used additionally.

Summarized data of the maximal toxicity of BLM-PEP compared with that of the present BLM are shown in Table XVI. In the 5 mg/kg BLM-PEP group, one dog became moribund at the termination of treatment and another died during treatment as follows: dog 77-1 was sacrificed moribund on day 37 of the treatment regime, while dog 77-2 died on day 33. Important clinical signs exhibited by these two dogs included anorexia, weight loss, and various mucocutaneous lesions. Major toxicity was associated with hepatic and renal damage as indicated by elevated SGPT and BUN. The changes in SGPT and BUN caused by BLM-PEP were stronger than for the present BLM. On the other hand, pulmonary toxicity was weaker than for the present BLM, as described later. Other toxicological changes were almost the same as those for the present BLM.

In the 2.5 mg/kg BLM-PEP group general toxicity was moderate, the same as for the present BLM. Summarized data on clinical symptoms, hematology, blood chemistry, and uranalysis are shown in Table XVII.

TABLE XVIII. Subacute Toxicity in Dogs Following Intravenous Administration of BLM-PEP and BLM: Histopathological Grade of Fibrous Change of Lung

Drug	Dose (mg/kg/day)	Dog no.	A/B[a]	Mean of fibrous grade[b]
BLM-PEP	5	1	15/17 = 0.88	0.85
		2	14/17 = 0.82	
	2.5	1	12/17 = 0.71	0.95
		2	20/17 = 1.18	
BLM	5	1	28/17 = 1.65	1.62
		2	27/17 = 1.59	
	2.5	1	24/17 = 1.41	1.30
		2	20/17 = 1.18	
Control	0	1	0/17 = 0	0
		2	1/17 = 0	

[a] $A/B = \dfrac{\text{Total score}}{\text{No. of specimens.}}$

[b] Grade: − (0) Indicating the absence of fibrosis; ± (1) the presence of areas with questionable fibrosis in alveolar septae; + (2) a few foci of fibrosis, often in subpleural area; ++ (4) scattered foci of fibrosis; +++ (6) diffuse fibrosis.

TABLE XIX. Absorption and Excretion [a]

Time after injection (hr)	BLM-PEP (μg/ml)		BLM (μg/ml)	
	Dog No. 1 (8.2 kg)	Dog No. 2 (9.8 kg)	Dog No. 1 (8.8 kg)	Dog No. 2 (8.8 kg)
0.5	18.0	8.2	8.4	11.6
1.0	6.7	3.8	2.9	2.5
2.0	2.2	2.9	1.3	1.1
4.0	1.0	0.5	0.5	0.3
6.0	< 0.2	< 0.2	< 0.1	< 0.1
8.0	Trace	Trace	Trace	Trace
10.0	Trace	Trace	Trace	Trace
Urinary recovery (48 hr)	21.73 mg (72%)	28.44 mg (95%)	26.63 mg (89%)	24.26 mg (81%)

[a] Dog, beagle, male; dose: 30 mg/dog; route: IV.

Summarized data on pulmonary toxicity of BLM-PEP compared with the present BLM are shown in Table XVIII. Pulmonary lesions were found for each drug in all dogs treated with 5.0 mg/kg or 2.5 mg/kg. The test method for pulmonary toxicity was the same as that used for mice. The grade of pulmonary fibrosis of BLM-PEP was about 1/2 that of the present BLM at a dose level of 5 mg/kg. The same trend of a lower pulmonary toxicity both in mice and dogs has been confirmed by the above described experiments. However, the decreasing ratio of pulmonary toxicity in mice was greater than in dogs; this probably resulted from the extended observation periods in mice, as pulmonary toxicity was time-related.

IX. ABSORPTION AND EXCRETION IN DOG

Blood level and urinary recovery of BLM-PEP compared with the present BLM in dogs are shown in Table XIX and Fig. 3. Intravenous administration of 30 mg/kg of BLM-PEP in two beagle dogs resulted in maximum serum concentration of 18.0 μg/ml (No. 1 dog) and 8.2 μg/ml (No. 2 dog) at 30 minutes, and thereafter decreased gradually. Urinary recovery was 72% (No. 1 dog) and 95% (No. 2 dog). Thus blood level and urinary recovery of BLM-PEP were almost the same as with the present BLM.

In one patient intravenous administration of 15 mg of BLM-PEP resulted in the following serum concentrations after injection: 30 min—2.7 μg/ml; 60 min—1.4 μg/ml; 120 min—1.1 μg/ml; and 180 min—1.1 μg/ml.

TABLE XX. Pyrogenicity in Rabbits [a]

Dose (mg/kg)	Drug	No. of febrile responders (> 0.6°C elevation)	
		1–3 hr	4–6 hr
0.3	PEP	0/6	0/6
	BLM	0/6	0/6
0.6	PEP	0/6	1/6
	BLM	0/6	3/6
0.9	PEP	4/6	4/6
	BLM	2/6	4/6

[a] Summary of 2 lots: BLM–U2100AS, U2200AS; PEP–Lot 101, 102.

X. PYROGENICITY IN RABBIT

Febrile response of BLM-PEP compared with the present BLM in rabbits is shown in Table XX. BLM-PEP was as pyrogenic as the present BLM. The pattern of temperature elevation of BLM-PEP was similar to that of the present BLM, but at a dose of 0.6 mg/kg it seems that the incidence of febrile responders may possibly be decreased.

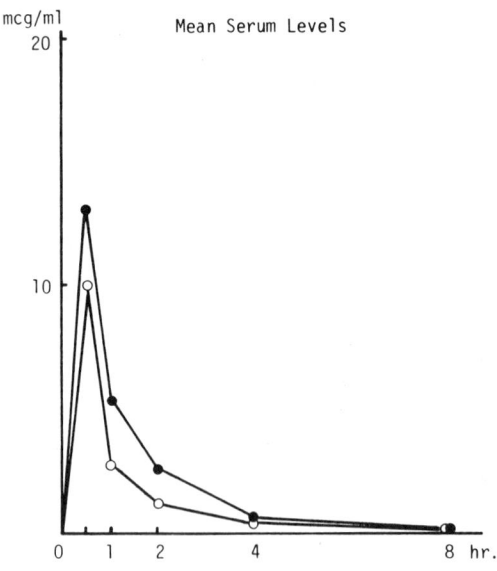

Fig. 3. Absorption and excretion. ●—● BLM-PEP: 25.09 mg (83.5%); ○––○ BLM: 25.45 mg (85.0%).

TABLE XXI. Incidence of Febrile Response in Patients [a]

	BLM-PEP	BLM
Single dose	10 mg [(w)]/man	15–30 mg [(p)]/man
$\frac{\text{Responders}}{\text{Patients}}$ (%)	10/52 (19.2)	459/1031 (44.5)

[a] Arranged by R&D Section, Nippon Kayaku, 3/10/77.

TABLE XXII. Incidence of Pulmonary Toxicity [a] in Patients [b]

	BLM-PEP	BLM
Mean total dose	ca. 150 mg [(w)]	ca. 200 mg [(p)]
$\frac{\text{Responders}}{\text{Patients}}$ (%)	3/52 (5.8)	137/1031 (13.3)

[a] Breathlessness, dyspnea, radiographical abnormality, pulmonary fibrosis, etc.
[b] Arranged by R&D Section, Nippon Kayaku, 3/10/77.

XI. MUTAGENICITY

Mutagenic activity of BLM-PEP in microbiological assay using *Salmonella typhimurium* TA 100 and TA 98 is shown in Fig. 4. These strains are histidine requiring base-pair change mutant (TA 100) and frameshift mutant (TA 98). Assay was carried out by the modified method of Ames described by Yhagi (1975). In both conditions, S-9 mixture added or not added, mutagenicity of BLM-PEP was negative.

XII. INCIDENCE OF FEBRILE RESPONSE AND PULMONARY TOXICITY IN PATIENTS (PRELIMINARY SURVEY)

Recent data on febrile response and pulmonary toxicity of BLM-PEP in patients compared with the literature on the present BLM are shown in Table XXI and XXII. It seems that the incidences of febrile response and pulmonary toxicity in the BLM-PEP group are smaller than for the present BLM. Further long-term studies on efficacy and adverse effect in patients are in progress as phase II and III studies in about 40 hospitals in the field of head and neck, larynx, skin, lung, malignant lymphoma, and others.

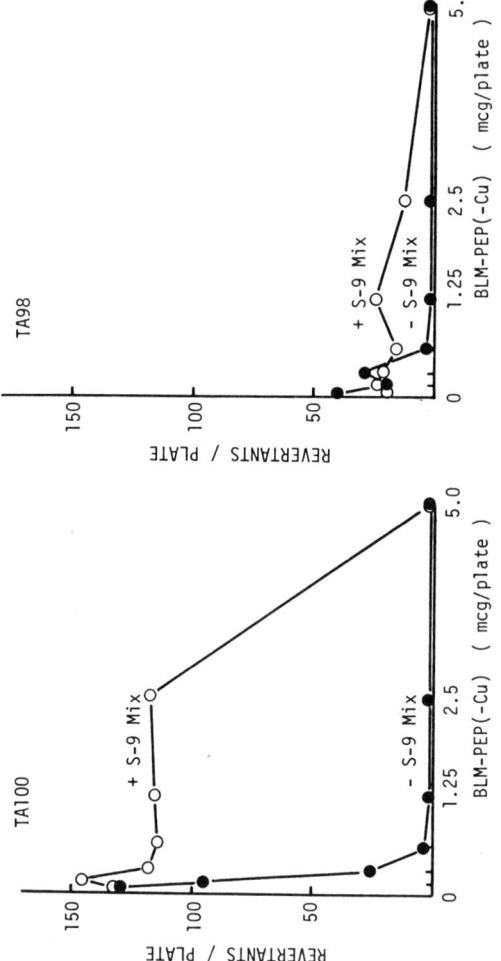

Fig. 4. Mutagenicity

XIII. SUMMARY

In summary, preclinical characteristics of BLM-PEP compared with the present BLM were as follows:

1. The antitumor effect of BLM-PEP was stronger than that of the present BLM in the following systems:
    a. HeLa S_3 cell
    b. Ehrlich carcinoma (solid) in mice
    c. AH66 ascites hepatoma in rats
    d. MNNG-induced gastric carcinoma in rats

2. The antitumor effect of BLM-PEP was the same as that of the present BLM in the following systems:
    a. Ehrlich carcinoma (ascites) in mice
    b. 20-Methylcholanthrene-induced squamous cell carcinoma in mice
    c. Dog and human gastric carcinoma heterotransplanted in nude mice
    d. Spontaneously grown Sticker Sarcoma of the dog

3. Pulmonary toxicity of BLM-PEP was lower than that of the present BLM as follows: mice: $1/2$-$1/4$; dogs: $1/2$.

4. LD_{50} of BLM-PEP in mice was smaller than that of the present BLM, but was similar in rats.

5. Systemic toxicity of BLM-PEP in dogs was slightly stronger than that of the present BLM; type of toxicity was reversible.

6. Organ distribution of BLM-PEP in mice was about 2-3 times higher than that of the present BLM.

7. Absorption and urinary recovery of BLM-PEP in dogs was the same as for the present BLM.

8. Pyrogenicity of BLM-PEP in rabbits was almost the same as that of present BLM.

9. Mutagenicity of BLM-PEP in microbiological tests was negative, as for the present BLM.

10. The trend of lower febrile and pulmonary toxic response of BLM-PEP which was observed in experimental animals was almost confirmed in phase I and II clinical studies.

ACKNOWLEDGMENT

We are pleased to acknowledge the considerable assistance of Mr. H. Inoue, Mrs. N. Amano, S. Yamaguchi, Miss Y. Ichoda, and S. Aoyagi.

REFERENCE

Yahagi, T. (1975). *Nucleic Acids and Enzymes 20*, 1178–1189 (in Japanese).

Chapter 28

BU-2231, A THIRD-GENERATION BLEOMYCIN: PRECLINICAL STUDIES

William T. Bradner

I. INTRODUCTION

BU-2231 is a complex of new glycopeptide antibiotics given the name tallysomycin. It was isolated and identified in the antibiotic screening program at the Bristol Banyu Research Institute, Ltd., Tokyo (Kawaguchi *et al.*, 1977). *In vitro* tests established that the BU-2231 complex was more active against bacteria and fungi than bleomycin and also had more potent lysogenic induction activity for *Escherichia coli* (lambda) phage. The complex was tested at Bristol-Syracuse (Bradner *et al.*, 1977) for effects on Walker 256 carcinosarcoma in ascitic form and found to have substantial activity with a minimum effective dose about one-quarter of that of bleomycin (Table I). Researchers in our Japanese laboratories proceeded with separation of the components and determination of structure. Individually isolated components were then tested for biological effects both *in vitro* and *in vivo*.

II. CHEMISTRY

The structures of BU-2231A and B are shown in Fig. 1. The nucleus of BU-2231 differs from bleomycin in two of the amino acids found on hydrolysis and in the unique amino sugar 4-amino-4. 6-dideoxy-L-talose. BU-2231A and B both have the spermidine side chain associated with bleomycin A_5 (Fujii *et al.*, 1973). However,

Copyright © 1978 by Academic Press, Inc.
All rights of reproduction in any form reserved.
ISBN 0-12-161550-2

TABLE I. Antitumor Activity of BU-2231, Walker 256 Carcinosarcoma, Ascitic form [a]

Material	Dose (μg/kg/day)	MST (days)[b]	Effect, MST T/C[c]	Survivors Day 5	Survivors (Day 44)
BU-2231	2560	26.0	289	6/6	
(crude)	640	>44.0	> 489	6/6	(5)
	160	>44.0	> 489	6/6	(4)
	40	9.0	100	6/6	(1)
	10	8.5	94	6/6	(1)
Bleomycin	2560	>44.0	> 489	6/6	(4)
	640	17.5	194	6/6	(1)
	160	10.0	111	6/6	
Control	Saline	9.0	–	10/10	

[a] Host: SDD rats; treatment: once daily, 8x, IP.
[b] Evaluation: MST = median survival time.
[c] Effect: T/C = MST treated/MST control x100. Criteria: T/C $\geq$ 125 considered significant antitumor effect.

TABLE II. Antimicrobial Activity of BU-2231A and B [a]

Organism	MIC (μg/ml) BU-2231A	BU-2231B	Bleomycin
Staphylococcus aureus 209B	0.05	0.2	6.3
Bacillus subtilis PCI 129	<0.003	0.006	0.4
Escherichia coli NIHJ	0.013	0.025	0.2
Pseudomonas aeruginosa D15	1.6	3.1	> 50
Proteus vulgaris A9436	0.4	0.2	12.5
Mycobacterium 607	0.2	0.2	1.6
Candida albicans IAM4888	12.5	6.3	> 100
Cryptococcus neoformans D49	0.8	0.4	3.1
Aspergillus niger vartieghem	1.6	3.1	> 100
Blastomyces dermatidis IFO 8144	6.3	3.1	6.3
Trichophyton mentagrophytes D155	12.5	3.1	> 100

[a] Kawaguchi et al., 1977).

TABLE III. Antitumor Activity against P-388 Leukemia (Results Shown in T/C%) [a]

Material	Test	Dose in mg/kg (IP), QD 1 →9 10	3	1	0.3	0.1	0.03
BU-2231A	No. 8	Tox	162	150	150	–	–
Bleomycin		148	148	125	119		
BU-2231A	No. 9	–	–	153	147	135	129
Bleomycin		–	–	141	141	112	
BU-2231A	No. 11	–	–	169	131	131	100
Bleomycin		–	131	131	106		

[a] Criteria: T/C $\geq$ 125 considered significant antitumor effect. Value underlined. Data from Bristol Banyu Research Institute.

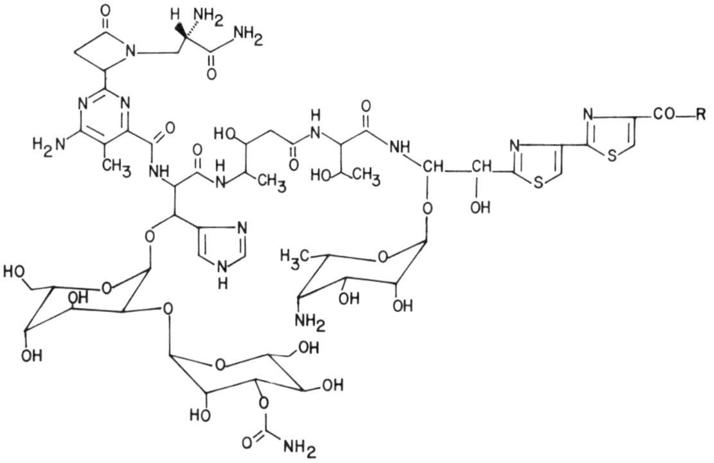

Bu 2231A: R=NHCH$_2$CH$_2$CH$_2$CHCH$_2$CONH(CH$_2$)$_3$NH(CH$_2$)$_4$NH$_2$
                                                NH$_2$

Bu 2231B: R=NH(CH$_2$)$_3$NH(CH$_2$)$_4$NH$_2$

Fig. 1.   Structural formula of BU-2231A (tallysomycin) and BU-2231B.

BU-2231A also contains a β-lysine molecule inserted between the spermidine and the nucleus. The structures of the new amino acids are shown in Fig. 2 along with their bleomycin equivalents using the original bleomycin numbering system (Takita et al., 1968, 1972). Number III is 4-amino-3-hydroxy-n-valeric acid and lacks the methyl group found in bleomycin amino acid III. The bisthiazole amino acid of BU-2231 (No. VI) contains two hydroxyls not present in the bleomycin counterpart. Natural tallysomycin products are isolated as copper chelates; however, the biological studies reported were performed using material from which most of the copper had been removed.

III. BIOLOGICAL EFFECTS, *IN VITRO*

The antimicrobial activity of BU-2231A and B is compared with that of bleomycin in Table II. In most cases, the tallysomycin products are more potent than bleomycin, ranging up to 100-fold with the gram negative bacteria shown. In tests for the induction of lysogenic phage production by *Escherichia coli* W-1709 (lambda)

TABLE IV. Toxicity, Activity, and Therapeutic Index

| | Toxicity (LD_{50} IP) | | P-388 Activity (ED_{125} IP), | Therapeutic index, |
	Single dose (mg/kg)	QD 1→9 (mg/kg/day)	QD 1→9 (mg/kg/day)	QD 1→9, LD_{50}/ED_{125}
BU-2231A	12.5	3.8	0.08	48
Bleomycin	70	15	0.92	16
Ratios:				
BLM/BU-2231A	5.6x	3.9x	11.5x	3

TABLE V. Effect of BU-2231A and Bleomycin in SC Implanted B16 Melanoma [a,b]

Material	Dose (mg/kg/day)	MST (days)	Effect MST T/C%	Survivors, day 50
BU-2231A	6	16.5	Tox [c]	0/10
	3.6	31.5	128	0/10
	2.2	42	170	0/10
	1.3	34.8	141	0/10
	0.8	36.8	149	0/10
Bleomycin	32	14.5	Tox	0/10
	16	45	183	0/10
	8	44.7	181	0/10
	4	38.3	155	0/10
	2	36	146	0/10
Control	–	24.7	–	0/40

[a] Data from Arthur D. Little, Inc.

[b] Treatment: QD 1→9, IP.

[c] Tox: Toxicity, T/C < 85.

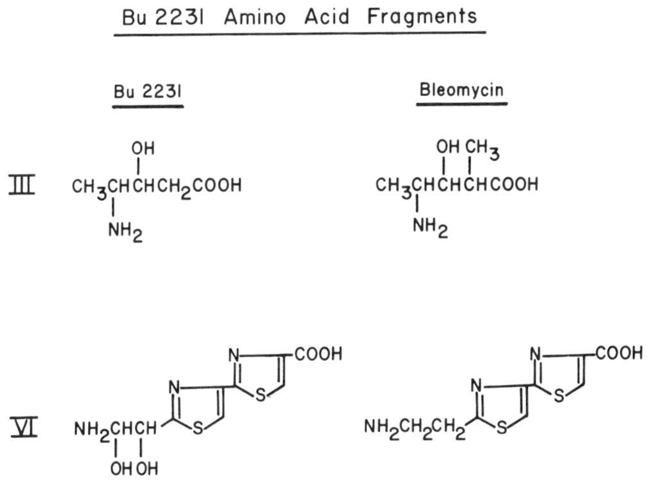

Fig. 2. Amino acid fragments of BU-2231 and bleomycin which are different.

BU-2231 A and B had minimum inducing activities of 0.0025 and 0.02 μg/ml, respectively, compared to 0.08 μg/ml for bleomycin.

IV. BIOLOGICAL EFFECTS, *IN VIVO*

In multiple tests of BU-2231A and bleomycin against P-388 lymphatic leukemia in mice, BU-2231A was consistently more potent (Table III). Table IV shows a comparison of acute and subacute (short-term chronic) toxicity in normal mice for the two drugs along with average therapeutic parameters for tests on P-388 leukemia. Based on the ratio of the subacute LD_{50} to the minimum effective dose for treatment of P-388, a therapeutic index can be generated. Although BU-2231A is 3.9 times more toxic than bleomycin, it is 11.5 times more active, thus representing approximately a threefold gain in therapeutic index.

BU-2231A and bleomycin were compared in tests on B16 melanoma implanted subcutaneously in mice (Table V). Although BU-2231A was the more potent drug, bleomycin developed somewhat better survival indices (T/C). In a test against Lewis lung carcinoma implanted intraperitoneally as a tumor brei, copper-containing BU-2231A was compared with copper-free. There was no difference between the two, as slight activity was observed with both forms (Table VI).

Since bleomycin is known to have inherent pyrogenicity both clinically and in laboratory animals, a test was performed in rabbits to examine the pyrogenicity of

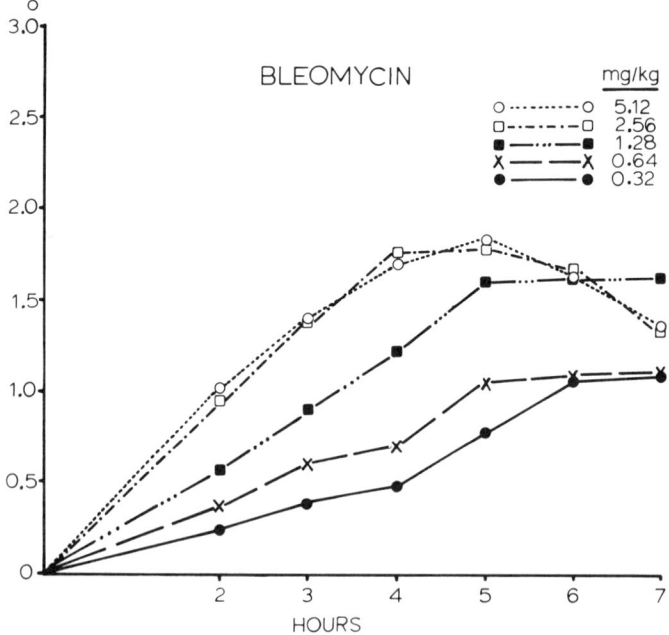

Fig. 3. Pyrogenic response of rabbits to single doses of bleomycin. Ordinate shows rise in ° C.

TABLE VI. Effect of BU-2231A on Lewis Lung Carcinoma [a]

Material	Dose (mg/kg/day)	MST (days)	Effect MST T/C%
BU-2231A	3.2	16.0	92
(with copper)	1.6	23.0	131
	0.8	21.0	120
	0.4	19.5	112
BU-2231A	3.2	19	109
(copper-free)	1.6	22.5	129
	0.8	21.0	120
	0.4	19.0	109
Control	–	17.5	–

[a] Inoculum: Tumor brei, IP. Treatment: QD 1 → 9.

BU-2231A. Dose-response titrations were performed with bleomycin given as a single IV injection over a twofold, five dose range and fever recorded as rise in degrees C (Fig. 3). Similarly, BU-2231A was tested but the doses were one fourth of the bleomycin doses based on toxicity differences (Fig. 4). A slow rise with delayed peak typical of bleomycin was observed with BU-2231A with a very similar titration pattern over all the doses.

Toxicity to the lung in the form of life-threatening fibrosis is the main course-limiting side effect of bleomycin therapy. Thus, we considered it particularly important to test BU-2231A for such action. Adamson and Bowden (1974) reported development of pulmonary pathology in mice following chronic bleomycin treatment. Preliminary studies of this model in our laboratory, (Bradner and Hirth, unpublished), suggested that the CDF_1 hybrid was the best of several strains tested and that delay of sacrifice for post mortem examination until one month after the end of therapy was necessary for development of lesions to their maximum. On this basis, groups of 10 CDF_1 mice were treated twice weekly for 6 weeks, three dose levels each of BU-2231A and bleomycin using the fourfold subacute toxicity criteria. Histopathology was performed on all surviving mice by Dr. Robert Hirth of our Toxicology Department (Bradner et al., 1977), and on moribund mice in good condition. Included were tissues from control animals receiving saline injections. Although the lesion developed in mice is not as intense as that observed with larger animals and humans, subpleural fibrosis was found in both groups of treated mice and not in controls. The number of animals manifesting subpleural fibrosis and/or pneumonitis was 7/28 for BU-2231A compared to 15/27 for bleomycin (Table VII). This suggestion that BU-2231A may have reduced toxicity to the lung is now being investigated in larger animal species.

TABLE VII. Lung Histopathology, BU-2231A–Bleomycin Comparison [a]

	Dose (mg/kg/day)	No. animals	Diffuse >basophilia or hyperplasia of pneumocytes	Interstitial fibrosis and/or pneumonitis	Subpleural fibrosis and/or pneumonitis	Focal epithelial hyperplasia	Foci macrophages
BU-2231A	4	9	1	2	3	1	3
	2	9	1	0	3	3	1
	1	10	1	2	1	2	0
Bleomycin	16	7	3	4	6	6	5
	8	10	10	3	3	8	1
	4	10	3	1	6	3	1

Totals: 7/28 BU-2231A
15/27 Bleomycin

[a] Mice: CDF$_1$. Treatment: 2x weekly, 6 weeks. Autopsy: One month after last dose.

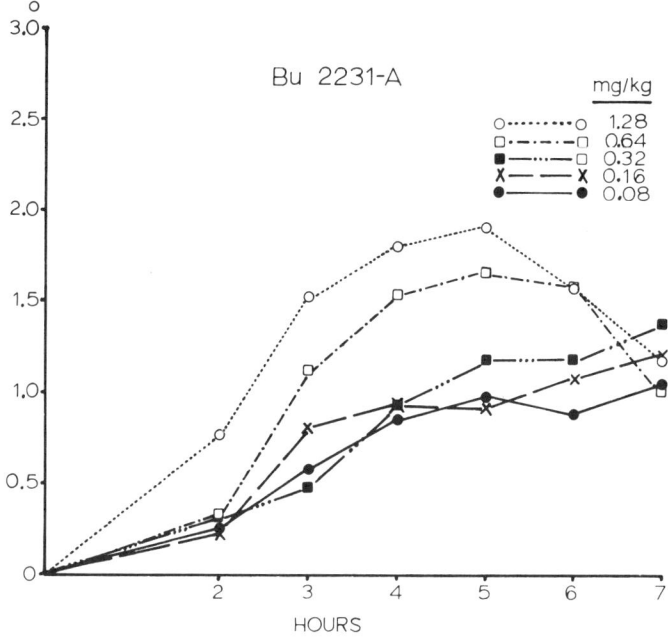

Fig. 4. Pyrogenic response of rabbits to single doses of BU-2231A. Ordinate shows rise in °C.

V. SUMMARY

1. BU-2231A is a new bleomycin-type antibiotic differing both in nucleus and side chain.

2. BU-2231A is four or more times as toxic as bleomycin in both single and chronic lethality.

3. BU-2231A is highly active on Walker 256 carcinosarcoma.

4. BU-2231A is more active than bleomycin on P-388 leukemia.

5. BU-2231A is less active than bleomycin on B16 melanoma.

6. BU-2231A is slightly active on Lewis lung carcinoma.

7. BU-2231A is pyrogenic and shows dose response similar to bleomycin when given at equivalent levels relative to LD_{50}.

8. BU-2231A appears to cause a lower incidence of pneumonitis/fibrosis in chronically treated mice than bleomycin when the two drugs are given at equivalent fractions of the LD_{50}.

REFERENCES

Adamson, I. Y. R., and Bowden, D. H. (1974). *Am. J. Pathol.* 77, 185.
Bradner, W. T., Imanishi, H., Hirth, R. S., and Wodinsky, I. (1977). *Proc. Am. Assoc. Cancer Res. 18*, 18–35.

Fugii, A., Takita, T., Maeda, K., and Umezawa, H. (1973). *J. Antibiot. 26*, 3.

Kawaguchi, H., Tsukiura, H., Tomita, K., Konishi, M., Saito, K., Kobaru, S., Numata, K., Fugisawa, K., Miyaki, T., Hatori, M., and Koshiyama, H. (1977). *J. Antibiot. 30*, 779-788.

Konishi, M., Saito, K., Numata, K., Tsuno, T., Asama, K., Tsukima, H., Naito, T., and Kawaguchi, H. (1977). *J. Antibiot. 30*, 789-805.

Takita, T., Muraoka, Y., Maeda, K., and Umezawa, H. (1968). *J. Antibiot. 21*, 79.

Takita, T., Muraoka, Y., Fugii, A., Itoh, H., Maeda, K., and Umezawa, H. (1972). *J. Antibiot. 25*, 197.

Chapter 29

MECHANISM OF ACTION OF TALLYSOMYCIN, A THIRD GENERATION BLEOMYCIN[1]

James E. Strong

Stanley T. Crooke

I. INTRODUCTION

The chemical and biological properties of tallysomycin have been previously described (Bradner, this volume). In this paper, recent studies on the mode of action of tallysomycin will be compared with bleomycin A_2. *In vitro,* tests indicate that even though tallysomycin is more potent than bleomycin in lysogenic phage induction, bacteriacidal activity, and against animal tumor systems including Walker 256 carcinosarcoma and P-388 lymphocytic leukemia in mice, the drug is less capable of inducing degradation of bacteriophage PM-2 DNA as well as DNA of Novikoff hepatoma ascites cells grown *in vitro.*

II. MATERIALS AND METHODS

A. Analysis of DNA Degradation

A fluorimetric assay was used to detect breakage of circular bacteriophage PM-2 DNA. Bacteriophage PM-2 DNA was isolated as previously described. (Salditt *et al.,*

[1] Supported by American Cancer Society Grant IN-27Q to J.E.S. and by Bristol Laboratories, Syracuse, New York.

1972; Strong and Hewitt, 1975). The assay consisted of incubating 50 μg PM-2 DNA with varying concentrations of drug in 0.5 ml borate buffer (0.05 M, pH 9.5) plus 25 mM 2-mercaptoethanol at room temperature. The reaction was terminated by adding 0.1 ml duplicate aliquots of the reaction mixture to 0.9 ml denaturation buffer (0.04 M Na$_3$PO$_4$, 0.01 M EDTA, 0.10 M NaCl, pH adjusted to 12.1 with 0.15 M NaOH) followed by addition of 0.1 ml ethidium bromide (Sigma) (22 μg/ml in denaturation buffer).

Fluorescence of the resultant mixture was determined on a spectrophotofluorometer (Aminco-Bowman) at 530 nm excitation and 590 nm emission. After subtraction of background fluorescence (without DNA), the amount of DNA degradation was indicated by the percentage decrease in fluorescence relative to control reactions not containing drug. No decrease in fluorescence of the control reaction was observed in any experiment.

B. Agarose Electrophoresis

Following reaction of covalent circular PM-2 DNA with either bleomycin or tallysomycin, as described above, the reaction was terminated by adding 10 μl of 50 mM EDTA to 50 μl of the reaction mixture. This was diluted with an equal volume of 0.1% bromphenol blue in 50% glycerol and 20 μl was electrophoresed on a 0.9% agarose gel. Electrophoresis was performed in 40 mM Trizma (Sigma), 5 mM sodium acetate, and 1 mM EDTA, pH 7.8 at 4 V/cm for 16 hr at room temperature. After electrophoresis, the gels were incubated for at least 2 hr in 500 ml electrophoresis buffer containing 0.5 μg/ml ethidium bromide. Under these conditions, the order of migration of DNA from fastest to slowest was: closed circular DNA, double-stranded broken linear DNA, and single-strand broken circular DNA.

C. Alkaline Sucrose Sedimentation

Novikoff hepatoma ascites cells were grown in RPMI-1640 medium (Gibco) with 10% fetal calf serum to a cell density of 5 x 10^5 cells/ml. These cells were next incubated with either [^{3}H]-TdR (3 μCi/ml, 360 mCi/mM) or [^{14}C]-TdR (0.1 μCi/ml, 57 mCi/mM) for 16 hr. The [^{3}H]-TdR-labeled cells were incubated with 50 μg/ml bleomycin or tallysomycin for 1 hr at 37°. Cells were then centrifuged (1000g, 5 min) and resuspended in SSC (0.15 M NaCl, 0.015 M sodium citrate) at a concentration of approximately 2 x 10^6 cells/ml. Cell suspensions (0.5 ml) were layered onto a 5–20% alkaline sucrose gradient (0.3 M NaOH, 0.7 M NaCl plus 1 mM EDTA) to which 1 ml of lysis solution (0.5 M NaOH, 0.02 M ADTA, and 0.1% Triton X-100) plus 0.5 ml [^{14}C]-TdR-labeled cells had been added. The cells were incubated 1 hr in lysis solution at room temperature and centrifuged in an SW 27 rotor for 2 hr (21,000 rpm, 20°). Fractions (1.2 ml) were collected from the top of the gradient and precipitated with 10% trichloroacetic acid (4°) following addition of 100 μg ovalbumin as coprecipitate. Precipitates were collected on glass fiber filters, dried and counted.

D. Precursor Uptake

Experiments measuring incorporation of $[^3H]$-TdR into trichloroacetic acid in-soluble material were performed as follows: Approximately 1×10^6 cells/ml growing logarithmically were incubated in fresh RPMI 1640 medium (plus 10% fetal calf serum) containing 25 μg/ml bleomycin or tallysomycin for the indicated time inter-vals. Tritium-labeled thymidine (2.5 μCi/ml, 360 mCi/mM) was then added to the cells and incubation continued for 1 hr. Following incubation, cells (0.5 ml) were filtered on glass fiber filters and washed with 10 ml salt solution (0.14 M NaCl, 0.005 M KCl, 0.008 M MgCl$_2$). The washed cells were then treated with 10 ml 10% tri-chloroacetic acid (4°C, 5 min) and washed with 10% trichloroacetic acid. Filters were dried and radioactivity determined in a liquid scintillation counter.

E. Affinity Constant Determination

The procedure of Chien *et al.* (1977) was used to determine affinity constants of bleomycin and tallysomycin for salmon sperm DNA. Estimates of total bleomycin and tallysomycin bound to DNA were derived from fluorescence quenching by add-ing increasing amounts of drug to a constant amount of DNA and measuring the fluorescence decrease at 300 nM excitation and 360 nM emission on an Aminco-Bowman spectrophotofluorometer relative to control without DNA.

F. Drugs

Bleomycin A$_2$ (lot U-18A$_2$S) and tallysomycin A (lot 34-F-12) obtained from Bristol Drug Company were used in comparison experiments. Blenoxane (Bristol Drug Co., lot J4106) was used in experiments involving development of PM-2 fluor-escence assay. Units of bleomycin could be converted to weight measurement by the formula 1.6 u/mg. All drugs were stored at $-20°$.

III. RESULTS

The estimation of PM-2 DNA breakage by bleomycin and tallysomycin was per-formed using the procedure as described in Fig. 1. Use of this technique for quantita-tion of bleomycin activity (Fig. 2) showed that decrease in fluorescence was directly related to concentration of bleomycin. Fluorescence decrease was also logarithmically proportional to incubation time, thus allowing first-order rate constant determina-tion. A comparison of bleomycin concentration with rate constants obtained by this procedure yielded a straight line passing through the origin (Fig. 3). The fluorimetric assay was used to investigate requirement of 2-mercaptoethanol and the pH optimum for bleomycin activity. It was found that maximum DNA breakage occurred at pH 9.5 with 25 mM 2-mercaptoethanol (Fig. 4). The same pH optimum and 2-mercap-toethanol requirement were found for both bleomycin A$_2$ and tallysomycin. How-ever, the rate of DNA breakage was consistently less for tallysomycin than bleomycin.

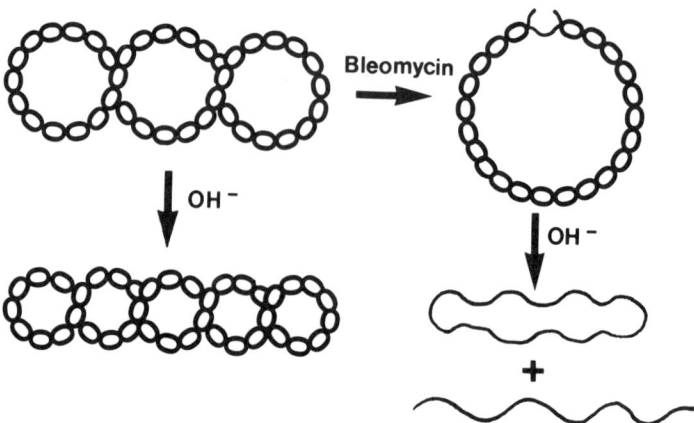

Fig. 1. Fluorescence assay for bleomycin activity. Bleomycin produces strand scission in PM-2 superhelical DNA. The broken DNA is rendered susceptible to alkaline denaturation. However, unbroken DNA remains double stranded under the same conditions. Addition of ethidium bromide to double-stranded DNA results in an increased quantum yield of fluorescence. Single-stranded DNA does not bind ethidium bromide under the assay conditions so that the amount of fluorescence above background is proportional to concentration of superhelical double-stranded PM-2 DNA.

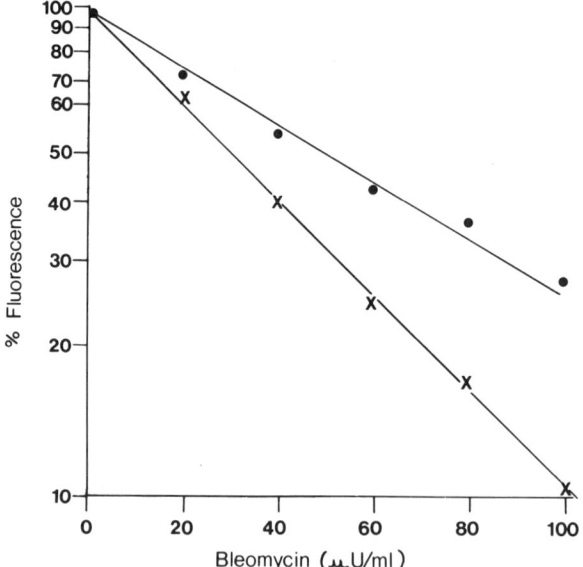

Fig. 2. Quantitation of bleomycin activity by fluorescence assay. Incubation of PM-2 DNA with Blenoxane® 30 min (●) and 60 min (x). The Blenoxane® concentration is expressed in $\mu u/ml$, which may be converted to ng/ml by the following relationship: 1.6 u/mg. The % fluorescence is relative to control fluorescence. No decrease in control fluorescence was observed during incubation.

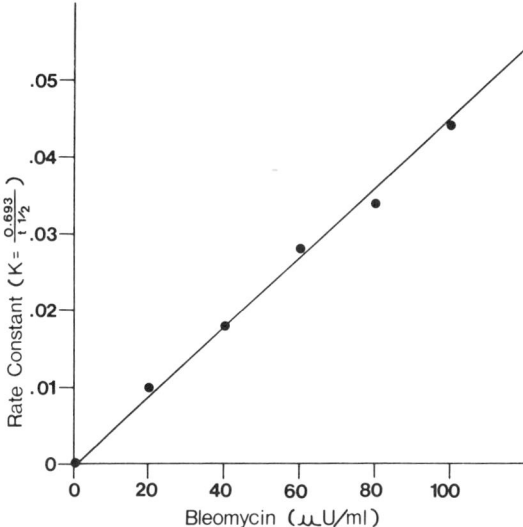

Fig. 3. Rate constants for various bleomycin concentrations. Rate constants for different concentrations of Blenoxane® were determined by dividing ln 2 by the time necessary to decrease fluorescence by 50% in the fluorescence assay.

More than fivefold higher concentration of tallysomycin was required to produce a similar rate of fluorescence decrease as in bleomycin A_2 (Fig. 5). The products of bleomycin and tallysomycin action upon PM-2 DNA were electrophoretically separated on agarose gels (Fig. 6). These results also indicated that tallysomycin produced less DNA breakage than bleomycin A_2. The temperature optimum for both tallysomycin and bleomycin was found to be 30–37°C. The energy of activation for DNA breakage by the two drugs was determined using the Arrehenius plot (Fig. 7). The activation energy for bleomycin-induced DNA degradation was 13,909 cal/mole, whereas that for tallysomycin was 33,547 cal/mole. This result was consistent with a decreased rate of tallysomycin-induced DNA breakage.

Degradation of cellular DNA by bleomycin and tallysomycin was also investigated. Novikoff hepatoma ascites cells grown *in vitro* were treated with varying concentrations of tallysomycin or bleomycin for 1 hr then lysed and centrifuged on alkaline sucrose gradients. As a control, untreated [^{14}C]-thymidine-labeled cells were mixed with drug-treated [^{3}H]-thymidine-labeled cells and lysed on top of alkaline sucrose gradients. There was a dose-related decrease in sedimentation of the [^{3}H]-thymidine-labeled DNA between 10 and 100 μg/ml tallysomycin or bleomycin A_2. However, at each concentration the DNA sedimentation for bleomycin A_2-treated cells was slower than for tallysomycin-treated cells. The results of 50 μg/ml bleomycin A_2 or tallysomycin treatment of Novikoff hepatoma cells are depicted in Fig. 8. The peak fraction of [^{14}C]-TdR-labeled control cellular DNA remained the same in each tube. However, both bleomycin A_2- and tallysomycin-treated cellular DNA species were shifted to lower sedimentation rates. This indicated that both tallysomycin

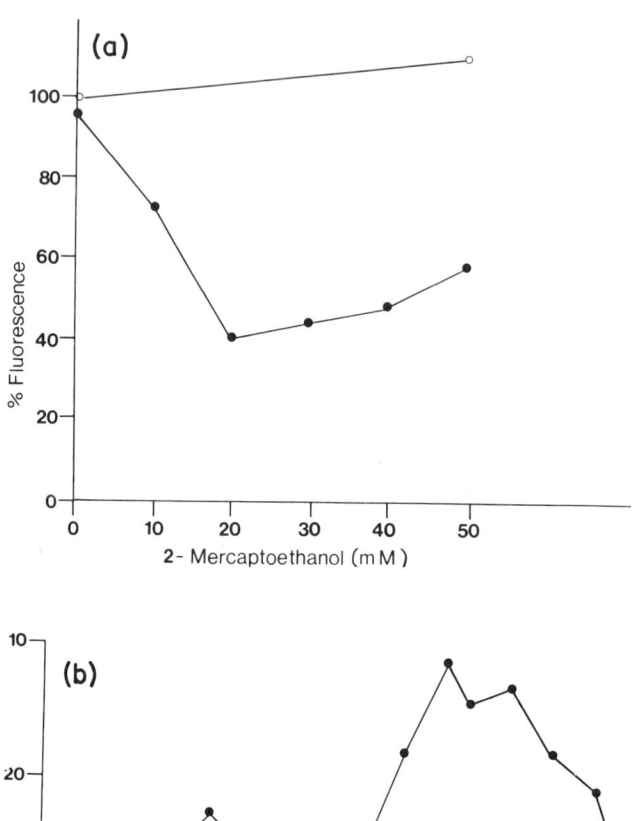

Fig. 4. (A) Effect of 2-mercaptoethanol on bleomycin activity. Indicated concentrations of 2-mercaptoethanol were added to buffer (0.05 *M* Tris, pH 8.0) containing 100 μu/ml Blenoxane® and incubated 60 min with PM-2 DNA. (B) Effect of pH on bleomycin activity. Blenoxane® (100 μu/ml) was added to incubation buffer (0.05 *M* phosphate + 0.05 *M* borate + 20 m*M* 2-mercaptoethanol) which had previously been adjusted to indicated pH and the solution incubated (60 min) with PM-2 DNA.

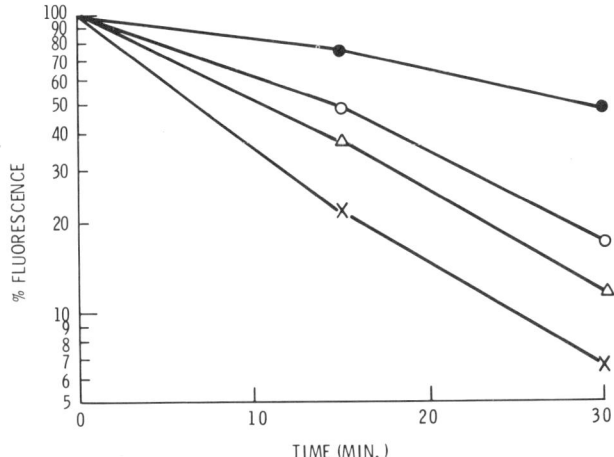

Fig. 5. Bleomycin and tallysomycin activity in fluorescence assay. Tallysomycin: (●) 10 ng/ml, (○) 25 ng/ml and (△) 50 ng/ml plus bleomycin A_2 (x) 10 ng/ml, were incubated for the indicated times with PM-2 DNA and activity determined in the fluorescence assay.

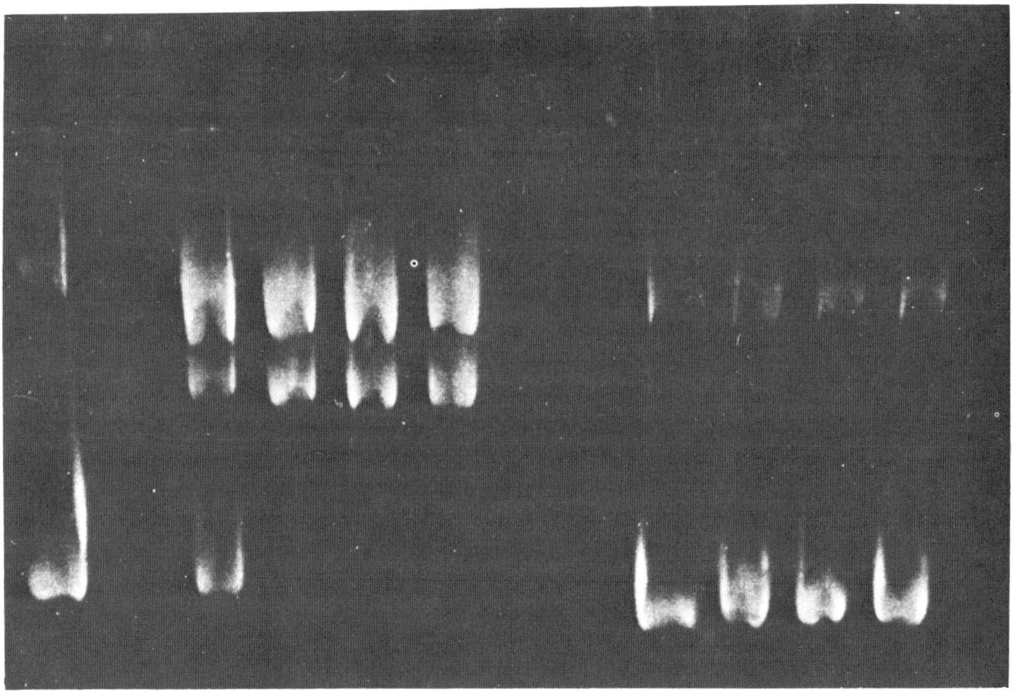

Fig. 6. Agarose gel electrophoresis of PM-2 DNA following incubation with bleomycin A_2 or tallysomycin. Both drugs (20 ng) were incubated with PM-2 DNA. Following the reaction, 1 μg PM-2 DNA was placed in each well and electrophoresed for 16 hr. Gels were viewed with ultraviolet light. From left to right patterns represent (1) control, (2) bleomycin A_2 10 min, (3) 20 min, (4) 40 min, (5) 60 min, (6) tallysomycin 10 min, (7) 20 min, (8) 40 min, (9) 60 min.

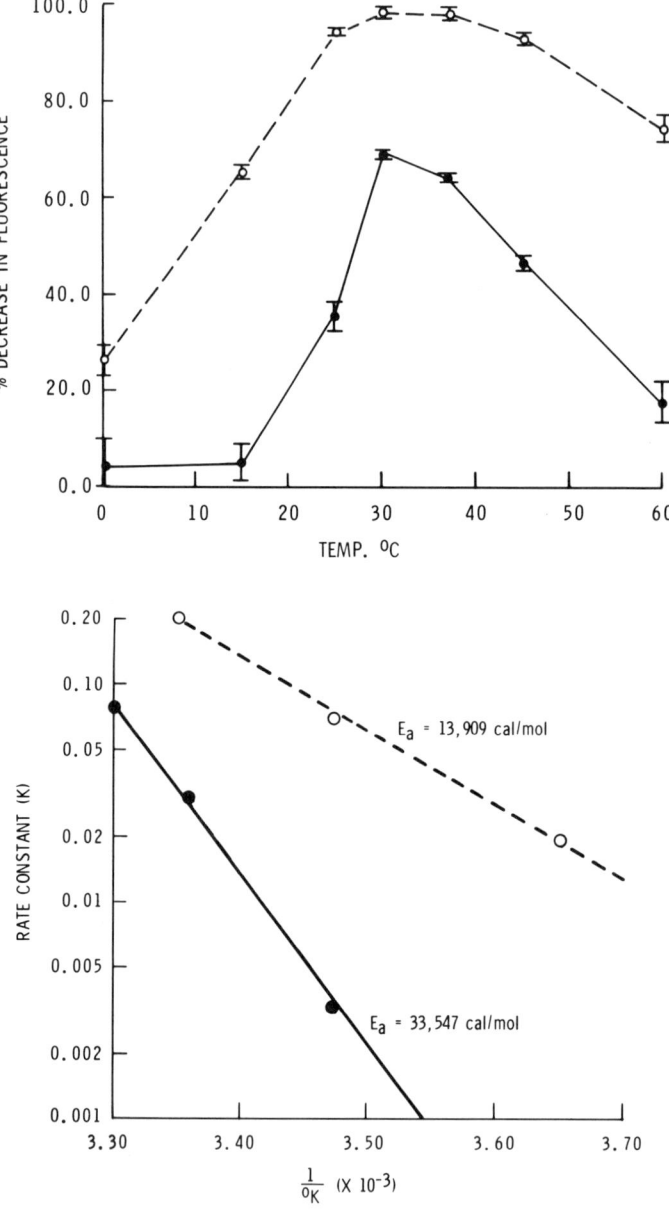

Fig. 7. Temperature effect on bleomycin A_2 and tallysomycin activity. The fluorescence assay was performed following incubation of 25 ng of each drug for 15 min with PM-2 DNA at the indicated temperatures. Bleomycin (○); tallysomycin (●). (B) Arrehenius graph for the determination of activation energy. Rate constants of activity in the fluorescence assay were determined for both drugs at the indicated temperatures. Energy of activation for bleomycin (○) was 13,909 cal/mole and for tallysomycin (●), 33,547 cal/mole.

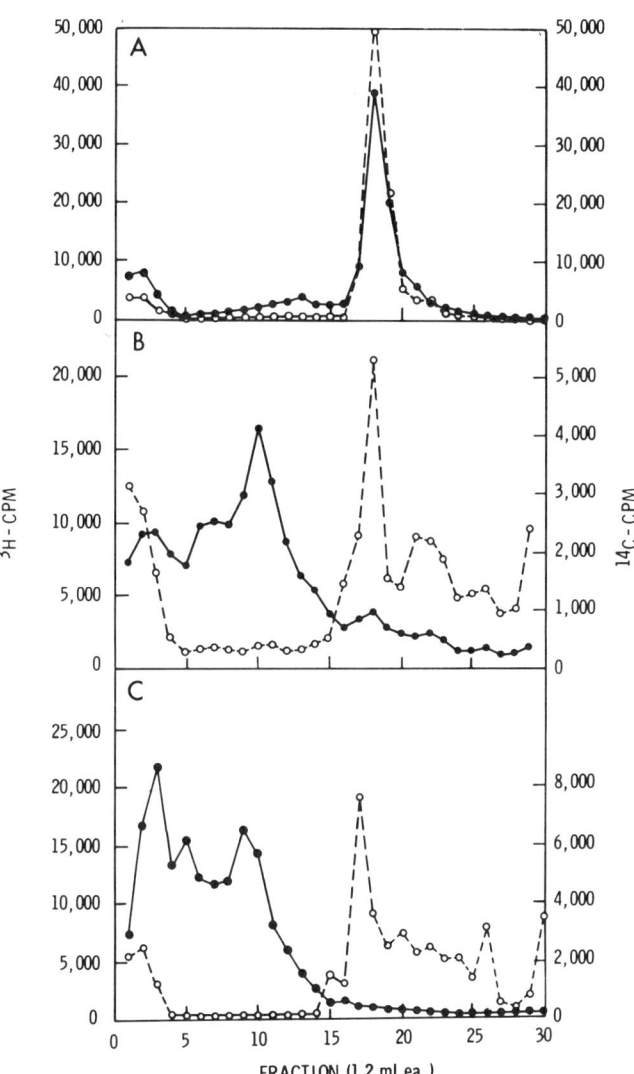

Fig. 8. Alkaline sucrose gradient centrifugation of tallysomycin- and bleomycin-treated cells. Control cells labeled with [^{14}C]-TdR (○) and [^{3}H]-TdR drug-treated cells (●) were included in each gradient tube. (A) No drug treatment of [^{3}H]-TdR-labeled cells; (B) tallysomycin (50 μg/ml, 1 hr)-treated [^{3}H]-TdR-labeled cells; (C) bleomycin (50 μg/ml, 1 hr)-treated [^{3}H]-TdR-labeled cells.

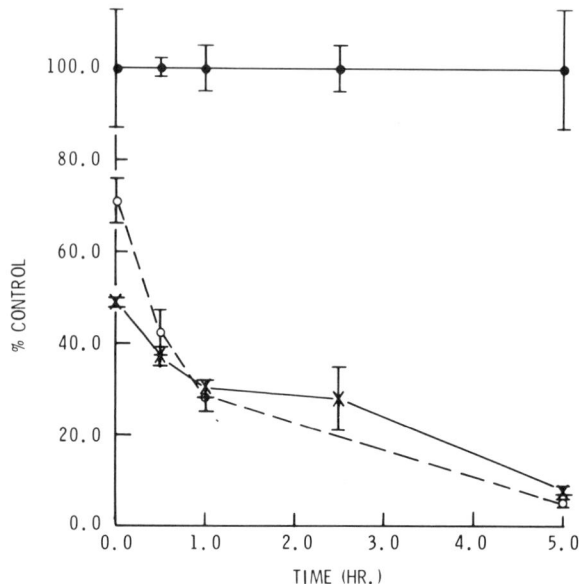

Fig. 9. Uptake of [^{3}H]-thymidine into bleomycin- and tallysomycin-treated cell DNA. The amount of radioactivity incorporated in 10% trichloroacetic acid-insoluble material relative to control, untreated cells following incubation with drug (25 μg/ml) for the indicated time intervals is indicated as percent control. The time intervals represent drug addition prior to incorporation of [^{3}H]-TdR for 1 hr. The standard deviations for duplicate samples are depicted. Bleomycin A$_2$ (x) and tallysomycin (o).

and bleomycin broke DNA *in vivo*. However, bleomycin A$_2$ caused a greater decrease in sedimentation of DNA than tallysomycin.

The incorporation of [^{3}H]-thymidine into trichloroacetic acid (TCA)-insoluble material was inhibited in both tallysomycin- and bleomycin-treated Novikoff hepatoma ascites cells. Figure 9 demonstrates that at 25 μg/ml drug concentration little difference in inhibition of [^{3}H]-TdR incorporation could be detected between bleomycin- and tallysomycin-treated cells. Increasing drug concentrations with a constant incubation time also did not reveal significant differences in inhibition of [^{3}H]-TdR uptake in Novikoff hepatoma ascites cells (data not shown). However, it was unclear whether the decrease in TCA-insoluble [^{3}H]-TdR radioactivity represented inhibition of DNA synthesis or uptake of labeled precursor by the cells since the ratio of trichloroacetic acid-insoluble radioactivity to whole cellular radioactivity was constant for both treated and control cells (data not shown).

Affinity constants of bleomycin and tallysomycin for salmon sperm DNA were determined using a fluorescence quenching technique (Pesce *et al.*, 1971). The maximum quenching by DNA of bleomycin fluorescence was found to be 50%. The maximum quenching of tallysomycin fluorescence by DNA addition was 70% (Fig. 10). The ratio of bound to free drug was calculated using these values for totally

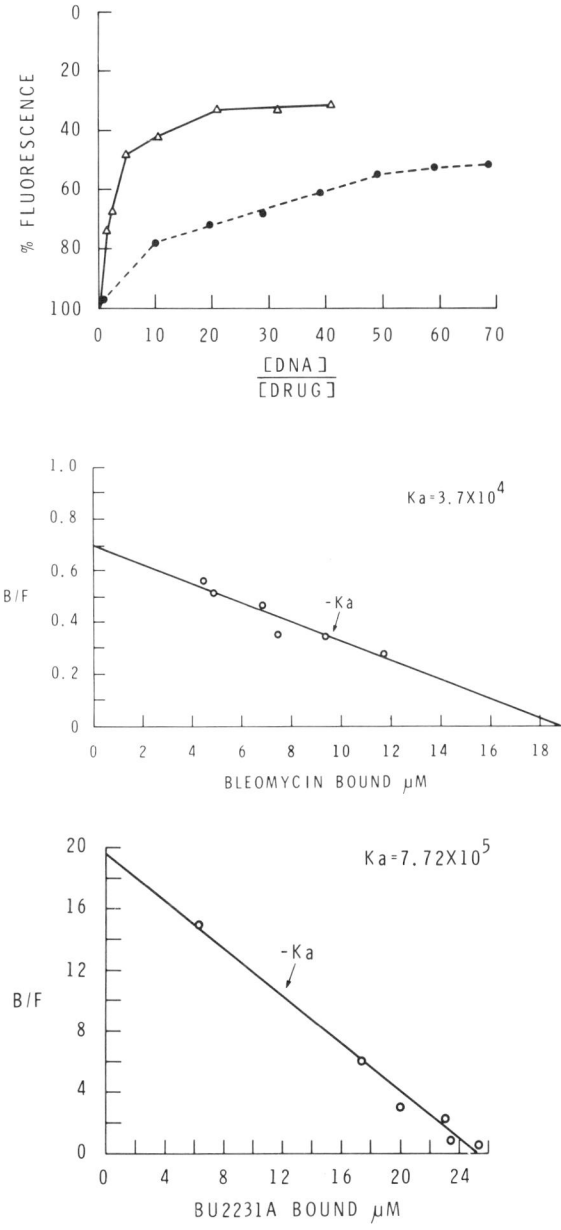

Fig. 10. Fluorescence quenching of bleomycin and tallysomycin. Fluorescence was measured at 300 nm excitation and 360 nm emission. Percentage fluorescence was determined relative to drug fluorescence without DNA. (A) Fluorescence quenching obtained by varying ratio of DNA nucleotide concentration to drug. (●) Bleomycin A_2, (△) tallysomycin. (B) Affinity constant determination for bleomycin A_2. (C) Affinity constant determination for tallysomycin (Bu2231A).

bound drug (Chien et al., 1977; Pesce et al., 1971). The affinity constant for the two drugs was determined by Scatchard analysis following addition of increasing quantities of bleomycin A_2 or tallysomycin to a constant amount of DNA (Fig. 10). Affinity constants so determined were 3.7 x 10^4 M^{-1} and 7.72 x 10^5 M^{-1} for bleomycin A_2 and tallysomycin, respectively. The stoichiometry of bleomycin and tallysomycin binding to DNA was also determined. One bleomycin molecule was bound per 3.74 nucleotides, whereas one tallysomycin molecule bound per 3.95 nucleotides.

IV. DISCUSSION

In addition to DNA strand scission, bleomycin causes release of free bases and production of aldehyde groups by opening the deoxyribose ring structure (Haidle et al., 1972; Muller et al., 1972). Depurinated DNA is sensitive to alkali treatment (Lindahl and Anderson, 1972) and it has been shown that bleomycin produces alkali labile sites in DNA (Muller and Zahn, 1976). We have performed experiments on DNA breakage by bleomycin in both neutral and alkaline conditions following incubation and found that the rate of strand scission was twice as great following alkaline denaturation (data not shown). Thus, the fluorimetric assay probably detects alkaline labile damage (free base removal) in addition to strand scission. However, the agarose gel electrophoresis was performed under neutral conditions and both methods demonstrated greater strand scission by bleomycin A_2 than tallysomycin.

The in vitro DNA breakage activity of bleomycin and tallysomycin was also demonstrated in drug-treated Novikoff hepatoma cells. Both drugs reduced the rate of sedimentation of cellular DNA on alkaline density gradient centrifugation. Bleomycin caused a greater decrease in sedimentation than tallysomycin at equal concentrations. The decrease in sedimentation of cellular DNA apparently did not occur after lysis of cells, as suggested by Cox et al. (1974), since untreated control cellular DNA did not show a decreased sedimentation rate following lysis of the cells in the presence of treated cells.

The affinity constant of tallysomycin and bleomycin A_2 corresponded to the drugs' biological activity. The affinity constant for bleomycin A_2–DNA interaction was 3.7 x 10^4 M^{-1}. This was lower than obtained by Chien et al. (1977) using fluorescence quenching (1.2 x 10^5 M^{-1}) but agreed with the value obtained by Sastry et al. (1977), using the perturbed gamma-ray angular correlation technique (6.2 x 10^4 M^{-1}). The number of nucleotide molecules per bleomycin was also less in this investigation (3.7) than obtained by Chien et al. (1977) (11 nucleotides per bleomycin) but agrees more closely with Sastry et al. (1977) (4.8 nucleotides per bleomycin). The tallysomycin affinity constant was approximately 20-fold greater than bleomycin A_2. This increased affinity corresponded to the approximately 32-fold increase in lysogenic bacteriophage induction by tallysomycin compared to bleomycin A_2 (Bradner, this volume). The number of nucleotides per bleomycin bound was not significantly different between bleomycin and tallysomycin (3.74 and 3.95, respectively) despite the increased affinity of tallysomycin for DNA.

Umezawa *et al.* (1976) utilized strand scission of superhelical SV40 DNA as a quantitative assay for bleomycin activity. A comparison of antimicrobial activity with strand scission capacity revealed little, if any, correlation between these two parameters for many bleomycin derivatives. The present investigation demonstrates that under the experimental conditions employed, increased DNA breakage of PM-2 DNA and Novikoff hepatoma cellular DNA cannot be demonstrated as the mechanism for increased potency of tallysomycin compared to bleomycin A_2.

ACKNOWLEDGMENTS

The authors wish to express appreciation to Dr. Roger Hewitt, M. D. Anderson Hospital and Tumor Institute, for his generous gift of PM-2 DNA and collaboration in developing the PM-2 breakage assay.

REFERENCES

Chien, M., Grollman, A. P., and Horwitz, S. B. (1977). *Biochemistry 16*, 3641.

Cox, R., Daoud, A. H., and Irving, C. C. (1974). *Biochem. Pharmacol. 23*, 3147.

Haidle, C. W., Weiss, K. K., and Kuo, M. T. (1972). *Mol. Pharmacol. 8,* 531.

Lindahl, T., and Anderson, A. (1972). *Biochemistry 11,* 3168.

Muller, W. E. G., and Zahn, R. K. (1976). in *Fundamental and Clinical Studies of Bleomycin,* Carter, S. K., Ichikawa, T., Mathe, G., and Umezawa, H. (Eds.). University Park Press, Baltimore, pp. 51–62.

Muller, W. E. G., Yamazaki, Z., Bretner, H. J., and Zahn, R. K. (1972). *Eur. J. Biochem. 31,* 518.

Pesce, A. J., Rosen, C. G., and Pasby, T. L. (1971). In *Fluorescence Spectroscopy, an Introduction for Biology and Medicine,* Marcel Dekker, New York, pp. 203–240.

Salditt, M., Braunstein, S. N., Camerini-Otero, R. D., and Franklin, R. M. (1972). *Virology 48,* 259.

Sastry, K. S. R., Hallee, G. J., Ottlinger, M. E., and Westhead, E. W. (1977). Paper presented at the 4th International Conference of Hyperfine Interactions, Madison, New Jersey.

Strong, J. E., and Hewitt, R. R. (1975). In *Isozymes III,* Vol. III, Markert, C. (Ed.). Academic Press, New York, PP. 473–483.

Umezawa, H., Asakura, H., and Hori, M. (1976). In *Chemotherapy,* Vol. III, Hellman, K., and Connors, T. A. (Eds.). Plenum Press, New York, pp. 165–168.

Chapter 30

BLEOMYCIN–FUTURE DIRECTIONS

Stanley T. Crooke

I. INTRODUCTION

The papers presented in this symposium and in previous symposia concerning bleomycin amply demonstrate the complexity of bleomycin and the questions it has generated. Certainly the chemistry of the bleomycins is complex. The bleomycin molecule is large and has numerous reactive groups. Morover, studies previously discussed demonstrate that modifications may be made in various parts of the molecule without loss of antitumor activity. Thus, the potential chemical manipulations remain, to a very significant degree, unexplored.

Although a great deal is known about the molecular pharmacology of bleomycin and analogs, many questions remain unanswered. Some of these may be answered as structure-activity relationships emerge from studies on various active and inactive analogs. The relationship, for example, of DNA degradation to antitumor activity and/or pulmonary toxicity may best be answered by studying a series of inactive, or minimally active analogs.

Equally complex are clinical questions concerning bleomycin. Although significantly more is now known about the clinical pharmacology of bleomycin than even a year ago, almost no information is available concerning tissue levels in human beings, and little is known about the metabolism of bleomycin. Are there, for example, pharmacogenetic differences which predispose patients to bleomycin pulmonary toxicity? Equally unclear are the proper doses, schedules, optimal combinations, and

Copyright © 1978 by Academic Press, Inc.
ISBN 0-12-161550-2

methods of administration of bleomycin for various malignancies.

The foregoing notwithstanding, however, enough is now known about bleomycin to suggest directions for future research. Of course any suggestions concerning directions of research in such a complex area are, by definition, incomplete, and reflect selection based in part on personal biases.

II. GOALS FOR NEW BLEOMYCIN ANALOGS

The goals which I would propose for future analog development are as follows:
Less pulmonary toxicity
Lower incidence of hyperpyrexia
Greater activity in adenocarcinomas
Less mucocutaneous toxicity
Longer serum half-life
Topically active-Non absorbed
Lower cost of goods
Single component

With one or two exceptions, these have been the goals of the analog development efforts for the past several years. Certainly, a great deal of effort has been expended toward the development of an analog with a broader spectrum of activity. However, relatively little attention has been directed to an analog with less potential for induction of hyperpyrexia. This could be particularly important for patients with lymphomas in whom hyperpyrexia is associated with acute hypotensive reactions. An analog with less mucocutaneous toxicity would be of particular value for patients with head and neck cancers treated with bleomycin in combination with radiotherapy.

Four goals which are perhaps of lower priority, but are nontheless of importance, are the development of analogs with a longer serum half-life, which are single components, and which are less expensive, and a nonabsorbed topically active analog. Accumulating evidence suggests that in certain diseases a prolonged infusion of bleomycin may be more active than intermittent bolus doses. Clearly, since bleomycin is cell-cycle phase specific, and has a short $t_{1/2}\beta$, an analog with a slower plasma clearance rate is potentially attractive. An analog which would be active when administered topically, but not absorbed, is of potential value in the treatment of neoplastic skin diseases, particularly since recent data suggest that the carcinogenicity of bleomycin may be surprisingly low (Benedict *et al.*, 1977). A compound which is a single component would allow better definition of the metabolism of bleomycin than the presently employed mixture, and clearly a less costly derivative would be of substantial benefit.

III. PRESENT STATUS

A. Models

1. Pulmonary

Critical to any analog development program is the availability of appropriate pre-clinical models. The pulmonary toxicity of bleomycin analogs is currently evaluated in mice or aged rats (Adamson and Bowden, 1974; Ohwada *et al.*, 1973; A. Matsuda, 1977, personal communication). Both systems are inadequate for at least two reasons. They are subacute models requiring several weeks and substantial amounts of compounds to complete. In neither model do 100% of bleomycin-treated animals develop pulmonary lesions. Thus the ability of each of the systems to detect differences between analogs is reduced.

Earlier studies suggested that the pulmonary toxicities of bleomycin were readily demonstrable in dogs (Schaeppi *et al.*, 1974). However, these studies are subacute, and require much more drug than the rodent models. Recent studies have demonstrated that the development of pulmonary toxicity in dogs is much less predictable, and requires longer treatment periods and higher bleomycin dosage than previously reported (J. Anderson, 1977, personal communication). Thus the dog is a relatively poor species for such studies.

2. Hyperpyrexia

The modified rabbit hyperpyrexia model currently employed at Bristol Laboratories would appear to be adequate for studies on new analogs. Inasmuch as the hyperpyrexia induced by bleomycin is delayed, it is necessary to extend the observation period to 8 hours postdose. Figure 1 shows a typical febrile response to tallysomycin (BU2231).

3. Activity against Adenocarcinomas

Several animal tumors thought to be closely related to human adenocarcinomas are currently available. Two models, the carcinogen-induced stomach adenocarcinoma in rats and the Colon 38 rodent adenocarcinoma developed at Southern Research Institute, have recently been employed to study bleomycin and analogs (A. Matsuda, 1977, personal communication; F. Schabel, 1977, personal communication). Although PEP-bleomycin was distinctly more active against the rat adenocarcinoma than bleomycin, it has, as yet, failed to demonstrate clinical activity against human adenocarcinomas (Umezawa, 1977, unpublished data). Against the Colon 38 adenocarcinoma, tallysomycin was more active than bleomycin (F. Schabel, 1977, personal communication). Whether tallysomycin is active against human adenocarcinomas remains to be determined.

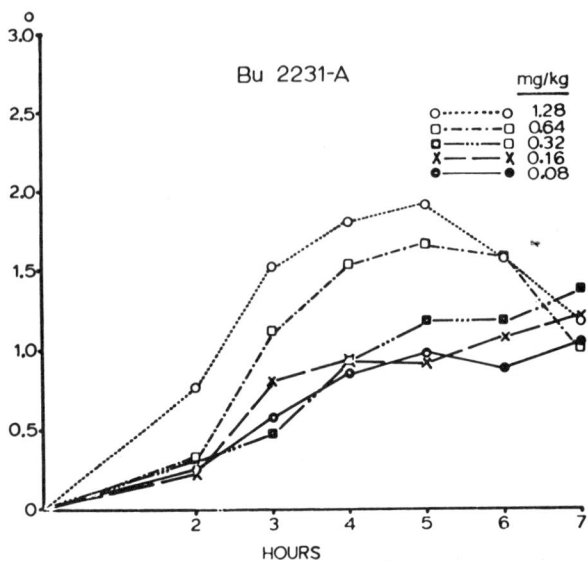

Fig. 1. Hyperpyrexia induced in rabbits by tallysomycin.

4. Prescreens

The PM2 DNA assay would seem an excellent prescreen for new bleomycin analogs. It is highly sensitive, rapid, requires minimal compound, and is simple.

IV. STRUCTURE-ACTIVITY RELATIONSHIPS

Figure 2 shows the structure of bleomycin with several areas of the molecule which have been modified in SAR studies. Umezawa and co-workers (1976b) have studied the effects of changes in the terminal amine position of the molecule (1). They have demonstrated that numerous alterations in this portion of the molecule may be introduced without loss of antitumor activity or the ability to degrade DNA. Morover, the presence of guanidino compounds as the terminal amine was shown to result in nephrotoxic compounds (Umezawa, 1976a). However, if no terminal amine is present a significant reduction in DNA degradative and antitumor activities is observed.

That reduction of the bithiazole portion of bleomycin (2) has no significant effect on antitumor activity was demonstrated by the activity of the phleomycins (Bradner and Pindell, 1971). Also, changes in area 3 which have resulted in tallysomycin and zorbomycin and the zorbonoycins suggest that this portion of the molecule may be altered substantially without loss of antitumor activity or DNA degradative activity (W. T. Bradner, 1977, unpublished data; J. Strong and S. Crooke, 1977, unpublished data). However, tallysomycin, for example, may have a spectrum

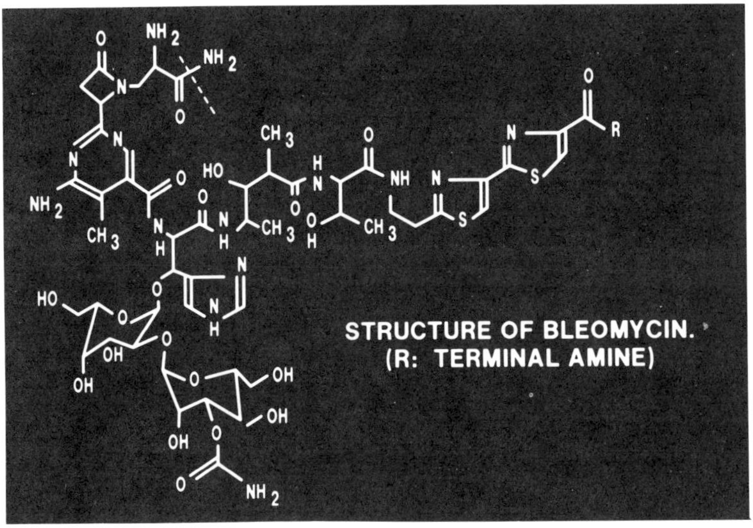

Fig. 2.   Structure-activity relationships of bleomycin.

of activity which differs from bleomycin.

Shift of the carbamoyl group (4) to give the iso-bleomycins has been reported to result in reduction of both DNA cleavage and antitumor activities (Nakayama *et al.*, 1973). Similar effects on antitumor activity were noted when epimerization at position (5) was effected. However, DNA degradative activity was unaffected (Umezawa, 1977, unpublished data).

Recently, a possible derivative of the amino group at position (6) has been prepared which has antitumor and DNA degradative activities equal to or greater than those of bleomycin A_2 (L. Galvan and S. Crooke, 1977, unpublished data). Finally, it has been reported that hydrolysis of the amide at position (7) results in a marked reduction in both activities (Umezawa, 1976a).

It is interesting that so many modifications may be introduced in various parts of the bleomycin structure without significant loss of activity, but even very minor modifications significantly alter the cross-reactivity to the antibodies employed in the radioimmunoassay for bleomycin (Strong *et al.*, 1977).

V. PROPOSALS FOR FUTURE RESEARCH

A. Models

1. Pulmonary Toxicity

Clearly, improved methodology is needed. The rodent models may be improved by the use of transmission and scanning electronmicroscopy. Bleomycin produces distinctive lesions which may be detected at an earlier stage by use of electron-microscopy, and thus shorten the time necessary for these studies.

Recently, the lung hydroxyproline concentration of mice treated with bleomycin has been reported to increase in a dose-related manner. This system would have the advantage of being much simpler, and more quantitative than the histologic methods presently employed, and should be explored thoroughly.

Other potential new methods include the possibility of serial determinations of serum angiotensin converting enzyme levels which have been reported to correlate with the development of pulmonary toxicity. Another potential method is the use of Type II alveolar macrophages in tissue culture. To employ this system, the effects of low concentrations of bleomycin on morphology, and biochemical parameters would need to be studied.

The use of aerosolized bleomycin in rodents has been suggested as a method of reducing the amount of drug required, and of increasing the incidence of pulmonary lesions. Unpublished data on guinea pigs, however, are not promising.

2. Adenocarcinoma Animal Models

Although the rat carcinogen-induced stomach adenocarcinoma model predicted that PEP-bleomycin would be active against human adenocarcinoma of the stomach, and preliminary data suggest it is not, the model should not be discarded until more definite data on PEP-bleomycin are obtained, and at least one more analog is evaluated in the model and in the clinic.

The activity observed for tallysomycin against the Colon 38 adenocarcinoma is promising, and if tallysomycin is active clinically this could prove a useful model.

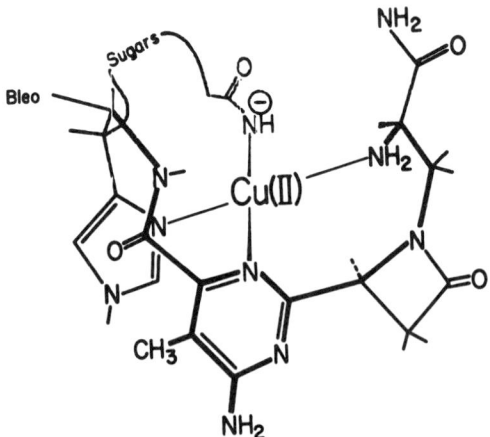

Fig. 3. Metal-binding site of bleomycin.

3. New Analogs

The elegant studies of Dr. Umezawa, Dr. Matsuda, and their co-workers have demonstrated that copper binding to bleomycin results in loss of antitumor activity, and that an intracellular mechanism exists for removing copper from bleomycin (Umezawa, 1976b). It is possible that tumors resistant to bleomycin lack the copper-removing system. The earlier studies of Umezawa and co-workers and more recent studies from our group have defined the chemistry of the metal-binding site (Dabrowiak *et al.*, 1977). Figure 3 shows the metal-binding site. Figures 4 and 5 show molecular models of bleomycin and copper-chelated bleomycin. Since an important group in metal binding is the amino group of the β-amino alanine group, it may be possible to prepare an active analog which has a reduced capacity to chelate metals. Such an analog might be active against certain bleomycin-insensitive cells.

The introduction of lypophillic groups in the bleomycinic acid nucleus (rather than a lypophillic terminal amine), might result in an analog with several potential advantages. A more lypophillic compound might attain higher intracellular concentrations. It might have better tissue penetration, and it might have a longer half-life.

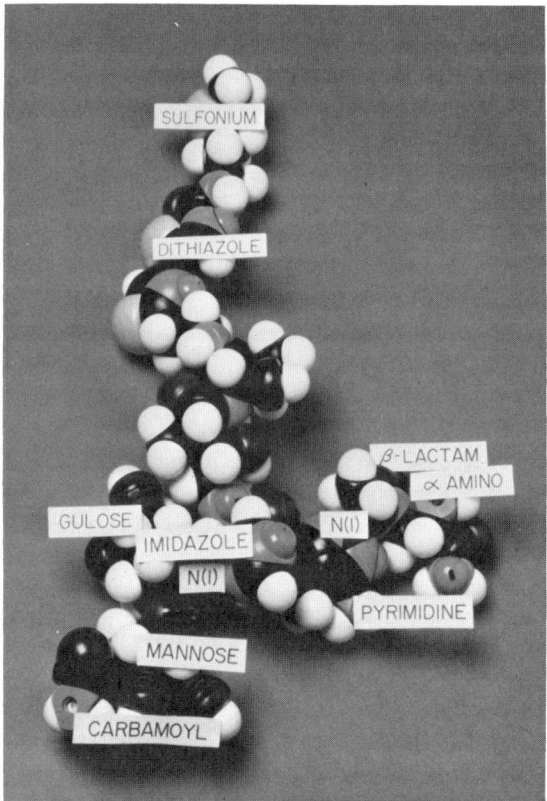

Fig. 4. Molecular model of bleomycin.

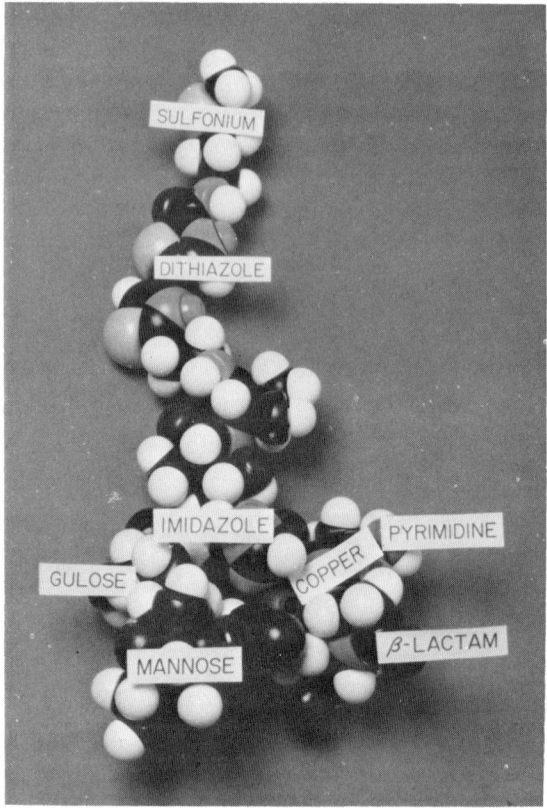

Fig. 5.   Molecular model of copper-chelated bleomycin.

It may in fact, be possible to prepare a prodrug which might replace the cumbersome prolonged bleomycin infusions.

Although the concept of linking active cytotoxic agents to tissue specific carriers has in general not yielded dramatic results, some of the lack of success may have been due to the very narrow therapeutic indexes of the alkylating agents and antimetabolites with which carrier compounds were coupled. Since bleomycin has a relatively large acute therapeutic index, a three- or fourfold increase in tissue selectivity might result in a significant gain. Thus, the potential linkage of hormones or tumor-selective antibodies to bleomycin might be of interest.

VI. CONCLUSIONS

As a result of the efforts of Dr. Umezawa, Dr. Matsuda, and their co-workers, and many other scientists, much is known about the bleomycins. As we enter the era of third-generation bleomycin analogs, there is promise of many interesting new developments.

REFERENCES

Adamson, I. Y. R., and Bowden, D. H. (1974). *Am. J. Path. 77,* 185–197.

Benedict, W. F., Baker, M. S., Haroun, L., Choi, E., and Ames, B. N. (1977) *Cancer Res. 37,* 2209–2213.

Bradner, W. T., and Pindell, M. H. (1971). *Nature 196,* 682–684.

Dabrowiak, J. C., Longo, W., Van Husen, M., Greenaway, F., and Crooke, S. T. (1977) *J. Am. Chem. Soc., Abstr., Medicinal Chemistry 51.*

Nakayama, Y., Kunishima, M., Omoto, S., Takita, T., and Umezawa, H. (1973). *J. Antibiot. 26,* 400–402.

Ohwada, H., Katsuki, H., and Hayaski, Y. (1973). *Bleomycin: New Drug Application.*

Schaeppi, U. H., Phelan, R., Stadnicki, S. W., Fleischman, R. W., Hegman, I. A., Ilievshi, V., and Redding, R. A. (1974). *Cancer Chemother. Rep. 58,* 301–310.

Strong, J., Broughton, A., and Crooke, S. T. (1977). *Cancer Treatment Rep. 61,* 1509–1512.

Umezawa, H. (1976a). *Gann Monogr. Cancer Res. 19.*

Umezawa, H. (1976b). In *Progress in Biochemical Pharmacology,* Vol. II, Caputo, A., and Paolite, R., (Eds.), Karger, Basel, Switzerland.

A
B
C 8
D 9
E 0
F 1
G 2
H 3
I 4
J 5